ORGAN TRANSPLANTATION RESEARCH HORIZONS

ORGAN DONATION AND TRANSPLANTATION – AN INTERDISCIPLINARY APPROACH

ORGAN TRANSPLANTATION RESEARCH HORIZONS

Additional books in this series can be found on Nova's website under the Series tab.

Additional e-books in this series can be found on Nova's website under the e-book tab.

ORGAN TRANSPLANTATION RESEARCH HORIZONS

ORGAN DONATION AND TRANSPLANTATION – AN INTERDISCIPLINARY APPROACH

MARY ANNE LAURI, Ph.D.
EDITOR

NOVA BIOMEDICAL
New York

For permission to use material from this book please contact us:
Telephone 631-231-7269; Fax 631-231-8175
Web Site: http://www.novapublishers.com

Library of Congress Cataloging-in-Publication Data

ISBN: 978-1-62948-257-6

Library of Congress Control Number: 2013949855

Published by Nova Science Publishers, Inc. † New York

To Josef, Beppe and Christina

CONTENTS

PREFACE

Organ transplantation is a relatively recent phenomenon. The first organ to be successfully transplanted in a human was in 1954 in Boston. Later in 1963 in Belgium and Denver and in 1966 in the Netherlands other transplants were carried out. However, organ transplantation only hit the media headlines in 1967 when Christian Barnard performed a heart transplant. Not many people had heard about organ donation and transplantation before that landmark in medical history. After the operation however, newspapers, radio and television crews flocked to South Africa to report this great medical achievement and people all over the world spoke about this "miracle". When the patient who received a heart transplant died a few days later, controversy followed. Members of both the medical and the lay community questioned the procedure of transplantation and felt that heart transplants could not and should not be carried out. The controversy continued even after successive successful transplants had been performed. However, once the experimental phases were over and the success rate of organ transplants increased, these operations were performed with relative frequency and became routine especially for kidney transplants.

The problem of organ shortage hits people of all ages, young and old, and is present in all countries whether rich or poor. No one has as yet succeeded in developing artificial kidneys, hearts and livers that work as well as human ones, therefore organs for transplantation must still be donated by human beings: either from deceased or from live donors. For some patients, organ donation is a matter of life and death. Many potential recipients of organs die when they could have lived a normal life for many more years. All this can change if there are enough organs for transplantation.

Decisions related to organ donation, whether personal or societal, are therefore very emotionally charged. How should governments legislate in order to increase the availability of donated organs? How should medical personnel approach relatives in order to ask them to donate the organs of a beloved who has just lost his or her life in an accident? How can the media help in order to encourage more organ donation? Should I give consent for a deceased relative if he or she never declared his or her views on organ donation?

In this book, a number of authors will grapple with diverse issues surrounding organ donation, such as medico-legal and ethical issues, attitudes and persuasion through communication campaigns, inter-personal communication, images people hold of the body, attitudes towards death and the role of religious beliefs in consenting to organ donation. Some of the authors have not only studied these questions academically but they are themselves organ donors or recipients, thereby giving us a unique insider's view of the issues involved.

Not all countries address the problems associated with organ donation in the same way. **Ellul**, a medical consultant who has also served on the Maltese Bio-Ethics Consultative Committee, in her chapter discusses in detail how legislation, mainly in Europe and in the US, addresses the issues of donor rights, allocation of organs, confidentiality, compensation, informed consent, opt-in and opt-out systems, advance directives, brain death and organ trafficking amongst others.

Cole, is the Dean of the Faculty of Wellbeing of the University of Malta and is herself a kidney donor .She uses a phenomenological approach to explore her own experience as a live donor. She describes the thoughts, emotions and decisions which she and her siblings went through prior to the donation. This chapter addresses issues which potential donors experience and can therefore help organ procurement coordinators identify the right strategies when helping family members in their decision of who to donate.

Procurement coordinators play a crucial role in the harvesting of organs for both live as well as deceased or cadaveric organ donation. **Camilleri-Zahra** is an organ recipient and has first-hand experience of the process of being diagnosed with kidney failure, searching for a living donor and going through the transplantation with all that such an experience entails before and after the operation. In her chapter she discusses the motivations that may guide live organ donors and believes that most donors donate organs primarily because they are altruistic and want to help the recipient. Unlike some psychologists she believes that altruism does exist.

Siegel, a social psychologist at Claremont University in the US, looks at organ donation from the point of view of the recipient. A renal patient considering whether to accept an organ from a live donor is making a decision that will have life-altering ramifications. Siegel argues that, ideally, such a decision should be made with a clear mind. He uses Goal Disruptive Theory to explain the psychological processes a patient goes through and how this theoretical framework can be used in practice to help increase the health and wellness of patients with renal failure.

Schweda and Wolke have researched organ donation from the ethical, medical, philosophical and anthropological perspective. In their chapter they examine the perceptions of lay and affected persons regarding the ways organ transplantation shapes and transforms relations between donors and recipients. From the perspective of donors in living donations, notions of self-transcendence and transfer play an important role in the relationship between the donor or donor family and the recipient as well as other family members. From the standpoint of the recipient, problems of acceptance, gratitude, indebtedness and even guilt may be present to different degrees both in living as well as deceased organ donation.

Shanteau was one of the first researchers who studied organ donation from a psychological point of view. In his chapter he cites several important studies conducted as part of a 30-year effort to understand organ donation behavior in the state of Kansas. Here he reports the results of two recent experiments exploring the impact of prior actions of signing or not signing organ donor statements on willingness to donate. The results of this study revealed that those who are opposed to signing such statements are willing to be donors if the organs will benefit immediate family members.

Another factor that helps increase family consent rates is the way that members of the donor family are approached and asked to donate the organs of a loved one who has just passed away. **Jansen**, a senior policy maker and researcher at the Dutch Transplantation Foundation argues that training provided by the Foundation to health care professionals was successful. The training helped professionals in broaching the subject of donation with potential donor families as well as positively influencing their consent rate.

The importance of the role of the family is confirmed by **Hyde**, a research fellow at Griffiths University, Australia. After giving a comprehensive review of the literature she concludes that the next critical step and key future research focus is to bring family back into the decision-making equation so that we may understand how family and individual factors work together to take informed decisions and to communicate organ donation wishes. Even **Anker**, a Research Assistant Professor in the Department of Communication at the University at Buffalo in the US, discusses how messages communicated by organ procurement coordinators during the donation requests stand to influence familial decision-making, and hence the lives of those on the national waiting list for transplantation. In this chapter, Anker reviews the context of donation requests and suggests four underlying approaches. She finds tentative support for the use of communication strategies advocated by the family-centred care approach. The chapter places emphasis on interpersonal communication during the request process between the procurement coordinator and the donor family.

Although organ shortage is present in all countries, the shortage is even more critical among certain ethnic groups and cultures. **Reinhart**, who has worked on projects examining the crafting of messages to promote organ donation, explores the complex reasons why there is a disproportionately low number of African American donors and investigates four overall barriers to increasing African American donors; lack of awareness and knowledge, medical distrust, religious and bodily concerns and medical missteps. She argues that often African American wait twice as long for an organ to be donated as any other racial or ethnic group. The fact that the waiting list is growing three times faster than the rate of available donors makes it imperative that one addresses the barriers to donating organs. She briefly discusses successful past efforts and campaigns addressing African Americans and proposes approaches for future campaigns.

The shortage of organs for transplantation is exacerbated by several factors. People live longer and therefore a greater number experience organ failure. The improvement of medical technology and the discovery of cyclosporine and similar substances, has increased the success rate of even difficult transplants such as hearts and livers. The supply of organs however has not increased at the same rate.

Many people, while acknowledging the need for organs and the benefits of transplantation, are afraid to sign donor cards pledging to donate their organs after their death. Most of their fears are unfounded and irrational. For example, some people are afraid that to donate one's organs is painful. The fact that, in cadaveric donation, organs are donated once the person is dead and therefore unable to feel pain is either misunderstood or discounted. Other fears are the result of beliefs, attitudes, myths and traditions. Religion plays a very important role in whether or not people donate. **Borg**, from the Department of Media and Communication Studies and who also lectures at the Faculty of Theology at the University of Malta analyses the position that three major religions, Christianity, Islam and Hinduism, have on this issue. He argues that the concept of afterlife and the theology of the body have particular relevance for the religious understanding of organ donation and consequently on policies and efforts at increasing donation rates. One example where religion has direct influence is the fear that the removal of some organs would hinder the process of resurrection or reincarnation of the body after death. He argues that the scientific community as well as policy makers and legislators must be fully aware of the stance taken by different religions and harness it in a positive way in order to address people's fears of donating organs.

Changing attitudes and behaviour of people is notoriously difficult. Change is sometimes resisted even by those who would benefit from it. Very often, adopting a new idea means adopting new beliefs, attitudes and values, or maybe modifying existing ones. This takes place within the framework of the lay theories which people construct in order to understand the world around them. Even a positive innovation can challenge a deep and complex set of beliefs. This may partly explain why people resist change. A new concept makes one evaluate one's lifestyle and value system. If the change being advocated has to do with core issues like life and death, as in the case of organ donation, then the difficulty is even greater.

Strategies to bring about change in public behaviour take into consideration how this behaviour is understood in the context in which it is being introduced or carried out. It must therefore take into consideration the wider social representations which might facilitate or hinder the proposed change. If this is not done, the resistance to adopting the new behaviour may be so great that the whole exercise of bringing about this change in society would be doomed to failure; a failure based on rejection. Both my chapter, which focuses on the Maltese context, and the chapter by Malony, Walker and Charlton, who discuss the Australian experience, use social psychological theories to make the point that for campaigns to be effective, change agents must be knowledgeable about how people perceive organ donation. Organ donation means different things to different people. In my chapter, I discuss the proposition of introducing the opt-out system in Malta and explore why some people were in favour while others were totally against. I propose that understanding the social representations the public has of organ donation is important in making the right policy decisions. In this context I discuss the different metaphors used by participants to make sense of organ donation and then discuss how these metaphors are rooted in one's identity of the body. Three social representations of the body are identified as being salient. I argue that understanding these complex representations is essential before legislating for organ donation.

Maloney, Walker and Charlton use the same theoretical framework of social representations to argue that the public can hold a consensual, but contradictory network of meanings associated with organ donation. They propose that the salience of the social context at any one time elicits different aspects of the representational field of organ donation and transplantation and, in so doing, accommodates the co-existence of these sometimes contradictory understandings. They carried out a word association task and in line with their previous studies found that the understanding of the issue of organ donation was marked by a tension between *life/death* and *self/other*.

The marketing of organ donation therefore presents some problems which the marketing of consumer goods does not present. Hence it is even more important for the change-agents to find out what comes to people's minds when they hear the phrase "organ donation". Organ donation leads people to confront an issue that goes right to the core of their existential anxieties. The simple act of carrying a donor card makes one ask questions like "Why am I living?", "What will happen to me when I die?" and "Is there life after death?" Some people would prefer to ignore these issues completely rather than think through these anxiety-provoking questions which have no simple answers. In this context choosing the right messages for a campaign may be important. **Alvaro**, whose applied research and evaluation activities involve studying persuasion in the context of health promotion, addresses how the mass media can be used to educate the public about organ donation and motivate donation-related behaviour. He proposes that future organ donation campaigns should be based on a solid messaging theory/base and concludes that the key to successful campaigns is to determine the relative impact of one messaging approach to another.

Feeley and Yang, have also researched the social influence processes in health related contexts and the impact of emotion on decision making. They review the goals of organ donation campaigns and, based on this review, they introduce critical elements of communication campaigns designed to promote cadaveric donation. They use Berlo's (1960) Source-Message-Channel-Receiver model as an organizing framework. The authors conclude the chapter by discussing challenges to organ donation campaign research and argue that while campaigns are well-intended, there are more questions than answers regarding why and when campaigns work in achieving their stated objectives.

This book brings together researchers from three different continents who present different perspectives on the complex issue of organ donation. I hope that this collection can help students, change agents and policy makers in their quest to increase the number of people willing to donate the gift of life. I also hope that these chapters show that organ donation is a rich and multi-faceted subject and it can best be understood by the cross fertilization of theories from diverse disciplines such as psychology, sociology, law, anthropology and medicine. Organ donation is a fertile area of research and findings can save people's lives.

Mary Anne Lauri

ACKNOWLEDGEMENT

I wish to thank my former student, now my research assistant, Amy Camilleri Zahra, without whose invaluable help I would not have been able to complete the editing of this book.

ABOUT THE AUTHORS

Eusebio Alvaro

Dr. Eusebio M. Alvaro is a Research Professor in the School of Behavioural and Organizational Sciences (SBOS) at Claremont Graduate University (CGU) and Co-Director of the Health Psychology & Prevention Science Institute (HPPSI). His basic research centers on the study of social influence processes with an emphasis on biased message processing, resistance to persuasion, indirect effects of persuasive messages, and mechanisms by which minorities can achieve change. His applied research and evaluation activities involve studying persuasion in the context of health promotion, disease prevention, and medicine with a particular focus on the development and testing of mass media messages targeting health behaviour change. These activities all draw on behavioural science theories in order to determine how negative health behaviours may be overcome and positive behaviours encouraged while also feeding back into theory development and refinement.

Ashley E. Anker

Ashley E. Anker is a Research Assistant Professor in the Department of Communication at University at Buffalo - The State University of New York. Her research has focused on the intersection of health promotion and persuasion, with a particular interest in communication surrounding organ donation.

Rev. Dr Joseph Borg

Rev Dr Joseph Borg read for a Masters in theology from the University of Malta and a PhD in communication studies from the University of Bolton. He lectures at the Faculty of Media and Knowledge Sciences and the Faculty of Theology.

Borg was one of the co-ordinators of the Organ Donation Campaign (2005/2006). For a number of years he was a member of the National Bio-ethics Consultative Committee and a member of the Malta Medical Council. Borg published several book chapters and peer reviewed papers mainly about media education and the media in Malta.

Amy Camilleri-Zahra

Amy Camilleri-Zahra graduated from the University of Malta, Malta with a Bachelor of Psychology (First Class Honours) and is currently pursuing a Masters degree in Disability Studies at University of Leeds, United Kingdom. Her research interests are disability issues particularly in relation to feminism and social attitudes, and psychological issues related to organ donation and transplantation. She is presently an Assistant Manager (UNCPRD) at the National Commission Persons with Disability in Malta.

Maureen Cole

Maureen Cole B.A, B.Soc.Wk. (Hons.) (Monash), Ph.D. (UEA) is a senior lecturer in social work, head of the Department of Social Policy and Social Work and Dean of the Faculty for Social Wellbeing at the University of Malta. Her main teaching responsibilities centre on social work theory and practice and on social work supervision. Her research focus is the practice and experience of social work supervision.

After she became a live kidney donor, she has also developed an interest in organ donation and transplantation.

Bridget Ellul

Dr. Bridget Ellul, MB.ChB., MRCPath., FRCPath., is the Head of the Department of Pathology, Faculty of Medicine and Surgery, University of Malta. She graduated in Medicine at the University of Glasgow, UK, in 1980 and specialized in histopathology and forensic medicine, returning to Malta in 1991 as a Consultant Histopathologist at the Health Department. In 2000, she moved to a full time academic post, becoming Head in 2005. She has provided forensic pathology services as a medical court expert since 1987 and has an interest in road traffic accidents and deaths by drowning. She chaired the Board of the Institute of Criminology, formerly called the Institute of Forensic Studies, University of Malta, from 2001-2012. She has an interest in medical law and ethical issues and lectures in the Masters in Bioethics. In 2006, she published the book, *Health, Ethics and the Law*, co-authored with Professor Maurice Cauchi and Professor Kevin Aquilina, published by the Malta University Press. She is a member of the national Health Ethics Committee, the Bioethics Research Programme of the Faculty of Medicine & Surgery and the Medicine and the Law Programme of the Faculty of Laws. She has served on the Medical Council, the Bioethics Consultative Committee and the Faculty Research Ethics Committee. She is the current President of the Malta College of Pathologists.

Tegan Charlton

Tegan Charlton recently graduated from Southern Cross University, Coffs Harbour, NSW, Australia with a Bachelor of Psychology (First Class Honours) and is currently pursuing a Masters degree in Organisational Psychology at Griffith University, Mt Gravatt, QLD, Australia. Her research interests lie in the Australian organ donation process and workplace Mavericks.

Thomas Feeley

Thomas Feeley is Professor and Chair of Communication at University at Buffalo, The State University of New York. His research interests are in the area of social influence processes in health-related contexts. He has published extensively on the topic of organ donation promotion.

Melissa Hyde

Melissa Hyde, Ph. D. is a Research Fellow with the Behavioural Basis of Health, Griffith Health Institute at Griffith University, Australia. Dr Hyde's primary interest is in research that has the capacity to save lives or improve quality of life. Since 2005 she has focussed on understanding people's decisions about organ/tissue donation, especially family communication about organ donation wishes. As well, she has an interest in altruism/helping behaviour (e.g., volunteering, charitable giving) as it relates to medical and health contexts.

Nichon Jansen

Mrs. Nichon E. Jansen is working as a senior policy maker and senior researcher at the Dutch Transplantation Foundation, in Leiden the Netherlands, since 1998. She finished her PhD in February 2012. The main subject of interest is the shortage of organ donors and how to improve donation rates in the Netherlands.

Mary Anne Lauri

Mary Anne Lauri studied at the University of Malta and at the London School of Economics, UK. She is a social psychologist. One of her research interests is the application of social representations theory to issues such as media and health. She has published several papers on organ donation. She presently is Pro-Rector at the University of Malta.

Gail Moloney

Gail Moloney is a senior lecturer in psychology at the Coffs Harbour campus of Southern Cross University in NSW, Australia. Her research interests are in the theoretical articulation of social representations theory & social identity in relation to varying social issues such as the resettlement of refugees, depiction of minority groups through political cartoons, blood donation, and organ donation & transplantation. She co-edited *Social representations and identity: Content, process, and power* (2007) with Iain Walker.

Amber Reinhart

Amber Marie Reinhart (Ph.D., University of New York at Buffalo) is an Associate Professor of Communication at the University of Missouri, St. Louis. Her research interests are in health communication, message design, and research methods. Past projects examined crafting messages to promote organ donation, how the Internet affects health decision making, and tailoring health messages for risky behaviours.

Mark Schweda

Mark Schweda is a researcher at the Department for Medical Ethics and History of Medicine at the University of Göttingen, Germany. He studied philosophy and German literature in Berlin and Nottingham. His research focus is on ethical, philosophical, and socio-cultural aspects of organ transplantation and of human aging.

James Shanteau

James Shanteau, Commerce Bank Distinguished Graduate School Professor, received his Ph.D. in Experimental Psychology from the University of California, San Diego. Since joining the faculty at Kansas State University (KSU), he has held visiting appointments at University of Michigan, University of Oregon, University of Colorado, Cornell University, National Science Foundation, and University of Toulouse. His research interests include analysis of expertise in decision makers (including air traffic control) and studies of consumer health-care choices (especially organ donation / transplantation decisions). Currently, he is Coordinator of the Judgment / Decision Making Laboratory at Kansas State University.

Jason T. Siegel

Dr. Jason T. Siegel is an associate research professor at Claremont Graduate University's School of Behavior and Organizational Science. His research utilizes classic and contemporary social psychological and communication frameworks to explain and influence a range of health behaviors including depression, drug abuse, and organ donation. Dr. Siegel has been studying living and non-living organ donation for nearly 15 years; he has been developing Goal Disruption Theory (GDT; see GDTheory.com) for over a decade. While GDT was not created with organ donation in mind, applying it to the domain of living donation allows unique insight into the psychological plight of people diagnosed with renal failure.

Iain Walker

Iain Walker is a senior research scientist with the Commonwealth Scientific and Industrial Research Organisation, Australia's national science body. His primary research interests focus on using social science knowledge to address sustainability issues. He has other research interests diffused across several areas, including relative deprivation theory, prejudice, social representations, and social identity. He co-authored *Social cognition: An integrated introduction* (3rd ed., 2013) with Martha Augoustinos and Ngaire Donaghue, co-edited *Relative deprivation theory: Specification, development, integration* (2002) with Heather Smith, and co-edited *Social representations and identity: Content, process, and power* (2007) with Gail Moloney. He is an adjunct professor of psychology at the University of Western Australia, Southern Cross University, and the University of the Sunshine Coast.

Sabine Wöhlke

Medical Anthropologist, with special interest to Gender Studies. She is research assistance in the Department of Medical Ethics and History of Medicine in Göttingen, Germany. Her research focus are: ethical and medical anthropological research on organ transplantation, especially living organ donation; Gender studies; Reciprocity and the gift in the context of organ transplantation; Body images and body concepts in medicine; qualitative socio-empirical research.

Z. Janet Yang

Z. Janet Yang (Ph.D., Cornell University, 2009) is an assistant professor in the Department of Communication at the State University of New York at Buffalo. Her research is primarily focused on science, health, environmental, and risk communication with an emphasis on the impact of emotion on decision-making.

In: Organ Donation and Transplantation
Editor: Mary Anne Lauri
ISBN: 978-1-62948-257-6

Chapter 1

MEDICO-LEGAL ASPECTS OF ORGAN DONATION

Bridget Ellul*
University of Malta, Malta

ABSTRACT

This chapter deals with medico-legal issues that must be addressed on a national, European, and international level to guarantee the organisation of a viable Organ Transplant Service, which besides offering professional high quality medical services ensures that the rights of both donors and recipients are upheld. The discussion focuses on the two main pillars of human organ transplantation, *availability* and *access*, whether the organs are procured from living or dead donors. The pivotal factor in *availability* of organs is the *voluntary consent* of the donor. In relation to consent for cadaver organs, there is a critical look at the legally accepted *definitions of death* that have evolved primarily in relation to establishing death in patients on life support systems. Analysis of the opt-in or opt-out system is accompanied by a look at the role of donor cards, proxy consent and advance directives. The success of limiting coercion in obtaining consent is examined by analysing the criminalisation of *organ trafficking*, regulation of medical tourism and promotion of altruistic donation. Finally, there is consideration of the *rights of donors* to confidentiality, to compensation and to good quality of life post donation.

In discussing *access*, the role of the state is more important in terms of measures to set up a service with the right *infrastructure*, including donor registries, adequate budgeting for medical transplant services, licensing of facilities, training programmes for personnel and accreditation systems. Adequate *data protection* of health records, including donor registries, is essential, particularly when we are enhancing access by promoting *cross-border* transplant services. Harmonisation of legislation is crucial in cross-border services. Last but not least the role of *education* is outlined. This is the key to ensuring availability and access, through public awareness, promotion of patient support groups and improved communication between healthcare professionals and patients, on a national and international level.

* E-mail: bridget.ellul@um.edu.mt.

INTRODUCTION

Organ transplantation hinges on the essential element of donation, from donor to recipient, so discussion in relation to medico-legal issues must primarily focus on the donor-recipient relationship.

There must be a clear delineation of the rights and duties of both parties, in the context of the role of the state in ensuring optimum health for its citizens by providing an equitable transplantation service coupled with the assurance of safety, and long term health cover, for both donors and recipients.

Therefore this chapter addresses medico-legal issues with regard to ensuring equitable availability and access without compromising those rights.

The shortage of organs is now felt even more acutely due to the ever increasing demand for organs from an ageing population, accompanied by a decrease in availability, both of living and deceased organ donors, in part due to the ageing of the pool of potential living donors. Another factor is the reduction in suitable deceased donors following improvements in medical care, coupled with an international effort to reduce traumatic deaths, particularly those following road traffic accidents, which primarily have in past years provided the highest rate of deceased organ donations.

This has led countries to work towards global co-operation in organ sharing. In the European Union, EU, a task force set up to examine these issues, produced a ten point Action Plan On Organ Donation and Transplantation (2009-2015) for co-operation between member states aimed at maximising donation. In the US, the United Network for Organ Sharing (UNOS), a private organization, has the federal contract to run the Organ Procurement and Transplantation Network, OPTN, in line with the *National Organ Transplant Act* of 1984.

Donor Organs

Advances in biotechnology and medicine, including sophisticated medical equipment used in harvesting and banking organs, and the development of new drugs to combat rejection have increased the types of organs that can now be transplanted.

However the main organ remains the kidney, plus or minus pancreatic tissue, both from living and deceased donors. The kidney was the first living organ to be successfully transplanted in a human, in Boston in 1954, from one male to his identical twin (Public Broadcasting Service: A Science Odyssey). The first successful deceased organ transplant operation was also that of a kidney, in Belgium in 1963, followed by a liver transplant in 1967 in the USA, a heart transplant in 1967 in South Africa and heart/lungs in 1981 in the USA (Eurotransplant 2012)..

Living donors are only able to donate one of a pair of organs or part of an organ with regenerative potential, thus initially limiting donation to a kidney, but they can now donate portions of pancreas and liver. Tissues, such as bone and tendons, and of course blood, can also be donated.

Living donor organs have a longer post transplant life) since the organs are in a better physiologic state than deceased donor organs. Therefore there has been a drive to encourage and promote living organ donation.

Living donations are primarily directed to a specific recipient, to relatives who are genetically related, to family members who are not genetically related or to recipients who are in a close relationship with the donor. Directed live donation is now acceptable beyond these confines through programmes of extended matching, as a paired donation or in even more complex patterns of pooled donation, involving more than two donor-recipient pairs. A live donor can also donate to an unknown recipient on the official waiting list, and this may be in combination with pooled donation, thus starting a so called donor chain. Complex patterns of donation are approved by an independent ethics body, such procedure being first recommended by the Council of Europe's *Additional Protocol to the Convention on Human Rights and Biomedicine, on transplantation of organs and tissues of human origin* (2002) in response to the divergent views as to possible recipients of living donation.

Since a live donor is not available for all recipients, deceased or cadaver donors remain the more common type of organs to be transplanted, with the primary organ donated still being the kidney (Global Observatory on Donation and Transplantation, 2011; OPTN, 2012). Cornea donation is also high but this organ is considered as a tissue donation under the US *National Organ Transplant Act 1984,* section 301, mainly due to the possibility of relatively late donation after death and the longevity of banking.

In recent years, pancreatic islet cell donation has increased, paralleling the increase in diabetic patients worldwide, particularly affecting third world countries as they move to a Western lifestyle. The rise in heart/lung operations has been rather slow. Surgeons can now transplant portions of the gastrointestinal tract and even parts of the body, such as face and limbs, with increasing successful outcomes. With improvements in medical management of organ harvesting and donor and recipient healthcare, it is now possible to transplant organs that are not a perfect match or that satisfy so called 'expanded criteria' whether in terms of disease status, age or less than optimal immunological typing. Moreover cross-border health care programmes and fast transport services, are facilitating an increase in the number of cadaver multiple donations and enabling matching of a donor to the best possible recipient, even if living far away from the donor. Some programmes are designed between countries to enable recipients to move to a more specialized centre for surgery to a neighbouring country, which also provides the donated organ. Such examples in Europe include Spain and Portugal, and Malta and Italy (European Commission, 2012).

AVAILABILITY

Organ donation is by definition an altruistic action and in fact there is an overwhelming worldwide consensus on this issue, which is central to ensuring respect for human dignity, the right to physical integrity and safeguarding self-determination through the exercise of free and informed consent. This is a general principle embodied in all international instruments relating to organ donation and transplantation, in particular those produced by the World Health Organisation, WHO, (2010), the EU *Directive 2010/45/EU* (2010) and the Council of Europe's *Additional Protocol* (2002), as well as in all national specific legislation such as in the US (1984), Canada (British Columbia 1996), Australia (Victoria 1982) and UK (England 2004, Scotland 2006) legislation. However it is by no means a uniform worldwide practice, even in our times; unfortunately there are countries that use less than ethical, or even criminal, means for organ procurement. These issues will be further explored in terms of limiting discriminatory practices to safeguard donor rights.

Consent

The main legal issue that underpins all donation for both living and deceased donors is informed consent while for the latter there is the added problem of a legal definition of death. Special arrangements in the case of living donors create specific legal problems relating to consent, such as in dealing with children as donors.

The traditional consent has been based on the willingness of the donor to gift his organ to a relative or, as stated in the Council of Europe's *Additional Protocol* (2002), article 10, to a person 'with whom the donor has a close personal relationship as defined by law'. However even in the Protocol a window is left open for non-related donors when it is stated, again in article 10, that in special cases, 'in the absence of such relationship, only under the conditions defined by law and with the approval of an appropriate independent body' donation can be accepted if approved by an ethics committee. There was strong debate at the drafting of the Protocol as initially the views were that living donation should be restricted but by 2004, the Council recommended (CM/AS(2004)Rec1611final) further 'distinctions on the basis of close personal relationships rather than blood relationships'. As already noted, this extended donation has now increased and is covered by local legislation. The rationale for ethical approval is to protect the donor and recipient from emotional attachments or expectations, which may lead to various degrees of persecution of recipients or to the undue burden of a sense of gratitude or responsibility suffered by the recipient towards the donor.

Informed Consent

The *Charter of Fundamental Rights of the European Union* in the first chapter on Dignity establishes the right to the integrity of the person, in article 3(2)(a), which 'in the fields of medicine and biology' requires due respect to the 'free and informed consent of the person concerned, according to the procedures laid down by law'. This is based on the basic ethical principle of guaranteeing individual autonomy.

Article 10 of the Council of Europe's *Convention for the Protection of Human Rights and Dignity of the Human Being with regard to the Application of Biology and Medicine: Convention on Human Rights and Biomedicine* (1997), generally known as the *Convention on Human Rights and Biomedicine*, states that 'everyone has the right to respect for private life in relation to information about his or her health' emphasising the right to informed consent. Hand in hand with the right to consent goes the right to refuse a procedure or to withdraw consent (article 13). This option must be mentioned to the potential donor at the initial consultation with regard to enrolment and an explanation given as to their legal rights and the possible implications of withdrawing consent for both donor and potential recipient. This is of particular importance with intended directed donation, where a relation or trusted individual withdraws consent at a late stage, with resulting devastating psychological effects on the recipient.

Though consent to living organ donation may initially appear no different from consent to a surgical operation, it must be appreciated that this is totally different as primarily it is not for the benefit of the donor. The emphasis must be on informed consent, such that the donor appreciates the quality of life to himself or herself after the loss of the kidney, both from a medical aspect but also from possible limits to social life. However there is definitely a psychological impact due to the emotional and ethical issues involved, and donors should be offered counselling pre and post donation. It is not the remit of this chapter to discuss the ethics of possible coercion in non-related donation, but counselling becomes more imperative here. Specifically, the Council of Europe stresses the requirement for 'free, informed and specific consent' either 'in written form or before an official body' (article 13).

Competency

From a legal aspect consent depends on the competence of the potential donor to agree to the donation. This implies that the donor can understand the issues involved and can take a decision based on an assessment of benefits and risks. This is no different from any other consent for medical or civil matters. Special attention should be given to communicate information in a language that the donor understands, and is also able to ask questions to clarify any doubts.

Adult incompetent donors are usually excluded from being donors. While article 6(3) of the Council of Europe's *Convention on Human Rights and Biomedicine* (1997) provides for 'protection of persons not able to consent' by ensuring their interests are covered by an official representative, the *Additional Protocol* (2002) provides for a donation only in the case of donation to close relatives, or if 'the donation has the potential to be life-saving for the recipient' (article 14) or if there is no other compatible donor available. In practice, in such situations, legislation in most countries does allow guardians, or nominated representatives, to consent instead.

Minors can also be considered as incompetent but the cut off point for donating organs varies. In the Dutch *Organ Donation Act 1989*, 'adults and minors aged twelve years or more who are capable of reasonably assessing their interests in such matters may consent to the removal of their organs or certain specified organs after their death, or may record their objection to such removal'. Children in the UK are only exceptionally allowed to be living donors, with the approval of the Human Tissue Authority once consent to the procedure of organ removal is authorised by a Court, in accordance with the *Children's Act 1989*. 'Where a child is deemed competent to consent to that decision, the necessary consent will be their own' (Human Tissue Authority, UK, Code of practice 2, 2009). However there is a grey area legally for 16-18 year olds, since the *Children's Act* only covers those below sixteen, while they are still considered as minors under the *Human Tissue Act*. In the *Human Tissue Act (Scotland) 2006* there are different provisions for children aged 16 years and above. In particular they are only allowed to donate organs as part of domino procedures, which involve medical treatment for the child. This also applies to incompetent adults.

Germany amended its legislation (*German Transplantation Act, 1997*) and as from 1st August 2012 allows 16 year olds to consent for organ donation; so the law provides for individuals with health insurance, aged 16 years and over, to be asked regularly if they consent to being organ donors.

The difficulty is in balancing the rights of the donor with those of the recipient. It is even more difficult to accept that it is in a child's best interest to be a living organ donor. However there have been minors who offered to donate, and were considered competent to give consent, for the benefit of a sibling. More contentious is the issue of obtaining consent from parents for donation of organs from one child to a sibling, not to mention the decision to have another child just to be a donor for one of the children, although these classically involve bone marrow transplantation from a neonate to a sibling with leukaemia. The Court may need to be invoked to take a decision.

Although not all countries have enacted legislation to cover consent for medical procedures, in guidelines for professional medical practice, specifically in relation to transplant legislation, consent is always addressed.

Opt-in System

Organs or tissues shall not be removed from the body of a deceased person unless consent or authorisation required by law has been obtained. The removal shall not be carried out if the deceased person had objected to it (Council of Europe, *Additional Protocol*, 2002, article 17).

States recognise two systems of obtaining consent. In the 'opt in' system, individuals may be pro-active and register their willingness to donate after death by explicit consent in life, but more often such consent is specifically obtained from the relatives on the death of the potential donor. In the 'opt out' system, one has to definitely register an objection to the state, during life.

Valid explicit consent can be provided by carrying an organ donor card, by official registration in a state approved register or other system and by an Advance Directive.

Donor Cards

Donor cards are easy to obtain but in most countries they have no legal status and can be overridden by the relatives' wishes, doctors opting to ask relatives prior to harvesting organs.

The Eurobarometer study of 2006 revealed that although 81% of Europeans supported donor cards only 12% actually had a card and in fact there were significant differences between countries, with Holland having the highest rate with four out of ten citizens carrying a donor card while in Eastern Europeans and Baltic states only 1% carried a donor card. Having a donor card helps relatives to make a decision as to whether to consent to the harvesting of organs, because they are comforted from an assurance that they have carried out the wishes of their loved one.

Registry

The decision to donate carries more weight if it can be officially documented, for example on a driving licence, which has the added bonus of being accessible at a time when the patient may be unconscious and when there is limited time to ascertain the views of the individual. This is an accepted practice in many US and EU states, in Canada, Australia and New Zealand.

More definite consent is exercised by enrolment in an official national register, particularly if this is regulated by law and not by NGOs. Care needs to be taken however to make sure that recipients are not on multiple waiting lists of different registries from the same or different countries. Co-operation between neighbouring organisations is therefore crucial. The EU has always aimed at such co-ordination, particularly in view of mobility of citizens and with the reality of cross-border organ exchange becoming more uniformly established. There has been a progression from the European Transplant Network, Eurotransplant, to a network of National Organisations and in the near future, in line with the new EU *Directive 2010/45/EU* to co-ordination of national Competent Authorities.

In the US, one can submit a Letter of Intent for organ donation, which is registered in the same way as an Advance Directive. The US Living Will Registry website informs applicants that 'Your family will ultimately decide whether or not to donate your organs. Being able to read your wishes about organ donation will make their decision-making much easier, and discussing your wishes with your family now is the best way to help them make this decision'.

Registries require an administrative back up to ensure the register is kept up to date. Confirmation on a periodic basis, ideally annually, allows also for the possibility of opting out of the original decision. The information on the register is available to healthcare facilities that can access the system electronically. The US *Revised Uniform Anatomical Gift Act, UAGA, 2006*, (originally enacted in 1987) establishes standards for donor registries, allows computerised registries of donors and accepts electronic signatures, but it makes no similar provision for individuals who opt out of being donors. It enables procurement organizations to gain access to donor registries, medical records, and records of the state motor vehicle department.

Advance Directives

An even more specific legal acknowledgement of the wishes of a potential donor, and a certain way of ensuring these wishes are respected after death, is an Advance Directive.

An Advance Directive is a legal instrument, introduced primarily in the US, although it is also being utilised in Europe and Australia, to address the wishes of the individual regarding their future healthcare should they be in a state of unconsciousness or with dementia, unable to take decisions at the time. Such a scenario is of course more plausible today as advances in healthcare have ensured long term survival through maintenance on life support systems.

An Advance Directive may include a) a Living Will dealing specifically with issues relating to healthcare; or b) a medical Power of Attorney, or a durable power of attorney for healthcare, which nominates a representative or proxy to take decisions instead of the patient, in relation to life-sustaining measures (this is separate from a proxy for financial transactions); or c) a Do Not Resuscitate, DNR, order, which indicates that the individual agrees to refuse cardiopulmonary resuscitation.

The US *Patient Self-Determination Act, 1991* makes it mandatory to inform patients on admission, or registration, to hospital or nursing homes, about their rights under state laws governing Advance Directives, including '(1) the right to participate in and direct their own health care decisions; (2) the right to accept or refuse medical or surgical treatment; (3) the right to prepare an Advance Directive; and (4) information on the provider's policies that govern the utilization of these rights. The act prohibits institutions from discriminating against a patient who does not have an Advance Directive' (Wilkinson, Wenger and Shugarman, 2007). The Act also obliges health institutions to provide education on Advance Directives.

However in the Report commissioned by the US Department of Health and Human Services, from the Rand Corporation, there is no mention of the use of Advance Directives for the procurement of organs (Wilkinson et al., 2007). It has been legally argued that an Advance Directive is only effective during life and so cannot regulate what happens after death. In fact, in traditional forms used in the UK and Australia, there is no mention of organ donation on the forms. However in the US, in line with the *Revised UAGA* and local state law, one may register as an organ donor via an Advance Directive, even on line, without obtaining legal advice, although legal advice is recommended. Not all Advance Directives include a section on views regarding organ donation but the applicant may indicate their wish to be a donor in the comments section of the form. Such a decision is often then automatically registered on the individual's driving licence.

Opt-Out System

In the 'opt out' system or presumed consent system everyone is considered as a potential donor unless they actually opt out of being donors, in which instance their wishes must be respected. The legal issues here relate to the right to health, the right to autonomy and taking your own decisions, as well as the right to privacy, that is, taking a decision without involvement from the state. On the other hand putting the onus on the individual to register lack of consent may cause discrimination to the individual. The German National Ethics Council (2007) has argued that if you refuse to be a potential donor than you should forfeit the right to be considered as a recipient, should you become ill and require a donation.

The UK had seriously considered such a move following the recommendation of the British Medical Association in 2000, but the UK Organ Donation Taskforce, set up in 2008 concluded that the time was as yet inopportune, arguing mostly against the system from the point of view of increased expense. Ironically, its report outlined findings that showed a definite association of an increase in donated organs with a presumed consent system; in the case of deceased donations, this amounted to up to six donations more, per million of the population (Bird and Harris, 2010).

On 2nd July 2013, the Welsh Assembly in the UK voted in favour of the Human Transplantation (Wales) Bill, which will introduce an 'opt out' consent system in Wales in 2015, for individuals over 18 years, who have been residents in Wales for at least one year. The Bill provides for objection by relatives or long term friends.

Opt-in vs. Opt-Out System

A presumed consent system appears to provide the possibility for more donations, since the pool of potential donors is much larger than that in the explicit consent system, where the percentage of the population actually enrolling in a register remains low. However the review by Coppen, Friele, Gevers, Blok and van der Zee (2008) of consent systems in ten European countries showed that a presumed consent system does not necessarily translate into a definite increase in donations. The study covered 1995-2005 and included Austria, Belgium, France, Italy, Spain, Sweden, United Kingdom with presumed consent and Germany, the Netherlands and Switzerland with explicit consent. In 2006, the *Human Tissue Act* introduced formal explicit consent in the UK, when previously organs could be harvested if it was established that the deceased had not objected to transplantation. The researchers actually compared the number of deceased who were potentially suitable organ donors to the number of actually transplanted organs, or for France and Sweden to the number of organs harvested, rather than looking at changes in stark figures of national donation rates.

Previous studies by Gevers, Janssen and Friele (2004) on European systems had found no significant differences in organ donation between the ‘opt in’ and ‘opt out’ systems. The answer may be in the role of relatives, whose involvement reduces the potential increase expected. The usual practice is for the medical authorities to obtain consent for harvesting organs, from the relatives of the potential donor, whether this is a legal requirement or not and in fact, even where the local legislation allows for presumed consent, at least in Europe, all doctors take into account the relatives’ wishes. The European Commission’s study group, ALLIANCE-O (2004-2007), came to the same conclusion that in day-to-day practice, the two concepts do not differ significantly. A significant difference does only exist when the next of kin of a potential donor is not identified.

The family is faced with the complex issues of accepting bereavement while agreeing to donation. For some, this is a straightforward logical procedure, as they see that their loved one’s wishes are respected, or that the death had not been in vain. On the other hand, it may mean that the relative sees the donor as remaining alive in the recipient, with ensuing psychological effects for both the relative, and if confidentiality as to donor identity cannot be maintained, possibly also for the recipient.

The Eurobarometer Report (2007) established that 23% did not know whether to donate a deceased relative’s organs as opposed to 18% that were unsure about donating their own organs, thus it appears to be more difficult to decide about donating a relative’s organs. The refusal rate for agreeing to donation of organs from a deceased relative was 23% as opposed to 26% refusal to donate your own organs after death. The study also showed a positive correlation of willingness to donate, whether your own or a relative’s organs, with the level of education, the work position, which also reflected education, and with age. Thus senior citizens and those looking after the home were less likely to give a definite answer in favour of donation.

Success in obtaining consent reflects also on the communication skills of the health carers, as much as it does on the wishes of the deceased being known to the relatives. They are much more likely to agree to donation if they know their relative’s wishes, which is why discussion with family members about being an organ donor needs to be promoted. Again in the Eurobarometer study, 41% of European citizens had discussed organ donation with their family compared to 58% who had never raised the subject. Significant differences between EU countries exist with 75% of Dutch citizens and 66% of Swedish citizens having discussed organ donation as compared to only 24% in Austria and 28% in Portugal.

In a study by Coppen, Friele, Gevers and van der Zee (2010) involving a questionnaire sent to the Dutch Health Care Consumer Panel in 2004 and 2007, respondents were more likely to consent to donation from a deceased relative if they knew the relative had explicitly wished this and two thirds of respondents (response rate 98% and 80% respectively for 2004 and 2007) wanted to be consulted, whatever the consent system was.

In fact there are variations in the application of the presumed consent system with some countries rigidly adhering to the law and in others like Italy, Sweden and Spain, the relatives are still allowed to object to organ donation. The Belgian Law on the *Procurement and*

Transplantation of Organs 1986, in article 10(1) dealing with deceased donors, states that 'Organs and tissue intended for transplantation' ….'may be removed from [anyone who is registered in the municipal register or has been registered as an alien for more than six months] unless it has been established that opposition to such removal has been expressed.' Article 10(4) emphasises that:

The physician may not proceed with removal:

- if opposition has been expressed in the manner established by the King;
- if opposition is expressed by the donor in another way and provided the physician is duly informed;
- if a surviving relative informs him of opposition. This opposition cannot be in contradiction of an explicit last will made by the donor.

In Spain, the system operates more along lines of informed, than presumed, consent and permission of relatives is routinely sought and the law requires the family to confirm, in writing, that the donor had not objected to donation. However the huge success that Spain has had in achieving and maintaining the best European rates for organ procurement is attributed more to the organizational aspect of a co-ordinated efficient service than to consent legislation.

In the US, the *Revised UAGA 2006* provides a combination of opt in and opt out systems, enhancing the rights of donors and making both donation and refusal legal. The Act enhances the rights of individuals in expressing their decisions as to their choice regarding organ donation. So it obviates the need to ask relatives for consent once the donor is enrolled in a registry, although relatives may be contacted for medical history and to see if they want feedback regarding the outcome of donation. For those who chose to opt out, the law provides for specifically barring other persons from making a gift of the individual's organs after the individual's death.

UAGA 2006 makes it illegal and irresponsible to disconnect a ventilator from a person declared brain dead without first making proper enquiry as to the possibility of harvesting tissues and organs, the policy being not to waste opportunities for organ donation. Therefore it also 'preserves the right of other persons to make an anatomical gift of a decedent's organs if the decedent had not made a gift during life', such persons being of course relatives or designated proxies. Federal law requires that hospitals have an agreement with an organ procurement organization, such that patient deaths or imminent deaths are reported for assessment as to potential donation. If the procurement organisation establishes that a deceased person who is medically suitable to be a donor is not registered as a donor, the transplant co-ordinators must, in line with legislation, contact the family and request consent for organ donation. The Act also provides for an individual to delegate a healthcare agent or proxy, to take the decision as to donation or not.

Coercion to Consent

The removal of organs without proper consent 'constitutes a serious violation of human dignity and physical integrity' (EU *Directive 2011/36/EU*). The issue of adequate communication and explanation to ensure informed consent has already been addressed. Here the focus is on limiting coercion to obtain consent.

Organ Trafficking

The worst possible scenario for this is organ trafficking, often accompanied by other crimes. In 1990, the *UN Convention on the Rights of the Child* became the first international legal instrument to urge states to prevent 'the abduction of, the sale of or traffic in children for any purpose or in any form', (article 35), which later became more explicitly referred to in the UN *Optional Protocol to the Convention on the sale of children, child prostitution and child pornography* (2002) with specific mention in article 3.1.(a)(i)b of the 'transfer of organs of the child for profit' as one of the offences to be considered as a criminal act in the state parties. The *2000 UN Trafficking Protocol* included removal of organs as a form of exploitation in its definition of trafficking, in article 3(a), which definition is also employed in the *Council of Europe Convention on action against trafficking in human beings* (2005). Trafficking in persons includes 'recruitment, transportation, transfer, harbouring or receipt of persons' and the use of 'the threat or use of force or other forms of coercion, of abduction, of fraud, of deception, of the abuse of power or of a position of vulnerability or of the giving or receiving of payments or benefits to achieve the consent of a person having control over another person, for the purpose of exploitation', including the removal of organs. Practically the same definition is found in article 2.1 and article 2.3 of the EU *Directive 2011/36/EU on preventing and combating trafficking in human beings and protecting its victims.* ,.)

In 2004, the World Health Organisation asked member states 'to take measures to protect the poorest and vulnerable groups from transplant tourism and the sale of tissues and organs, including attention to the wider problem of international trafficking in human tissues and organs' (WHA Resolution 57.18, 2004). Recently this resolve was re-iterated at the *Declaration of Istanbul on organ trafficking and transplant tourism, 2008* developed through The Transplantation Society and the International Society of Nephrology.

EU *Directive 2011/36/EU*, article 8, provides for victim protection, emphasising that victims of trafficking should not be prosecuted 'for their involvement in criminal activities which they have been compelled to commit as a direct consequence of being subjected to' any threats. Article 12.4 states that they should 'receive specific treatment aimed at preventing secondary victimisation' and further trauma during the criminal proceedings; this may also encourage victims to come forward and report abuses.

Figures with regard to trafficking are not easy to obtain but it is likely that abduction for forced removal of an organ through criminal action, when the donor cannot resist, is rare. There is sporadic documented evidence of criminal organisations that kidnap people, particularly children, with a view to stealing their organs, but many of the reports are thought to be unfounded (Caplan, Dominguez-Gil, Matesanz and Prior, 2009; Pearson, 2004). More likely is the removal of organs, mainly a kidney by deceit, such as removal of a kidney while in hospital for some other operation or enticing persons to a job in another country and then exerting pressure for the sale of a kidney (Pearson, 2004).

However poverty remains the main driving force, as concluded in a study by Shimazono (2007), published in the WHO Bulletin, which estimates that in 2005, 5% of all recipients had travelled overseas for an organ transplant. The study identified India, Pakistan and the

Philippines as organ exporters while the organ importing countries were listed as 'Australia, Canada, Israel, Japan, Oman, Saudi Arabia and the USA' according to Organs Watch, a research unit set up at Berkeley, University of California. Organs Watch, quoted by Pearson (2004), also claims that there is significant organ trafficking in Argentina, Brazil, Cuba, India, Iran, Israel/West Bank, Moldova/Romania, Philippines, Russia, Turkey, USA and South Africa. The UN estimates 5-10% of all kidney transplants are the result of trafficking (Caplan et al. 2009). This is facilitated by a shortage of organs in a country linked with poor regulatory frameworks in another and backed by organized criminal syndicates that act as intermediaries and brokers offering various packages, nowadays openly on the internet.

Poor individuals are enticed to sell a kidney through sheer necessity, lured by the promise of substantial monies, which then either never materialize or are considerably less and in most cases the payment to the donor is completely mismatched with the payment to the recipient. Some ethicists, such as Savulescu (2003) and do argue in favour of the right of a person to choose to sell an organ as an answer to poverty, which is considered as a greater evil. However such a practice cheapens the value of the body, which becomes a commodity, while it also encourages a clandestine market which primarily favours the more well to do prospective recipients.

Other forms of deception include the lack of provision of adequate health care; in fact donors caught in the illegal trade are often victims of poor health, since the surgery may be less than safe or adequate and there is no post transplant care. The recipients may also be at risk since the donor may not reveal all health information and adequate safety of organs and medical management cannot be ensured; however the chance to obtain a living organ by fast track may be enough enticement for such potential recipients.

The position in Europe appears to be changing. In the questionnaire sent by the Council of Europe to EU members in 2002, six states were aware of recipients travelling to other countries to obtain organs, identifying Turkey and India as places for transplant tourism; Turkey and some eastern European states did acknowledge cases of illegal removal of organs in their own country as well as the receipt of illegal organs (Council of Europe, 2004, 2nd June). There are now recent claims that the illegal organ trafficking is increasing in Europe due to the financial crisis with people in Greece, Italy, Spain and the Balkans attempting to sell organs , including a kidney, bone marrow, lungs or corneas (Bioedge, June 2012).

A group of people who are more likely to be exposed to coercion to being organ donors are 'prisoners or persons deprived of their liberty', from whom 'any donations must be subject to guaranteed absence of pressure, to be checked by the appropriate bodies independent of the prison authorities' (Council of Europe, 2004, 21st June). It has long been alleged that China utilised organs from executed prisoners, with an apparently unwritten agreement between the medical and legal authorities for this to occur, putting into question the professional ethics as well as the human rights issues. In fact the World Medical Association, WMA, had condemned such practices at the 173rd WMA Council Session in 2006. There were also questions as to how many foreigners actually were recipients of such organs, although in 2007 the State Council of China legislated in favour of prohibiting commercial transplantation (Caplan et al., 2009). It is therefore heartening to finally have the state run agency, Xinhua, report that China's vice minister of Health has pledged 'to abolish organ donations from prisoners' and to set up a regulated organ procurement and transplantation system (Bioedge, March 2012).

The way to control illegal trade in organs is by robust regulation of medical practice, transplant procedures and facilities and procurement institutions; it is here that EU *Directives2010/45/EU and 2011/36/EU* and domestic legislation play an important part. Most developed countries have stringent laws and guidelines to regulate the healthcare professions and medical practice, and any unprofessional or unethical behaviour warrants disciplinary action, including the withdrawal of a licence to practice. The World Health Organisation (2010) guidelines for healthcare workers in relation to organ procurement and transplantation were endorsed at the 63rd World Health Assembly.

A national framework with payment for organs has apparently been legalized in Iran, since 1998. Donors are granted a one year medical insurance, the price is fixed by the Government and there is an annual fee by the recipient to the living donor. National organs cannot be used for foreigners (Caplan et al., 2009). Iran claims to have no waiting list, but there is still discrimination in accessibility in relation to ethnicity.

Definition of Death

The Council of Europe *Additional Protocol* (2002) is specific, stating that harvesting of organs from the deceased must not occur 'unless that person has been certified dead in accordance with the law' (article 16). In the US this fundamental principle is commonly referred to as the 'dead donor rule'.

Most countries have legislation for registration of deaths following Death Certification by a medical practitioner but not all countries have established a definition of death, preferring to leave this to the medical profession. This state of affairs was undisputed right through the mid 20th century but with the advances of life support systems, it has been possible to maintain unconscious individuals alive through the use of artificial ventilation. This has put pressure on legislators to define death in such individuals and so allow healthcare professionals to terminate artificial support without the claim of medical negligence being incurred.

Pellegrino, chairman of the President's Council on Bioethics, issued a personal statement in the white paper, *Controversies in the determination of death,* of 2008. He states that the 'definitions' of death:

> fall into two categories: the philosophical and the empirical. The first seek a conceptual understanding of the essential differences between life and death. The second seek to determine the clinical signs, tests, or criteria which separate life and death most accurately. Ideally, a full definition would link the concept of life (or death) with its clinical manifestations as closely as possible. So far, this linkage has been the subject of controversy because of its pivotal role in ethically justifying the removal of vital organs from donors in transplantation protocols.

Gómez-Lobo, also in a personal statement, in the same report, affirmed that 'the definition of death as 'the irreversible cessation of life' is a definition by exclusion'.

In this chapter we are only interested in the empirical definition of death and how it affects the legal acceptance of death. However the President's report was instrumental in confirming the ethics of the legally established 'dead donor rule' prior to transplantation, which had been undermined by some bioethicists arguing that since criteria for diagnosing death were not perfect, consent remained the only necessary ethical issue. Indeed Veatch (2008) argues that donors or relatives could choose the criteria that suit them best for defining death.

From time immemorial death has always been diagnosed following cessation of cardiac and respiratory functions, easily diagnosed by absence of heart sounds and breath sounds respectively. However this is no longer possible with a patient on a ventilator, which is aimed to ensure a supply of oxygen to maintain a circulation with perfusion of all organs, which therefore continue to function, irrespective of the function of the brain. In fact such a medical intervention is primarily used for patients with brain damage. It is in these patients that the concept of brain death was developed.

The study of neuroanatomy and neurophysiology has enabled mapping of neural pathways and delineation of brain function, such that we can distinguish the *'higher brain'* composed of (a) the cerebral hemispheres, responsible for action that is based on conscious awareness, including perception, emotion, thought, and language, and the cerebellum, which co-ordinates movement and (b) the *'lower brain'*, composed of the brainstem, which houses the vital respiratory centre and also the reticular activating system, which is the regulatory switch for consciousness, whether the cerebral hemispheres are functioning or not.

In the US the definition of death has always favoured *whole-brain death*, which is commonly just referred to as *brain death*, that is the death of the entire brain including the cerebral hemispheres, cerebellum and brainstem, which is based on the idea of the brain as the motor that integrates all bodily functions, a view pronounced by the President's Commission for the Study of Ethical Problems in Medicine and Biomedical Behavioral Research in 1981. The Commission noted that 'the neurological standard for death requires an irreversible loss of all brain functions, not complete anatomical destruction of the tissue. Members of the President's Council on Bioethics in the White Paper of 2008, took the explanation even further stating that:

> the patient with total brain failure is no longer able to carry out the fundamental work of a living organism. Such a patient has lost—and lost irreversibly—a fundamental openness to the surrounding environment as well as the capacity and drive to act on this environment on his or her own behalf.

In fact all US states have incorporated the whole-brain standard, as part of the definition of death, together with the cardiopulmonary standard, which now reads in the *Uniform Determination of Death Act, 1981* as: '(1) irreversible cessation of circulatory and respiratory functions, or (2) irreversible cessation of all functions of the entire brain, including the brain stem'.

Veatch (1989), basing his arguments on the philosophy of personhood has even contended for limiting definition of death to death of the higher brain, rather than the whole brain. Another reason put forward for adopting the 'higher brain standard' is that patients diagnosed as brain dead may still have some somatic integrative functions or even minor brain function, such as some localized electroencephalographic activity. However a diagnosis limited to death only of the higher brain means that patients with persistent vegetative state, who have a functioning brainstem but no higher brain functions would be diagnosed as dead.

In the UK, the Royal College of Physicians in 1995 developed a definition of death as 'the irreversible loss of the capacity for consciousness, combined with irreversible loss of the capacity to breathe' and equated 'brainstem death' to death of the individual. In the UK there is no statutory definition of death, although this definition has been recognized in court cases. The term 'brainstem death' was formally adopted in 1995 by the Royal College of Physicians although the concept had been first laid out by Pallis in 1982. However criteria for testing brain stem function had been in use since 1976, as established by the Conference of Medical Royal Colleges, when they were first indicated as tests for assessing prognosis of severely comatose individuals with brain damage. The tests would identify those in whom there was no possibility of recovery and so the ventilator could be switched off and the patients declared dead.

The definition of brain death is established following rigorous testing of brain function. The first set of criteria was laid out in 1968 by the Ad Hoc Committee of the Harvard Medical School to Examine the Definition of Brain Death and have evolved with just minor changes. It has been argued by Capron (2001) that this committee started the confusion in terminology by using the word 'death' to 'describe the loss of function in an organ -the brain'. This idea was again stressed by Pellegrino, in a personal statement, in the President's Council White Paper (2008) when he argued that equating death with total loss of mental capacity is essentially identifying 'death of the organism with death of one organ - the brain'.

The criteria for establishing brain death rely on the concept of irreversible brain damage. Before tests are carried out, the patient must be comatose with diagnosed structural brain damage and there must be exclusion of hypothermia, drugs and metabolic diseases as a cause of coma. The tests must show absence of spontaneous breathing, absence of motor responses and of brainstem reflexes. They are also performed by more than one doctor and repeated once after a time interval. Such a protocol is considered for diagnosing brainstem death but for whole brain death, other tests need to be carried out. These include an electroencephalogram, EEG, to demonstrate loss of cortical function, and radionuclide scanning or intracranial 4-vessel cerebral angiography or ultrasonography, to ascertain loss of cerebral blood flow.

The whole brain standard has spread throughout the world while the brainstem standard is only accepted in the UK and some countries with a past British connection, e.g. India, although Canada and Australia have also embraced the whole brain standard. Wijdicks (2002) has argued for standardization of the criteria required for diagnosis; based on a study comparing the methods employed in diagnosing brain death in 80 countries, he revealed that even in countries with the same legal definition, practices varied. Only 88% had guidelines and they all provided for absence of respiration, motor responses and brainstem reflexes. Only 59% of all countries recommended the apnoea test. The confirmatory tests were in fact only compulsory in 40% of the guidelines. Wijdicks, Varelas, Gronseth and Greer in 2010 reviewed the 1995 guidelines of the American Academy of Neurology on the diagnosis of brain death. They concluded that there was not enough evidence to establish if the new tests could determine the loss of function of the entire brain.

The use of neurological criteria has never been uniformly accepted as a means of declaring death. Controversy is still present from religious groups, notably the Jewish faith as Torah law accepts death only with the absence of cardiac and respiratory function. Section 5 of The State of New Jersey *Declaration of Death Act*, prohibits medical diagnosis of death by neurological criteria for patients who have religious objections.

It is therefore almost ironic that we are now seeing a return to using the cardiopulmonary standard of diagnosing death, that is, death due to the irreversible loss of the circulation with the advent of organ donation following cardiac death or the so called non-heart beating donor, or controlled donation after cardiac death. This type of donation was introduced at the University of Pittsburgh, US in 1992. Donations, with informed consent, are being accepted from patients dying following irreversible cardiac and circulatory arrest, without such patients having previously been on life support systems. However death must occur in a medical environment such that an established minimal time elapses before harvesting of organs. Organ harvesting occurs within a short time of the declaration of death and it has the advantage of providing organs in a better state of circulation than those from the dead donor.

Donation after cardiac death is increasing at a faster rate than that from brain dead individuals, at least in the UK, as reported by the NHS Blood and Transplant Health Authority in 2012. The cardiopulmonary standard is easier to comprehend by the lay person but unfortunately the practice of the procedure is not always dignified, if not bordering on the unethical. These patients are fulfilling the legal requirements for death but in an effort to obtain organs, there is an intense vigil to restart the perfusion process just after five minutes of the diagnosis to fulfill the requirement for a minimum warm ischaemia time, to ensure the viability of the organs. Adding to the contentious ethical issues is that in an effort not to lose precious seconds, there is preparation of the potential donor by medication and insertion of vascular cannulas and other medical equipment in the agonal patient, to be ready to switch on perfusion within five minutes of death. This is an undignified way to die.

The issues of donation from anencephalic neonates is being addressed here because it depends on the definition of death. Anencephalic infants are born with a neural tube defect resulting in failure of closure of the skull. They usually have limited cerebral cortex and cerebellum but the brain stem is present, and so they can breathe spontaneously, have newborn reflexes and variable autonomic function but they lack consciousness. Such children may live for just a few seconds but many survive without life support for hours or days. These neonates are not aware of their existence,

However Shewmon (1989) thinks that the brainstem in anencephalics can actually exhibit function usually attributable to the cortex, due to neuroplasticity.

Organs would only be beneficial to infants of a similar age. This makes a match difficult to obtain, and organ shortage is a real issue unless there is adequate co-operation between centres. In children, using medical criteria to define brain stem death is difficult. Guidelines for brain death in infants were formulated in 1987 by a Task Force composed of representatives from the American Academy of Pediatrics, the American Academy of Neurology, the Child Neurology Society, the American Neurological Association, the American Bar Association, and the National Institute of Neurological Diseases and Communicative Disorders and Stroke. These are similar to adult guidelines but protocols depend on age, e.g. for children between 7 days and 2 months of age, 2 sets of examinations and an EEG separated by 48 hours are recommended. However the criteria did not apply to infants below 7 days as there was insufficient data available. In anencephalics, there are greater problems because they can maintain an irregular function of the brain stem for up to 3 weeks (Parisi, Squiteri, Carottie, Dicarlo and Gagliardi, 1999). Also EEG and cerebral blood flow may be inappropriate tests as there are no cerebral hemispheres.

Ashwal and Serna-Fonseca (2006) recommend using the 1987 criteria for neonates, but emphasise that cranial nerve function is difficult to assess in term and preterm neonates and moreover these reflexes are still not fully developed. Sekar (2007) also suggests that the guidelines could be applied to neonates.

There is the added problem of deciding on viability of organs, to avoid unnecessarily endangering the safety of recipients. There is concern as to the viability of organs from anencephalics who were not on a life support system at the time of death because of gradual deterioration of already poor cardiorespiratory function, giving rise to ischaemia. If the infants are maintained on a life support system from birth, the organs are not ischaemic but, according to the Canadian Paediatric Society, 2005, 'while organ function may be maintained with life support, as brainstem function deteriorates, multisystem organ failure develops before sudden death.' In fact the Society does not recommend organ donation from anencephalics. This statement was reaffirmed in 2009 and 2013.

Donor Rights

Integrity

The *Charter of Fundamental Rights of the European Union* (2010) highlights the integrity of the person in article 3(1): 'Everyone has the right to respect for his or her physical and mental integrity'.

The Council of Europe's *Convention for the Protection of Human Rights and Fundamental Freedoms* (2010) provides protection of human rights and fundamental freedoms for all individuals, including the right to life and protection of health interests. Article 5, the 'Right to liberty and security' provides for the right to security of the person. Being a donor and giving away an organ can be arguably construed as violating this right unless this is a definite act of will, that is, it is accomplished with full consent in keeping with ensuring one's autonomy.

Article 1 of the Council of Europe's *Convention on Human Rights and Biomedicine* (1997) provides for protection of 'the dignity and identity of all human beings'; 'respect for their integrity and other rights and fundamental freedoms' in medical matters'. One can argue from a psychological standpoint that losing an organ damages the individual's identity.

Confidentiality

Consent is likely to be given only if the donor is convinced of the legality of the process and that his/her rights are being protected. The EU *Directive 2010/45/EU* considers confidentiality important. In the preamble, paragraph 22, it is stated that 'As a general principle, the identity of the recipient(s) should not be disclosed to the donor or the donor's family or vice versa'. A close relationship between donor and recipient has, albeit only known of anecdotally, led to the recipient being almost stalked by relatives of the deceased. On the other hand patient associations have in general been in favour of a relationship being forged between donors and recipients and have acted as a go-between for bringing about meetings between the parties. It is also worth noting that confidentiality is extremely difficult to ensure in small states where the media is easily the first to disseminate information about victims of major trauma accidents.

The protection of personal data and confidentiality is emphasised with respect to both donors' and recipients' personal data, in the context of traceability, registries, records of procurement organisations and transplantation centres as well as data processing, all in line with *Directive 95/46/EC on the protection of individuals with regard to the processing of personal data and on the free movement of such data*. Confidentiality in relation to data is also repeated in article 23(1) of the *Additional Protocol on Transplantation* (2002).

Health

According to the *Charter of Fundamental Rights of the European Union* (2010), article 35, 'Everyone has the right of access to preventive health care and the right to benefit from medical treatment under the conditions established by national laws and practices'. Living donors also have a right to expect adequate health care after the donation. The Council of Europe's *Additional Protocol on Transplantation* (2002), article 7, states that 'appropriate medical follow-up shall be offered to living donors and recipients after transplantation'.

Early problems include post-operative complications but these are minimal. Living donor surgery has a 0.03% mortality in the US (National Kidney Registry, 2012). Living donors have the same lifespan and end stage kidney disease as the age / sex / ethnicity matched population (Ibrahim, Foley, Tan, Rogers, Bailey, Guo, Gross and Matas, 2009).Where health services depend primarily on insurance, the donor from a low socioeconomic class is disadvantaged with regard to post donation healthcare.

Compensation

The principle of voluntary unpaid donation of tissues and cells was recognised for the first time in Spain in 1979 and in Luxembourg, Belgium and Finland in the early 1980s (European Commission, 2006). The same report states that donors cannot be remunerated but may receive compensation strictly limited to making good the expenses and inconvenience related to the donation. The principle that the body or body parts should not be a source of financial gain was formally established in article 21 in the *Convention on Human Rights and Biomedicine* (1997) and repeated in article 21(1) in the *Additional Protocol* (2002), which does allow 'compensation of living donors for loss of earnings and any other justifiable expenses caused by the removal or by the related medical examinations; payment of a justifiable fee for legitimate medical or related technical services rendered in connection with transplantation' and 'compensation in case of undue damage resulting from the removal of organs or tissues from living persons'. This would include remuneration for travel, time off work and healthcare costs. There could be a system of compensation by the recipient's insurer to make up for the savings in terms of healthcare for the recipient. Living donors may also have to travel abroad to be with their relative recipient if the transplant operation is not possible in their country of origin; they should also qualify for compensation.

Advertising for an organ with an offer of money is illegal in most countries and is mentioned in the Council of Europe's *Additional Protocol* (2002) in article 21(2): 'Advertising the need for, or availability of, organs or tissues, with a view to offering or seeking financial gain or comparable advantage, shall be prohibited'. This view was to emerge again in article 13.3 in the EU *Directive, 2010/45/EU*. However advertising for organs on the internet is now a reality for pooled donation schemes, which are meant to be voluntary non compensated schemes. Such schemes are now officially organized either on a national basis or by charities.

ACCESS

The *Charter of Fundamental Rights of the European Union* (2010), article 35 emphasises that: 'Everyone has the right of access to preventive health care and the right to benefit from medical treatment under the conditions established by national laws and practices. A high level of human health protection shall be ensured in the definition and implementation of all Union policies and activities.'

Allocation

Protocols

One of the main tenets of Human Rights law is protection of individuals from discrimination. Most countries have legal provisions to respect patient rights in the field of organ donation and transplantation, in particular with regard to ensuring justice in the allocation of organs and resources. WHO (2010) in its Guiding Principles on human cell, tissue and organ transplantation states that 'The allocation of organs, cells and tissues should be guided by clinical criteria and ethical norms, not financial or other considerations. Allocation rules, defined by appropriately constituted committees, should be equitable, externally justified, and transparent'. Yet it is extremely difficult to get a standard response to the question of how recipients are prioritized to allocate donor organs from deceased donors. The issue of course does not arise with a living donor as there is a one to one approach or at least in the chain system there is the best match possible approach.

The decision has always been, rightly so, left in the hands of the medical practitioners, yet there is no uniform harmonised standard by WHO. In the US, the Organ Procurement and Transplantation Network, OPTN, is empowered through the *National Organ Transplant Act* to produce allocation guidelines and these are available on their website. All major guidelines address the health status of the recipient and put this at the top of their list, based on an assessment of urgency in relation to chance of cure. Recipients may be assessed in terms of QUALYs, Quality-Adjusted Life Years, where one year of perfect health amounts to one (1) QUALY. There are of course objective ways of assessing QUALYs and these depend on potential income lost. Is that right for assessing whether to receive an organ or not? This would put a rich recipient ahead on the list, way above the patient from a lower socioeconomic group. On the other hand the social class may have adverse influence on the possibility of success of the transplant because the potential recipient is envisioned as one who may not be able to keep up with the healthcare required, if the state is not in a position to assist with funds; this further disadvantages the poorer recipients. Patients on dialysis actually cost more in terms of healthcare than transplant recipients, so it may be beneficial for the state to invest in funding transplantation rather than treatment for end stage renal disease. As WHO (2010) states: 'no recipient should be excluded solely for financial reasons'.

Medical issues limiting donation relate principally to medical assessment of suitability of an organ for donation. The first criterion is naturally for the organ to be healthy and free of transmissible infective diseases. Tests for immunity, blood grouping and HLA typing (six antigen matching) are used, especially for kidneys. There are no contentious issues here as naturally one needs to ensure safety to recipients. Legislation across Europe is now in the process of standardisation as the EU *Directive 2010/45/EU* is being transposed into domestic legislation.

UNOS, the United Network for Organ Sharing in the US, has been the national US operator of OPTN, since 1986. OPTN has a policy laying down minimum standards for screening donors, easily accessible on its website. In all protocols donors need to be free of infectious diseases that are transmitted by blood, primarily hepatitis B and C and HIV. In the US, there is current scientific evidence advocating infected individuals to agree to be donors to infected recipients, in a move to increase the pool of donors (UCSF, 2012). Studies show that the grafts have been accepted without significant problems (Morales, Campistol, Dominguez-Gil, Andrés, Esforzado, Oppenheimer, Castellano, Fuertes, Bruguera and Praga, 2010). The main advantage for the recipient is the enhanced quality of life; taking people off dialysis early gives them a better quality of life than waiting on the transplant list (Tonelli, Weibe, Knoll, Bello, Jadhav, Klarenbach and Gill, 2011). However the practice has as yet not been uniformly incorporated in medical guidelines.

One factor that is not nowadays a barrier, is age, provided the individual's health is good. Most recognized criteria delineate an age cut off point for organs, based on the well established fact that increasing age of the donor organ, particularly well established for kidneys, is associated with shorter post transplant survival then for kidneys donated from younger donors. However there is no reason why older recipients cannot be matched to older donor kidneys, which satisfy the 'expanded criteria' for donors. Of course concomitant disease increases the morbidity, so a transplant would not be considered. However corneas can be donated in patients with systemic cancer.

On the other hand age is a limiting factor in relation to matching the size of the donor organ to the recipient. The size of the organ is important for transplants from children to children. For child to adult donation, traditionally kidneys donated from young children were both given to the same recipient but now a single kidney has been successfully transplanted. Kidneys have been donated even from a deceased infant as young as 9 months and transplanted into adults (Zhang, Paramesh, Florman, Yau, Balamuthusamy, Krane and Slakey, 2009).

Living Donors for Non-Related Recipients

The issue of whether donations from living non-related donors should be uniformly available is slowly gaining acceptance and it must be seriously considered as a real choice to increase donations. The main objections are ethical but with robust legislation to ensure infrastructure and confidentiality to preserve the donor's rights, there should be no major objection. In fact there are now chain systems run by NGOs as well as by some US states that foster this type of donation built on the deceased donor donation best match. With improvements in computerized data systems, it has become increasingly easy to identify, locate and prepare recipients for transplant without running risks of losing viability and wastage of organs. Now, organs can be sent to any country in the world with a minimum delay and in conditions that can preserve viability. This is the concept used in chains but here the match is the important bottom line.

Health of the Recipient

The main issue is always to ensure that having undergone the emotional and psychological trauma of receiving an organ, there is only the most minimal likelihood that rejection occurs. The EU has been at the forefront of ensuring transplant safety and has directives dealing with this issue for blood (*Directive 2002/98/EC*), tissues and cells (*Directive 2004/23/EC*) and solid organs (*Directive 2010/45/EU*). These directives all ask for testing of the donors prior to making them eligible to be donors. This includes testing for infectious diseases, that may be absolute contraindications to being a donor, such as HIV, hepatitis B and C, although even now this practice is changing as infected individuals may be donors to infected recipients.

With a view to ensuring that health authorities have complied, there is emphasis on the traceability of the organ (*Directive 2010/45/EU,* article 10) such that any adverse events can be linked to the possibility of a problem in the donor. In rare instances this may be a genetic problem.

Matching is of course crucial for kidneys; the better the match the more likely is the success of this transplant but the heart does not need to be matched. HLA typing is often farmed out to laboratories that may not be part of the hospitals offering the transplant services and it falls to the competent Transplant Authority to ensure the laboratories are in line with the local legislation regulating laboratories, including relevant ISO accreditation and professionalism in laboratory scientists.

In an attempt to ensure safety within the EU, *Directive 2010/45/EU* requires adverse event reporting (article 4(g), article 11 and article 17(d)) and post transplant results (article 17(e)), including adverse reactions of drugs used to prevent rejection and pharmacovigilance. However data is not easily available from all countries, although mechanisms for reporting exist, such as the NOTIFY Library of Adverse Events and Reactions, co-ordinated by the WHO and the Italian National Transplant Centre, with the collaboration of the EU funded project SOHO V&S, Vigilance and Surveillance of Substances of Human Origin. More emphasis must be placed on organisational structures to ensure data collection. Member states in Europe must have a Competent Authority to organise the transplant system and this must report to the Commission every three years to confirm compliance with the EU *Directive 2010/45/EU*, article 17 and article 22. UNOS, is the responsible body in the States.

Data Protection

The duty of a state to keep records must be in compliance with Data Protection laws, for sensitive health data. In the EU, the *Data Protection Directive 95/46/EC*, has been transposed into national legislation for member states. In the US, similar provisions are available through the *Privacy Act, 1974* and the *Electronic Communications Privacy Act*. The Council of Europe's *Convention on Human Rights and Biomedicine* (1997) states in article 10 that: 'Everyone is entitled to know any information collected about his or her health. However, the wishes of individuals not to be so informed shall be observed'.

The *Charter of Fundamental Rights of the European Union* (2010), article 8 states:

1. Everyone has the right to the protection of personal data concerning him or her.
2. Such data must be processed fairly for specified purposes and on the basis of the consent of the person concerned or some other legitimate basis laid down by law. Everyone has the right of access to data which has been collected concerning him or her, and the right to have it rectified.

Directive 2010/45/EU lays down the minimum data that must be collected to ensure the quality and safety of organs, including a register of donors, demographic details and medical history of the donors and recipients. Article 16 emphasises the need for protection of all personal data collected. Data has to be kept secure over the years to allow traceability of organs (article 10) should a safety issue arise. Data has to be up to date to avoid the stress of contacting relatives or donors themselves who have opted out of being organ donors or who have changed their wish to donate through an Advance Directive. States must ensure that the stored data is easily available to the authorised personnel who are providing the transplant service, that is the competent authority or its delegate. For an efficient service, access to donor registries, including the list of those who have opted out, must be available to procurement organisations and transplant centres, so that donor – recipient matches are made possible in the shortest available time. Proper maintenance of data also ensures that there is no accidental contact with relatives of deceased individuals who have opted out, mistakenly to ask for consent and thus causing undue emotional stress on the relatives. Electronic data has made storage and retrieval much easier but has also led to the need for more electronic security measures.

Organisational Structures

In the 10 point policy of the EU (2008), it was recognized that to increase organ donation there is a need to employ certain strategies. Experience from countries with an actual increase in the number of donations and successful operations, has shown that the success story devolves around a sound administrative set up. Spain has actually been on record to explain her progress in this field. Initially thought to be due to presumed consent, it became obvious that with a soft presumed consent policy and no register for opting out, this was not the full explanation. It soon became evident that the dedicated medical transplant co-ordinators were responsible for the success. As the personnel liaisoning with families, they were in a key role to explain the organ donation process; naturally they had to be properly trained.

In the EU, *Directive 2010/45/EU*, article 17, provides for a competent Transplant Authority, to be a regulatory body, which can delegate its powers to another body on a national level. The Authority must oversee the whole sequence from donation to transplant and beyond to post transplant surveillance of the health of both parties. The administrative duties include the responsibility for identifying an organizational structure adequate for the country. The Authority is to authorise, maybe through licensing, the functions of procurement organisations that retrieve and transport the donor organs, and to oversee the function of transplant centres, directly involved in the surgery.

The Transplant Authority's role extends to ensuring that all hospitals are adequately licensed for the service they provide. They have to inspect premises on a regular basis. Such licence usually includes accreditation of premises and adequate resources, and mandates employment of fully trained professional healthcarers, whether doctors or paramedics. It must be in a position to recommend adequate training for personnel, including training for the administrators of the system.

One important aspect is the funding of the service. It is to the benefit of all if these services are centrally funded on a national basis out of the health budget. *Revised UAGA* in US also establishes standards for donor registries, allows computerized registries of donors and accepts electronic signatures, but it makes no similar provision for those who do not want to be donors. It enables procurement organizations to gain access to donor registries, medical records, and records of the state motor vehicle department. There is introduction of regulations relating to cooperation and co-ordination between procurement organizations and coroners or medical examiners.

Mobility

Competent Transplant Authorities that maintain robust organizational structures are in a unique position to promote and facilitate transplant medicine and research as they form relations with counterparts in neighbouring and distant countries in an effort to maximise resources and knowledge through the set up of international organ exchange systems. On a national level, countries do have specific arrangements with neighbouring states for cross-border movement and healthcare but it would be beneficial to all if this were on a European basis. Though it is mainly organs that are transported, where more practical, as in heart and lung transplants, it is the recipient who travels.

The EU *Directive 2011/24/EU* on cross-border healthcare specifically states in article 1(3)(b) that it does not apply to 'allocation of, and access to, organs for the purpose of organ transplants'. However for organ procurement there is a specific transplant policy, involving cross border co-operation, as outlined in the EU Action Plan on Organ Donation and Transplantation (2009-2015). Of course if a country is not in a position to offer specialised services, it has the human rights duty to allow its citizens to travel abroad and to pay for the healthcare services accessed in the other state. The Directive does allow organ exchange with third party countries (article 20) and European organ exchange organisations (article 21), under the supervision of the competent Transplant Authority.

Education

EU directives always insist on dissemination of the law but this is only a small step towards increasing knowledge and awareness about organ donation. Much work has to be done by the competent Transplant Authority to educate the public if we are to see an increase in the availability of organs. Successful programmes have invested in involving the public via media programmes and patient support groups. The latter are always proactive in meeting with relatives of both donors and recipients, offering counselling and advice and long term support. However counselling should be provided as part of the hospital based transplant services, or else farmed out to the procurement agencies, who are ultimately responsible for ensuring that informed consent is obtained.

Increased deceased donation depends on the communication skills of the person requesting organ donation from relatives. So training in this field is mandatory for all doctors who will be in such units but also for transplant co-ordinators who have to train others how to approach potential donors and their relatives. With regard to professionals, it is recognized that there are full time specialists in some countries, who are primarily involved in just transplant work but in many countries the services are offered, when the need arises, by professionals with a specialised interest. This emphasises the need for professional qualifications of personnel but also continual in house training for the specialists. The competent Transplant Authority should ensure that there is funding for these activities.

Accreditation schemes for laboratories should be in place in all laboratories, whose services are used to carry out tests on donor samples. All hospital facilities must be run according to accepted standards and guidelines. Last, but not least, research on transplant medicine has to continue on a national level, as well as throughout networks, such as Eurotransplant, the European Transplant Network.

CONCLUSION

Legislation is obviously necessary to ensure health and safety in the procurement and use of organs, to ensure equity in access to transplant services and to keep a check on abuse of the system. Its role in increasing availability of organs is in establishing proper guidelines for the medical professional responsible for obtaining consent,or for declaring death and in regulating professionals and institutions. It is however only one step; the way forward involves more international harmonisation and standardisation to ensure efficient use of resources in an attempt to provide early access to suitable organs for all those on a waiting list.

We are seeing a change in the type of organs available, with living donation being increasingly available for non-directed transplantation and deceased donor organs obtained from non-heart beating cadavers. It is now possible to engineer simple biological tissues, such as trachea or urinary bladder, from one's own stem cells, and though building complex solid organs will probably not be available for some years yet, the research may provide alternative pathways for repairing organs.

REFERENCES

Alliance-O: European Group for Coordination of National Research Programmes on Organ Donation and Transplantation. (2004-2007). *White Paper*. ERA-NET scheme, EC 0011853.

Critical Care Nurse, 26(2), 117-128.

Is it ethical for patients with renal disease to purchase kidneys from the world's poor?.Bioedge. (2012) *European crisis boosts illegal trade in body parts*. Retrieved 9 June 2012 from http://www.bioedge.org/index.php/bioethics/bioethics_article/10107.

Bioedge. (2012). *China to stop harvesting convict organs*, Retrieved 31 March 2012 from http://www.bioedge.org/index.php/bioethics/bioethics_article/10008.

Bird, S. M., Harris, J. (2010). *Time to move to presumed consent for organ donation*. British Medical Journal, 340.

British Medical Association Medical Ethics Committee. (2000). *Organ Donation in the 21st Century: A Time for a Consolidated Approach*. London. BMA.

Canadian Paediatric Society (CPS). Bioethics Committee, 2003-2004. (2005). *Use of anencephalic newborns as organ donors*. Paediatrics & Child Health 2005;10(6):335-7,

Ref. No. B05-01, Reaffirmed January 2009 and January 2013. Retrieved from http://www.cps.ca/documents/position/anencephalic-newborns-as-organ-donors.

Caplan, A., Dominguez-Gil, B., Matesanz, R., Prior, C. (2009). *Trafficking in organs, tissues and cells and trafficking in human beings for the purpose of the removal of organs*. Joint Council of Europe/United Nations Study, DG of Human Rights and Legal Affairs, Council of Europe.

Capron, A.M. (2001). *Brain death-well settled yet still unresolved*. New Engl J Med, 344(16), 1244-46.

Charter of Fundamental Rights of the European Union, 2010/C83/02, OJ L, 30.03.2010, C83/392, p.389-403.

Coppen, R., Friele, R. D., Gevers, S. K., & van der Zee, J. (2010). *Imagining the Impact of Different Consent Systems on Organ Donation: The Decisions of Next of Kin*. Death Studies, 34(9), 835-847.

Coppen, R., Friele, R. D., Gevers, S. K., Blok, G. A., & van der Zee, J. (2008). *The impact of donor policies in Europe: a steady increase, but not everywhere*. BMC health services research, 8(1), 235-244.

Council of Europe. (2002). *Additional Protocol to the Convention on human rights and biomedicine, on transplantation of organs and tissues of human origin*, Strasbourg: Council of Europe, 24.1.2002.

Council of Europe. (1997). *Convention for the protection of human rights and dignity of the human being with regard to the application of biology and medicine: Convention on human rights and biomedicine*. Oviedo:4.4.1997.

Council of Europe. (2005). *Convention on action against trafficking in human beings*. Warsaw, 16.5.2005.

Council of Europe. (2005). *Convention for the protection of human rights and fundamental freedoms* as amended by Protocols No.11 and No.14. Rome, 4.XI.1950.

Council of Europe. (2004). CDBI/INF/2004/INF(2003)11rev.2e. *Replies to the Questionnaire for member states on organ trafficking*, 2 June 2004.

Council of Europe. (2004). CM/AS(2004)Rec1611 final 21 June 2004.. *Trafficking in organs in Europe*. Recommendation 1611 (2003). Reply adopted by the Committee of Ministers on 16 June 2004 at the 888th meeting of the Ministers' Deputies.) Retrieved from http://assembly.coe.int/ASP/Doc/XrefViewHTML.asp?FileID=10574&Language=EN

Declaration of Death. L.1991, ch.90. (NJSA 26:6A-5) (US).

Declaration of Istanbul. (2008) Istanbul summit on organ trafficking and transplant tourism.

EU Directive 95/46/EC of the European Parliament and of the Council of 24 October 1995 on the protection of individuals with regard to the processing of personal data and on the free movement of such data. OJ L 281, 23.11.1995, p. 31-50.

EU Directive 2002/98/EC of the European Parliament and of the Council of 27 January 2003 on setting standards of quality and safety for the collection, testing, processing, storage and distribution of human blood and blood components, OJ L 33, 8.2.2003, p. 30-40.

EU Directive 2004/23/EC of the European Parliament and of the Council of 31 March 2004 on setting standards of quality and safety for the donation, procurement, testing, processing, preservation, storage and distribution of human tissues and cells. OJ L 102, 7.4.2004, p. 48-58.

EU Directive 2010/45/EU of the European Parliament and of the Council of 7 July 2010, on standards of quality and safety of human organs intended for transplantation. OJ L 207, 6.8.2010, p.14-29.

EU Directive 2011/24/EU of the European Parliament and of the Council of 9 March 2011 on the application of patients' rights in cross-border healthcare. Official Journal of the European Union, OJ L88, 04.04.2011, p.54.

EU Directive 2011/36/EU of the European Parliament and of the Council of 5 April 2011 on preventing and combating trafficking in human beings and protecting its victims, and replacing Council Framework Decision 2002/629/JHA, OJ L101, 15.4.2011, p1-11.

European Commission (2007). Special Eurobarometer 272, Europeans and Organ Donation. Brussels Directorate General Health and Consumer Protection, SANCO.

European Commission. COM(2008) 819/3. Communication from the European Commission. Action plan on Organ Donation and Transplantation (2009-2015): Strengthened Cooperation between Member States, Brussels, 8.12.2008.

European Commission. COM/2006/0593 final. . Report from the Commission to the Council and the European Parliament, on the promotion by Member States of voluntary unpaid donation of tissues and cells. Brussels.

European Commission. Journalists' Workshop. (2012). Organ Donation and Transpl*antation.* Facts and Figures. Retrieved at http://ec.europa.eu/health/blood_tissues_organs/docs/ev_20121009_facts_figures.pdf

Eurotransplant. (2012). Transplantation Timeline. Retrieved from http://www.eurotransplant.org/cms/index.php?page=about_timeline

German National Ethics Council. (2007) *Opinion: Increasing the number of organ donations: a pressing issue for transplant medicine in Germany.*

Gesetz über die „Spende, Entnahme und Übertragung von Organen und Gewebe, The German Transplantation Act, TPG. 1997 . (Germany).

Gevers, S., Janssen, A., & Friele, R. (2004). *Consent systems for post mortem organ donation in Europe*. Eur. J. Health L., 11, 175.

Global Observatory on Donation and Transplantation. (2012). *Facts*. Retrieved from http://www.transplant-observatory.org/Pages/Facts.aspx

Gómez-Lobo, A., personal statement, (2008) *Controversies in the determination of death*, a white paper by the President's Council on Bioethics, Washington DC.

Harvard Medical School. (1968), *A definition of irreversible coma* Ad Hoc Committee to examine the definition of brain death.. JAMA 205, no.6, 1968, p337-40.

Human Tissue Act 1982 (Vic) (Australia).

Human Tissue Act 2004 (UK). *Human Tissue (Scotland) Act 2006*.(UK, Scotland).

Human Tissue Authority, UK, Code of practice 2, *Donation of solid organs for transplantation*, 2009, paragraph 86.

Human Tissue Gift Act1996. (RSBC) (Canada) and *Consent to Donation Regulation 1999.* (B.C. Reg. 65/99).

Human Transplantation (Wales) Bill. (2013). Retrieved at http://www.senedd.assemblywales.org/ documents/s18966/Bill,%20as%20passed.pdf

Ibrahim, H.N., Foley, R., Tan, L., Rogers, T., Bailey, R.F., Guo, H., Gross, C.R., Matas, A.J. (2009). *Long-term consequences of kidney donation*. N Engl J Med, 2009;360:459-69.

McCullough, K. P., Keith, D. S., Meyer, K. H., Stock, P. G, Brayman, K. L. & Leichtman, A. B. (2009). *Kidney and pancreas transplantation in the United States, 1998-2007: access for patients with diabetes and end-stage renal disease*. Am J Transplant. Apr 2009;9(Pt 2):894-906.

Medical Royal Colleges, UK. (1976). *Diagnosis of brain death.* Statement issued by the honorary secretary of the Conference of Medical Royal Colleges and their faculties in the United Kingdom. BMJ 1976,2:1187-8.

Morales, J. M., Campistol, J. M., Dominguez-Gil, B., Andrés, A., Esforzado, N., Oppenheimer, F., Castellano, G., Fuertes, A., Brugera, M. & Praga, M. (2010) *Long-term experiencer with kidney transplantation from hepatitis C-positive donors into hepatitis C-positive recipients.* Am. J. Transplant. Nov:10(11):2453-62.

National Kidney Registry, New York. (2012). Retrieved from http://www.kidneyregistry.org/living_donors.php#overview

National Organ Transplant Act 1984 Pub.L. 98-507 (US).NHS Blood and Transplant (NHSBT) Health Authority. (2011-2012). *National Transplant Statistics, UK*. Retrieved from http://www.organdonation.nhs.uk/statistics/transplant_activity_report/current_activity_reports/ukt/kidney_activity.pdf

NHS Blood and Transplant (NHSBT) Health Authority. (2012). *Transplantation milestones.* Retrieved at http://www.organdonation.nhs.uk/about_transplants/transplantation_milestones/.

Organ Procurement and Transplant Network, OPTN. (2012). *About transplantation, history.* Retrieved from http://optn.transplant.hrsa.gov/latestData/rptData.asp.

Organ Procurement and Transplant Network, OPTN. (2012). *Identification of transmissible diseases in organ recipients*. Retrieved from http://optn.transplant.hrsa.gov/PoliciesandBylaws2/policies/pdfs/policy_16.pdf

Organ Donation Act (Wet op Orgaan Donatie) (1989) (the Netherlands) Section 9(1).

Organ Donation Taskforce. (2008). *The Potential Impact of an Opt Out System for Organ Donation in the UK: An Independent Report from the Organ Donation Taskforce.* London. UK Department of Health.

Pallis, C. (1982). *From brain death to brain stem death.* Br Med J (Clin Res Ed). 1982; 285(6353):1487-1490.Parisi, F., Squitieri, C., Carottie, A., Dicarlo, D. & Gagliardi, MG. (1999). *Heart transplantation on the first day of life from an anencephalic donor.* Pediatr Transplant 1999; 3: 150–151.

Patient Self-Determination Act, 1991 (US)

Pearson, E. (2004). *Coercion in the kidney trade?, A background study on trafficking in human organ worldwide, Sector project against trafficking in women*, Deutsche Gesellschaft für Technische Zusammenarbeit (GTZ) GmbH.

Pellegrino, E.D., personal statement,(2008). *Controversies in the determination of death*, a white paper by the President's Council on Bioethics, Washington DC.

President's Commission for the study of ethical problems in medicine and biomedical and behavioral research. (1981). *Defining death: A report on the medical, legal and ethical issues in the determination of death*. Washington, DC.

President's Council on Bioethics. (2008) *Controversies in the determination of death, a White Paper*. Chapter 7, Washington DC. Retrieved at http://ldysinger.stjohnsem.edu/@books/Pres_Council_2008/03_ch_7-end.htm.

Procurement and Transplantation of Organs 1986 (Belgium)

Public Broadcasting Service. A Science Odessey: People and Discoveries: First successful kidney transplant performed. Retrieved from http://www.pbs.org/wgbh/aso/databank/entries/dm54ki.html

Royal College of Physicians. (1995). *Criteria for the diagnosis of brain stem death*. J Roy Coll Physns of London 29:381-2.

Savulescu, J. (2003). Is the sale of body parts wrong?. *Journal of medical ethics*, *29*(3), 138-139.

Sekar, K.C. (2007) *Brain death in the newborn*. Journal of Perinatology. Supplement, Vol.27,Ps59-62,1p.2charts.Shewmon, D. A. (1989). *The Use of Anencephalic Infants as Organ Donors*. 261 JAMA 1773, 1776.

Shimazono, Y. (2007). *The state of the international organ trade: a provisional picture based on integration of available information*. Bulletin of the World Health Organization, *85*(12), 955-962.

SOHO V&S: *Vigilance and Surveillance of Substances of Human Origin*. Retrieved from http://ec.europa.eu/eahc/documents/health/conference_27-28_06_2013/SOHO _V_ Improving_Vigilance_of_Tissues_and_Cells.pdf

Task Force for the determination of brain death in children. (1987). *Guidelines for the determination of brain death in children*. Annals of Neurology 21(6): 616-617.

The New Jersey Declaration of Death Act PL 1991. c90 (NJSA 26:6a)

The NOTIFY Library of Adverse Events and Reactions. Bologna Initiative for Global Vigilance and Surveillance (BIG V&S) co-ordinated by the WHO and the Italian National Transplant Centre (CNT), with the collaboration of the EU funded project SOHO V&S, Vigilance and Surveillance of Substances of Human Origin. http://www.notifylibrary.org/

The Transplantation Society and the International Society of Nephrology. *Declaration of Istanbul*. (2008). Istanbul summit on organ trafficking and transplant tourism.

Tonelli, M., Wiebe, N., Knoll, G., Bello, A., Browne, S., Jadhav, D., Klarenbach, S. & Gill, J. (2011). *Systematic review: kidney transplantation compared with dialysis in clinically relevant outcomes*. American Journal of Transplantation, 11(10), 2093-2109.

UN *Convention on the Rights of the Child*. (1990). General Assembly Resolution 44/25, 20 November 1989, entered into force 2 September 1990.

UN *Optional Protocol to the Convention on the Rights of the Child, on the sale of children, child prostitution and child pornography*. (2002). General Assembly Resolution A/RES/54/263, 25 May 2000, entered into force 18 January 2002.

UN *Protocol to Prevent, Suppress and Punish Trafficking in Persons, especially women and children*. (2000). Adopted by General Assembly resolution 55/25, is supplementing the UN Convention, entered into force on 25 December 2003.. article 3(a).

Uniform Anatomical Gift Act, UAGA, 1987. (US). Revised 2006.

Uniform Determination of Death Act, 1980. (US)

United Network for Organ Sharing, UNOS. http://www.unos.org/

UCSF, University of California, Transplant Surgery, (2012). Hepatitis C Donor Program. Retrieved from http://transplant.surgery.ucsf.edu/conditions--procedures/kidney-transplantation.aspx

US Living Will Registry. Organ Donation Information and Registration, http://www.uslivingwillregistry.com/organdonation.shtm

Veatch, R. M. (1989). *Death, dying, and the biological revolution: Our last quest for responsibility*. New Haven, Connecticut: Yale University Press.

Veatch, R. M. (2008). *Donating hearts after cardiac death—reversing the irreversible*. New England Journal of Medicine, 359(7), 672-673.

WHO. (2004). *Human organ and tissue transplantation*. World Health Assembly Resolution 57.18. (22 May 2004).

WHO (2010). *Guiding principles on human cell, tissue and organ transplantation*. Endorsed by the 63rd World Health Assembly, May 2010, in Resolution WHA63.22. Geneva, Switzerland. World Health Organization.

Wijdicks, E. F. (2002). *Brain death worldwide: Accepted fact but no global consensus in diagnostic criteria*. Neurology, 58(1), 20-25.

Wijdicks, E. F., Varelas, P. N., Gronseth, G. S., & Greer, D. M. (2010). *Evidence-based guideline update: Determining brain death in adults*. Report of the Quality Standards Subcommittee of the American Academy of Neurology. Neurology, 74(23), 1911-1918.

Wilkinson, A., Wenger, N., Shugarman, L.R. (2007). *Literature Review on Advance Directives*, commissioned by U.S. Department of Health and Human Services. *RAND Corporation*.

World Medical Association. (200-65). *Council Resolution on Organ Donation in China*. Adopted at 173rd WMA Council Session at France, Divonne-les-Bains, 20.05 2006.

World Medical Association. (2012). *Statement on organ donation and tissue donation*. Adopted by the 63rd WMA General Assembly. Bangkok, Thailand.

Zhang, R., Paramesh, A., Florman, S., Yau, C. L., Balamuthusamy, S., Krane, N. K., & Slakey, D. (2009). *Long-term outcome of adults who undergo transplantation with single pediatric kidneys: how young is too young?* Clinical Journal of the American Society of Nephrology, 4(9), 1500-1506.

In: Organ Donation and Transplantation
Editor: Mary Anne Lauri

ISBN: 978-1-62948-257-6

Chapter 2

LIVE DONATION AND THE EXPERIENCE OF THE DONOR: A PERSONAL PERSPECTIVE

Maureen Cole*
University of Malta, Malta

ABSTRACT

This chapter first presents an overview of the pertinent research literature on live kidney donation and the experience of the donor. The author, herself a live kidney donor, then uses a phenomenological approach to explore her own experience as a live donor. This experience is then compared and contrasted to experiences as drawn from the literature with a special focus on the decision to donate and the psychosocial impact on the living kidney donor. In the final part of the chapter best practices are highlighted drawing on both the literature and the author's personal experience.

INTRODUCTON

The focus of this chapter will be on the experience of the donor in the context of live donation. As a live kidney donor myself, I will be overseeing the research literature and comparing some of the notions which emerge in the literature to my own experience. These experiences have been explored from a number of perspectives and focuses: in general terms, from an ethical perspective, in attempts to try to understand the motives and decision making process involved, as gift exchange, as examples of altruism and with a focus on the psychosocial impact on the donors, amongst others. The literature to be reviewed will be considered under two of these focuses, namely the decision to donate and the psychosocial impact on the living kidney donor. I have selected these specific focuses as they seem most pertinent to the analysis of my own experience and also because some of the other perspectives will be drawn upon in other chapters of this book. The literature to be reviewed refers to western lifestyles and contexts as this is closest to my own situation. The method I

* E-mail: maureen.cole@um.edu.mt.

will be using to analyse my experience is a qualitative phenomenological approach. I am hoping that my account goes sufficiently beyond the personal to allow others going through a similar experience and professionals working with live kidney donors to gain from it. In the final part of the chapter some best practices will be underscored using both the literature and my experience.

The Decision to Donate

The motives underlying live kidney donation have been studied fairly extensively. Lennerling, Forsberg and Nyberg's study (as cited in Lennerling, Forsberg, Meyer and Nyberg 2004, p. 1600) was an in-depth study of 12 potential kidney donors where seven categories of motives for the donation were identified. The motives which were articulated were the following:

- a wish to help;
- a feeling of moral duty;
- self-benefit from the relative's improved health;
- improved self-esteem from doing good deeds;
- identification with the recipient;
- external pressure; and
- logic - knowing that you can live a normal life with one kidney.

Lennerling, Forsberg and Nyberg (2003) state that these identified categories interacted to create a perception that donation is the only option (p.1243).

In a follow-up quantitative study, also of potential kidney donors who were being evaluated for donation in two Transplant Units, one in Sweden and the other in Norway, 154 questionnaires were returned with a response rate of 74% (Lennerling et al., 2004, p. 1601). The respondents consisted primarily of relatives but also included friends. The wish to help, self-benefit and identification with the recipient emerged as the strongest motives. On the other hand, a sense of guilt, pressure from others, the religious motive and increased self-esteem were rare or weak incentives for donation. The logic and duty motive emerged as moderately strong however differences were noted with respect to the moral duty motivation for respondents from the two countries. The long waiting time for kidneys from cadaveric donors was also an important reason to donate. Women were observed to score slightly higher for the logic motive and men for the sense of duty (Lennerling et al., 2004, p. 1600).

Similar motives to donate were identified in a study of persons who had undergone a donor nephrectomy at Sahlgrenska University Hospital between May 1965 and December 2005. Of the total 1112 donors, 692 participants responded to the questionnaire which included questions about living donors' motives "The most common motives for donation was (*sic*) the wish to help, worries about the recipient not receiving a transplant and the knowledge that one could live a normal life with one kidney" (Lennerling, Qureshi, Fehrman-Ekholm, 2012, p. 45). Comparable motivations were also noted in a study of 114 individuals by de Groot et al. (2012), however these authors mention the fact that other donors were not possible and that "anticipated regret" for not doing so, proved important motivators to donate (p.6).

In a qualitative study of 12 living kidney donors, in Ontario, Canada, who were chosen from a larger quantitative sample, the following themes emerged in relation to the decision to donate:

- how witnessing their loved ones' experience of illness and threat of losing the recipient influenced the participants' decision to donate,
- interpersonal and intrapersonal factors influencing the living kidney donor's decision to be tested as a potential donor and the actual process of donation … (Brown et al., 2008, p. 95).

These motives identified by Brown et al. (2008) reflect some of those mentioned by Lennerling et al. (2004) in that they do include a wish to help however, the additional factor of concern for losing the recipient is introduced here. This added to both the urgency and sheer magnitude of the decision.

The lead up to the decision regarding who was going to donate a kidney also involved the process of determining who was the most eligible donor. This too was noted as an important part of the decision making process. However, living kidney donors also spoke of "a sense of determination and commitment…" once they had taken the decision to donate (Brown et al., 2008, p. 95). This did not nonetheless exclude concerns about their own wellbeing. Amongst the concerns expressed were a fear of surgery, fear of long-term consequences, objections from others, concern for the recipient both without the transplantation and after the transplantation (Lennerling et al., 2004, p. 1602).

Participants in Brown et al.'s (2008) study said that their philosophy of life had influenced their decision to donate and the authors noted that the majority of them had "a strong sense of faith and spirituality, including an appreciation of the cycle of life…." (p.95-96). Altruism was also noted as an important feature of the philosophy of life of many of the participants in this study.

The decision to donate a kidney was supported and approved by family, friends, employers and the community at large. This proved a very important feature for participants in the Brown et al. (2008) study. Similarly in the Lennerling et al. (2004) study few donors stated that they had experienced objections to the donation from other persons. Gill and Lowes (2008) who explored the experience of twenty families who were undergoing live transplantation in a regional renal transplantation centre in South-West England state that donors' decision-making processes were quite straight-forward. The research participants asserted that their decision was voluntary with little time spent weighing things up and that they had not experienced pressure to donate. For most it was regarded as the "natural thing to do" and they did not regard the decision as "brave or heroic" (Gill and Lowes, 2008, p. 1611).

THE PSYCHOSOCIAL IMPACT ON THE LIVING KIDNEY DONOR

Live kidney donation is a complex issue which is not without its risks for the donor in terms of health and safety (Manyalich et al., 2009). There is however an expectation that these risks to the donor are outweighed by the psychosocial benefits that are obtained from improved relationships and increased self-esteem. These do not rule out the possibility of depression, anxiety and marital stress which have also been documented (Clemens et al., 2006, p. 2965). This was done through a systematic review of 51 English language studies from 19 countries, which were published between 1969 and 2006. The 51 studies examined 5139 donors who were assessed an average of four years after the donation. The question which drove this review was "what impact does living kidney donation have on a donor's social functioning, self-concept, body-image, psychological well-being and quality of life?" (Clemens et al., 2006, p. 2965).

I will now attempt to briefly articulate each of these aspects drawing primarily on this systematic review. The focus for determining *social function* was through the "donor's perception of the quality of their personal relationships" where the "majority reported no change or an improved relationship with their recipient (83-100%), spouse (82-98%), family members (83-100%) and nonrecipient children (95-100%)".

The notion of *self-concept* referred to as "…a donor's feelings of self-esteem and sense of accomplishment", was reported by some of the donors as having increased (Clemens et al., 2006, p. 2965).

This was not reported across the board in all the studies reviewed, as a matter of fact in one study, donors stated that they did not feel better about themselves after the donation, and a small percentage "felt that they had given up something for nothing in return" (p. 2971). Interestingly, the "…majority (83-93%) expressed no change in their attractiveness" this especially, in the light of their nephrectomy scar (Clemens et al., 2006, p. 2971).

Psychological well-being was interpreted as including "…stress, depression, anxiety, emotions and other psychiatric symptoms" (Clemens et al., 2006, p. 2965). Stress related to the donation was noted by donors.

This was linked to the surgery and recovery, to physical distress at work, to having one kidney and worrying that it might fail, to possible complications for their health, to concern about medical costs and about loss of income, to difficulties about obtaining insurance and to recipient outcomes.

Clemens et al. (2006, p. 2972) state that "across five studies, 77 to 95% of donors experienced no symptoms of depression after donation…." and "across 2 studies, 86 to 94% of donors experienced no undue anxiety after donation…". On the other hand, another study, reported that scores on the Beck Depression Inventory were significantly worse three months after the nephrectomy and in yet another study, "six percent of donors experienced an increase in pre-existing depression or anxiety" (Clemens et al., 2006, p. 2973). Three of the studies reviewed, indicated that a vast majority were generally happy with a substantial number in two of the studies indicating that they felt happier after the donation. In two of the studies, the reviewers state that "after surgery, 35% and 55% felt that they were treated as special people" (Clemens et al., 2006, p. 2972). On the other hand, though few in number, some donors expressed less positive outcomes such as:

- disappointment with the emotional experience of donation;
- that they had felt ignored or unappreciated;
- feelings of abandonment; and
- sadness and loss.

Brown et al. (2008) also describe this sense of loss or grief after donation. One of the participants in their qualitative study stated "When you have a child, you're going to come out of the operating room with something. And now you're coming out of there without something" (p.96). In the case of donors whose recipients had experienced negative outcomes, "13% felt the procedure had been a waste and 5% felt guilty and of those whose recipient died, only 50% felt their experience had been worth it" (Clemens et al., 2006, p. 2972). Two of the studies reviewed, reported no concerning mental health problems in the majority of donors however less positive outcomes were also identified. In one study, "of those who faced adverse recipient outcomes, 11% experienced suicidal ideation" (Clemens et al., 2006, p. 2973).

The concept of *quality of life* was defined as "affected in a complex way by the person's physical health, psychological state, personal beliefs, social beliefs and their relationship to salient features of their environment" (Clemens et al., 2006, p. 2965). This was assessed in 29 of the 51 studies reviewed and donors reported a high satisfaction with their quality of life. In 22 of the studies, versions of the Short Form Health Survey were used and in 17 of these many donor scores were similar or better than the general population. On the other hand less positive outcomes were also noted (Clemens et al., 2006, p. 2973).

The authors conclude that when all the studies they reviewed were considered, the psychosocial health of most donors appeared as unchanged or positively improved by donation. Although negative outcomes were reported, the proportion of donors who experienced these situations was small and most importantly, the majority stated that they would undergo the experience again (Clemens et al., 2006, p. 2974).

Andersen et al.'s (2007) research re-affirms some of the features highlighted in the Clemens et al. (2006) systematic review. The Andersen et al. (2007) study explored the physical and psycho-social health of twelve living kidney donors the first year after donor surgery. This was done through two interviews, one carried out a week after donation and another one year later. The authors used "a phenomenological method to reach an understanding of the essence of being a living kidney donor the first year after donor surgery" (Andersen et al., 2007, p.703). They found that "all participants expressed an overall positive experience about being a donor a year after transplantation" however the experiences differed for the ones who had been involved in a successful transplantation and the others who had experienced a transplantation failure (Andersen et al., 2007, p.702). This positive global experience was also confirmed in a study carried out drawing on living kidney and liver donors who had been assessed by the Veneto Regional Authority's Third Party Commission between February 2002 and December 2006. Of the 69 who participated, 96% expressed "a positive global opinion of the experience" (Feltrin et al., 2008, p. 466).

METHOD

I have used a qualitative phenomenological approach to explore my experience, feelings and ideas as a live kidney donor. I chose to use a first-person approach following in "…the path of the original philosophers like Husserl who pioneered phenomenology as the reflective study of structures of consciousness as experienced from the first-person point of view" (Finlay, 2011, p. 149). As suggested by Finlay, (2011) I chose to interrogate my personal account as though a transcript. This would help me to provide a rich and hopefully interesting description of the experience. In order to do this I recorded myself as I related my experience of being a live kidney donor. The question that guided my narrative was simply 'Describe your experience of being a live kidney donor'. Once this recording was transcribed I could engage with the transcript and through narrative descriptions of significant events could begin to present what is the essence of being a live kidney donor. Another important aspect of this engagement with the transcript was that I could also do what Giorgi descirbes as "…reading a sense of the whole" (Wertz, 2011, p. 145). This helped me to not only identify significant events but also begin to read story-lines into the narrative of my experience.

SOME BACKGROUND[1]

I donated a kidney to my brother on the 31st December 2005. My brother had suffered kidney failure and had been on dialysis for a few years before the kidney transplant. He suffered kidney failure as a result of Type I diabetes which he had been diagnosed with from the age of thirteen. He had a kidney and pancreas transplant which have to date both been successful. At the time of the donation I was 49 years of age and my brother was 47.

Reflections

I have chosen to structure my reflections around two somewhat contrasting story-lines which have helped me to make sense of this experience. The first of these story-lines is that I consider the decision to be a live kidney donor is an integral and natural sequence in my life process. In many ways I perceive the decision as very much part of who I am. The second of these story-lines is that of a certain surprise at myself at having taken such a decision because I do not view myself as particularly courageous; on the contrary, I am starkly aware of my fragility and became more so during the donation process.

A Natural Sequence in a Life Process

My reading of this experience as a natural and integral sequence in a life process can be understood in the context of various themes that I have identified in the narrative of the experience. I view my decision as motivated by the same values which have inspired my choices in life such as the choice of my profession, social work. I will now draw on the different themes to help articulate this narrative.

I see two important intertwining themes in this process and these are *relationship* and *responsibility*. In my view they were both key determinants in my eventual decision to donate a kidney to my brother and both emerge in the excerpt below:

> I must explain that my brother is a year and a half younger than I am. I am the oldest of five siblings. And …as the eldest daughter, I have always been quite responsible for my

[1] My family have authorised my disclosure to the public of our personal story.

> brother and sisters. So we're very close in age and also very close in terms of relationship. I always felt that my brother was almost like my twin, although I always felt the responsibility as the eldest sister …

The quotation below illustrates two other themes, that this is *a family affair*, and the strict regime to be adopted has to be for one and all. Closely linked to this is the *special status one gains when one needs care*. These too proved influential in this life process which eventually led up to my decision.

> Once my brother was diagnosed (with diabetes), there was an immediate change in regime in the family and we just were not allowed to eat sweets at home. I remember my mother emptying the larder and saying we wouldn't have sweets, when he was around definitely and also when he wasn't around. It became quite a strict regime in terms of the food we ate, to support him. He also in some ways took on a status of being special……So I remember that quite distinctly as well, that he was suddenly, or perhaps not so suddenly, in my eyes as a young person, he gained this special status, special status in terms of needing care. And also I think, I'm not sure whether this was communicated to me, that I had some responsibility to care for him.

Linked to this notion that one gains a *special status* when needing care, is the fact that my brother's diabetes was never easily controlled and from a fairly young age he started to suffer the consequences of diabetes. This introduced a certain element of *vulnerability and uncertainty* in his life, but also in our lives as his family.

> So somehow there was this notion that he was vulnerable. I'm not sure whether this was something that was communicated to us by our parents, but there was this message that reached me, that he was vulnerable.

Another theme which I think emerges in this 'natural sequence in a life process' was the *sanctioning of the kidney donation* by my father. My father was a medical doctor and I consider his words to have been very influential in my decision.

> I think in the late eighties, early nineties, my brother started experiencing problems with his kidneys. I recall that his creatinine levels started to rise. I don't know how bad this was, however I recall that it was bad enough for my father to, at the time, mention that he would probably require a kidney transplant. So this is early nineties, I don't know how early in the nineties, but my father passed away in 1994 so it would have definitely been before then…...
>
> Another thing which I recall about these first symptoms of kidney failure, was that my father had categorically said that if his (my brother's) kidneys fail and he needs a transplant he would donate a kidney.

The kidney failure process came to a head and my brother had to start dialysis in 2002. After unsuccessful attempts at Continuous Ambulatory Peritoneal Dialysis (CAPD), he started hospital haemodialysis. This resulted in *a restricted life-style* which really began to affect him and I became aware that this was really serious.

> I must also mention something about my brother's personality. Although my brother had diabetes for a number of years and has had quite a lot of problems coping with his condition, it has never stopped him from leading as normal a life as possible. Not only that, I think more than that. He's travelled and done everything he's always wanted to do. The kidney failure was the first time when his life became quite restrictive. Having to go for dialysis 3 times a week meant his life became quite conditioned by the dialysis, he couldn't do the things he really wanted to do...... Again I mention this because I think this had really put a damper on things for him and it really changed how he was living his condition.

The real *wake up call* for me came later. This came when I, together with my three sisters, first approached my brother's nephrologist to explore the possibility for one of us to donate a kidney to him.

> .....we all went together the four sisters, told him that we were all willing to give my brother a kidney. It was quite clear from the outset that one of my sisters would not be a possible match because of her blood group. The other three of us are all O+ and so is he so it was clear the three of us could be potential donors. .....when we spoke to the nephrologist he made no bones about saying, unless you give your brother a kidney quite soon, there is no time to waste, he might be dead in a couple of years. I think we left that appointment quite nervous in some ways saying this it, we just have to take this decision and keep going. And that's when the process started. This would have been mid-2004.

Another key theme that runs through my experience is *support*, this came from many sources, my husband, my mother, my siblings, friends, work colleagues, the transplant team at the hospital, the supporting nurse just before the operation, from reading about the procedure, from other live kidney donors I encountered, from a kidney recipient and from the judge who interviewed me to ascertain my free and informed consent. I think that it was primarily this all pervasive support that has helped me to view my experience as a natural and integral part of my life process.

> How can I do this? How could I have done this?

I will now turn my attention to the second story-line which I could read into my narrative. As I explained above, the decision to donate a kidney to my brother did not come easy, it was a tortuous decision punctuated with this view of myself as not being particularly courageous. Even after my experience I still contend that I am not an especially brave person. This fragility of mine was expressed in a number of ways. I will now identify some of the themes that illustrate it.

One of the ways this was expressed was in my initial *reluctance to face the situation* and to acknowledge just how serious my brother's condition was and to take action about it.

> When he (my brother) started dialysis the talk about his need for a transplant became more frequent, and one of my sisters who is a medical doctor, started broaching this idea amongst us. I recall a number of occasions where she'd say to me we really have to start thinking about giving Pierre a kidney. And what I can recall in myself is a certain initial reluctance to face this. I wasn't the first to come forward to say look we just have to give him a kidney let's get on with it. I think I was the one who was stepping on the brakes in some way, in that I said we're not going to get ourselves checked before we're clear that we will

give him the kidney if it's us. We eventually did all decide that we would be ready to give him a kidney.

This *reluctance to face the situation* was also shown by certain *irrational expectations* I had.

Although I had rationally accepted that fact that this was serious, somehow because my brother has always managed to bounce back whatever had been wrong with him, I somehow thought this was something he would bounce back from. So although rationally I knew that this was something very serious, I think emotionally I hadn't grasped just how serious it was.

Even after my two sisters and I did our blood tests and the process of cross-matching started, I was still thinking will it be *me or not me*.

We had gone for the blood tests and urine tests together, and then went to collect our results together, so there was myself and my two siblings. I think at that point, I was still hoping in some ways it wasn't going to be me, so this proved quite difficult, in saying I was hoping it wasn't going to be me, I was somehow feeling I was saying I was hoping it was going to be one of my sisters.

As things turned out my sister who was the best match could not proceed to give my brother a kidney on account of a condition which was discovered during the pre-donation tests she underwent. Once this was determined it was clear that I was going to be the donor. As I explained above, I felt that I had taken the decision in agreeing to be tested however now it was the real thing, I had to re-take the decision to be a donor. A thought that kept going through my head was the *kidney could be lost, this is a big risk for small returns*. I felt that I needed to take my decision fully cognisant of this possibility. An *important influence* during this critical period was a conversation I had with close a friend of mine who had just lost her brother to leukaemia.

....she said look, for me this would be very clear, if there had been anything I could have done to save my brother I would certainly have done it. You are in the lucky position to be able to do something to save your brother. I remember this so, so, so clearly. It suddenly seemed to fall into place. How can I not do this if by doing it I was going to save my brother?

In this difficult decision-making process some instances stand out as particularly supportive. I found having the *freedom to opt out* of my decision to donate a kidney to be one of these instances, although I also, in some ways, view this instance as an indication of the strength of my fears.

During this period of testing I also had to meet with a judge[2] and had to sign my consent to giving my kidney. This proved a very important experience for me. What happened was, I had to meet with this person, and he asked me whether I was doing this of my own free-will, whether I had in any way been coerced to give my kidney, and I explained that I hadn't. But one thing which I then later on found very comforting was that he said, look although you are

[2] The transplant operation was carried out at the Azienda Ospedaliera Universitaria Pisana and the meeting with the judge (giudice) I refer to was held at the Pisa Courts of Justice.

> going to be signing these papers today, you may, till the very last moment decide not to do this, there is nothing to force you to take this decision. I think this message of self-determination that I felt, that I was completely free to take the decision, proved very helpful. It was in some strange way an opt-out clause which was left open to me, so having that opt-out clause was a help. So I did that, I signed the papers, and then discussions started as to when this operation was likely to take place.

A *concern* I had in the days leading up to the operation was whether my brother was well enough to face the operation and come through it.

> Another thing I'd like to mention which did haunt me in the days leading up to the operation was, what if something went wrong during the operation. Not so much for myself, I felt that I was healthy, and though an operation is always an operation, I somehow would make it through. But this thought kept plaguing me, what if my brother passed away during the operation. Connected to this was this feeling that somehow I would have provoked this event, in that giving him the kidney meant that he could get the kidney and therefore the operation could take place, and if he died during the operation it was somehow my fault. I knew, even at the time, that this thought was completely irrational but it just kept coming back to my mind.

Perhaps the most poignant illustration of my fragility was just before the surgery when my brother had to support me.

> My last memory just before the operation was in the operating theatre, and lying side by side by my brother just before I was given anaesthetic, and there was I crying and my brother was saying "come on, we're here now, this is it, it's going to be fine".

DISCUSSION

Now that I have presented my experience in the form of two story-lines, I will attempt to compare and contrast it with experiences of live donors as drawn from the reviewed literature. Even a cursory look at the literature I have referred to above indicates that there are many similarities between my experience and that of other live donors as obtained from a number of research studies. I will explore these similarities first.

The realisation and conclusion that donation was the only option, which donors in the Lennerling, Forsberg and Nyberg (2003) study reached, is similar to my *wake up call* when we approached my brother's nephrologist to discuss a possible live donation. Like the participants in the Brown et al., (2008) study, "....the threat of losing the recipient" very much influenced my decision to donate (p.95). My "identification with the recipient" (Lennerling et al., 2004, p.1600) is reflected in the importance I gave to my *relationship* with my brother as a key determinant in the decision making process. This identification did not simply develop when he experienced the kidney failure; it was long-standing and is best described through my words "I always felt that my brother was almost like my twin…".

I did not refer to "external pressure" (Lennerling et al., 2004, p.1600) in my narrative although this was nonetheless present. There was certainly some peer pressure which resulted from our reasoning, as siblings, that we should all be tested to find out who was the best match. Although not articulated as such, this decision did exert some pressure on each of us. The other pressure, though very subtle, came from our belief that this was *a family affair*. Just as supporting my brother when he was diagnosed with diabetes was *a family affair*, giving him a kidney was also so. The other pressure came from my brother's nephrologist and the stark message he communicated to us about my brother's imminent death if he were not to receive a kidney.

In my case the logic motive, that is the knowledge that one can live a normal life with one kidney, (Lennerling et al., 2004) was buttressed by my father's *sanctioning of the kidney donation*, not only as a father but more so as a medical doctor. It was quite clear to me at the outset that once my father had stated that he would be the donor should the need arise then it was safe for me to do so and lead a normal life afterwards.

I likewise experienced a "… sense of determination and commitment…" (Brown et al., 2008, p. 95) once I had taken the decision to donate, this for me was very much linked to the decision to be tested. Once that decision was taken the process was going to take its course. This did not mean that the decision was easy or a forgone conclusion, as can be clearly manifested from the comfort I gained from knowing that I would still have the *freedom to opt out* up to the very last moment before the actual surgery.

The participants in the Brown et al. (2008) study stated that their philosophy of life had influenced their decision to donate and that altruism was an important feature of the philosophy of life of a number of the participants in their study. This link to my philosophy of life is manifested through my view that my decision to donate a kidney is a natural sequence in my life process which has been motivated by the self-same values which have guided my choices in life. Altruism is likewise an important value for me and is best expressed through my decision to become a social worker and eventually a social work academic.

Like the participants in the Gill and Lowes (2008, p.1611) study, I do not view myself as particularly "brave or heroic", on the contrary there were many junctures during the process when I felt quite weak and fearful. I think that the stress of my experience is manifest through the second story-line which I read into my narrative. This is where all my concerns are illustrated in my *reluctance to face the situation,* in my *irrational expectations* about my brother's condition and in my thinking that it *might not be me*. This was linked to many of the issues referred to by Clemens et al., (2006). I was concerned about the surgery and recovery and that I would have to stay away from work for some time and that this would be disruptive, about having one kidney and that it might fail, about the fact that the kidney could be lost and most of all about my recipient's outcome. I can really empathise with the respondents in the Andersen et al. (2007) study were a difference was noted in their view of the experience depending on whether the transplantation had been a success or a failure.

Some differences can be noted between my experience and that of participants in the research studies referred to above. The Lennerling et al. (2004, p.1600) study refers to "self-benefit from the relative's improved health" and "improved self-esteem from doing good deeds" amongst the motives expressed by the participants. I did not express these in my narrative. In my case, my brother and I did not live in the same household so although I did experience some benefit from his better health, this did not have a direct day to day impact on my life. I do not consider myself as having been motivated to improve my self-esteem through the good deed of donating an organ. This may have been a deep seated motive which was not expressed as such however I think that my fears and concerns far outweighed the draw of improved self-esteem. Furthermore, my reading of this is that as a person who values altruism, I had far less challenging opportunities to do good deeds which would have similarly improved my self-esteem.

Unlike the few donors who experienced less positive outcomes and referred to by Clemens et al. (2006), I was not disappointed with the emotional experience of donation, on the contrary it proved a powerful and positive spiritual experience. There was no point when I felt ignored, unappreciated or abandoned. Nor did I experience sadness and loss.

In conclusion, perhaps what stands out as different in my experience to the research studies referred to above is simply that the advantage of a first-person approach gave me the benefit of viewing the experience of a live kidney donor in the context of the life processes of both a donor and a recipient.

Some Pointers for Best Practices

I would now like to highlight what I consider some useful pointers for best practices drawing on both my experience and the literature about live kidney donation.

The feature that stands out mostly in the narrative of my experience as a natural sequence in a life process is the importance of understanding the uniqueness of each donor and that how they approach the donation needs to be understood within the larger context of their life process. This could be explored through a psychosocial assessment which Brown et al. (2008) suggest should be part of the routine workup for live kidney donation. The participants in their study had undergone a psychosocial assessment which explored "psychological and emotional stability, family history and family dynamics, absence of coercion, relationship to the recipient, understanding of and attitude to donation, and support networks" (p.98). Such an assessment could help identify the specific support needs of the individual donor and also recognise the very personal meaning the decision making process has for the donor.

One of the most important aspects of my experience as a live donor was my freedom of choice which I described as my *freedom to opt out.* This was strongly supported by the fact that the judge I encountered was extraneous to the Transplant Co-ordinating team and that he told me that even though I had signed the papers declaring that I was ready to be a live kidney donor I could still not go ahead with this even up to the last moment. Feltrin et al., (2008, p. 466-467) explain that living donors are also assessed for "*...the sincerity of their free and informed consent*" and that in compliance with national Italian guidelines on kidney and liver transplantation from living donors, what they describe as a 'Third-Party Commission' was established by the Veneto Regional Authority. This commission was formed of a specialist in forensic medicine, a clinical psychologist and a bio-ethicist. They examine the medical records and interview potential donors to then express a joint opinion. This is in addition to the clinical and immunological assessments and a psychological exam. Regardless of how it is implemented I consider this separation of responsibilities as very important in allowing a potential live kidney donor as full a freedom of choice as possible.

Another important notion related to the decision-making process and also in allowing full freedom of choice to the potential donor is the notion of a 'cooling-off' period. Rodrigue et al. (2007, p. 2329) who conducted a survey of 132 US kidney transplant programmes to find out how they evaluate and select potential kidney donors found that "A small proportion (11%) of programs require all potential donors to exercise a 'cooling-off' period to ensure that they have the adequate time to consider the information gathered during the evaluation process".

In effect the majority of programmes do not require a 'cooling-off' period. Difficult as this might be in the context of the urgent need for the kidney by the recipient; this use of a 'cooling-off' period is a pointer for a best practice that is respectful of the donor.

I was fortunate to have had my kidney donation *sanctioned by my father* who was a medical doctor and who had expressed a wish to donate a kidney to my brother well before the circumstances of his need for a kidney arose. This process facilitated things for me on various counts as it appeased many of my concerns although I nonetheless sought out information about the potential consequences of my donation. The recommendation by Clemens et al. (2011) that it is an ethical imperative for living kidney donors to be provided with "full and accurate knowledge of the potential risks and benefits that they may face" should be heeded in all instances of live kidney donation (p.463).

Special attention needs to be given to donors when the transplantation fails. Andersen et al. (2007) point out that their study confirmed that as expected " …poor recipient outcomes evoke physical and emotional reactions in the donor" (p.707). They also note that their study highlighted that in cases of transplant failure it was not easy for the donors to obtain sufficient help from healthcare personnel. The authors suggest the need for careful follow up of the donor in all instances however more so when there is transplant failure. The development of a follow-up methodology for live donors based on recipient outcomes is one of the aims of the European project Euro Living Donor Psychosocial Follow-Up (ELIPSY). This project, which ends in 2013, is intended to help develop " a protocol that can be used in the future for living donor follow-up in every European country". This is certainly an important pointer for best practices.

I would like to add another pointer to best practices. The live kidney donor must be assured at all junctures that their best interests will always be safeguarded. Although this is communicated to potential donors at the outset of the assessment process it should be re-iterated throughout the process.

This did not prove a concern for me because I witnessed the fact that my sister, who was the best match, was stopped from proceeding with the donation on account of a condition she was diagnosed with during the pre-donation tests. This decision by the Transplant Co-ordinating team made it clear that my interests would be safeguarded.

In conclusion I would like to support projects such as the European Living Donor (EULID) project (Euro Living Donor EULID - What is EULID?, n.d.) which is a project which received funding from the European Union. The main objective of this project was to analyse the European situation regarding legal, ethical, protection and registration practices related to live organ donation with a view to setting standards and giving recommendations that guarantee the health and safety of the live donor.

CONCLUSION

In this chapter I have focussed on my experience as a live kidney donor. I chose to review the research literature which focused on the decision to donate and the psychosocial impact on the living kidney donor as I considered these two perspectives to be particularly relevant to my experience.

This is manifest from the many similarities which emerged between the literature and my experience. Differences were nonetheless noted and these were highlighted in the discussion. The advantage of a first-person qualitative approach meant that I could reflect about my experience as part of a life process and not simply as a discrete event. In the final part of the chapter I drew on both my experience and the literature to suggest pointers for best practices.

REFERENCES

Andersen, M.H., Bruserud, F., Mathisen, L., Wahl, A.K., Hanestad, B.R., & Fosse, E. (2007). Follow-up interview of 12 living kidney donors one yr after open donor nephrectomy. *Clinical Transplantation*, 21, 702-709. doi:10.1111/j.1399-0012.2007.00726.x

Brown, J. B., Karley, M.L., Boudville, N., Bullas, R., Garg, A. X. & Muirhead, N. (2008). The Experience of Living Kidney Donors. *Health & Social Work,* 33 (2), 93-100.

Clemens, K., Boudville, N., Dew, M.A., Geddes, C., Gill, J.S., Jassal, V., Garg, A. for the Donor Nephrectomy Outcomes Research (DONOR) Network. (2011). The Long-Term Quality of Life of Living Kidney Donors: A Multicenter Cohort Study. *American Journal of Transplantation,* 11, 463- 469. doi:10.1111/j.1600-6143.2010.03424.x

Clemens, K.K., Thiessen-Philbrook, H., Parikh, C.R., Yang, R.C., Karley, M.L., Boudville, N., Garg, A.X. for the Donor Nephrectomy Outcomes Research (DONOR) Network. (2006). *American Journal of Transplantation,* 6, 2965-2977.

de Groot, I.B., Schipper, K., van Dijk, S., van der Boog, P.J.M., Stiggelbout, A.M., Baranski, A.G., & Marag-van de Mheen, P.J. (2012). Decision making around living and deceased donor kidney transplantation:a qualitative study exploring the importance of expected relationship changes. *BMC Nephrology,* 13:103. doi:1471-2369-13-103/1471-2369-13-103

Euro Living Donor EULID- What is EULID? (n.d.) Retreived from http://www.eulivingdonor.eu/eulid/what-is-eulid.html.

Euro Living Donor Psychosocial Follow-Up –ELIPSY. (n.d.) Retreived from http://www.eulivingdonor.eu/elipsy/what-is-elipsy.html.

Feltrin, A., Pegoraro, R., Rago, C., Benciolini, P., Pasquato, S., Frasson, P., Buizza, V., Ermani, M., Rupolo, G., (2008). Experience of donation and quality of life in living kidney and liver donors. *Transplant International* 21, 466-472. doi:10.1111/j.1432-2277.2007.00632.x

Finlay, L. (2011). *Phenomenology for Therapists: Researching the Lived World.* Chichester, UK: Wiley-Blackwell.

Gill, P. & Lowes, L. (2008). Gift exchange and organ donation: Donor and Recipient experiences of live related kidney transplantation. *International Journal of Nursing Studies,* 45, 1607-1617.

Lennerling, A., Forsberg, A., & Nyberg, N. (2003). Becoming a living kidney donor. *Transplantation,* 76, 1243-1247.

Lennerling, A., Forsberg, A., Meyer, K., & Nyberg, N. (2004). Motives for becoming a living kidney donor. *Nephrology Dialysis Transplantation,* 19, 1600-1605.

Lennerling, A., Qureshi, A. R., & Fehrman-Ekholm, I. (2012). Spouses who donate seem to be the winners - A questionnaire study of kidney donors long-term. *Open Journal of Nephrology,* 2, 44-48.

Manyalich, M., Ricart, A., Martinez, I., Balleste, C., Paredes, D., Vilardell, J., … Walaszewski, J. (2009). EULID Project: European Living Donation and Public Health. *Transplantation Proceedings,* 41, 2021-2024.

Rodrigue, J.R.Pavlakis, M., Danovitch, G.M., Johnson, S.R., Karp, S.J., Khwaja, K., …Mandelbrot, D.A. (2007). Evaluating Living Kidney Donors: Relationship Types, Psychosocial Criteria, and Consent Processes at US Transplant Programs. *American Journal of Transplantation,* 7, 2326-2332.

Wertz, F.J. (2011). A Phenomenological Psychological Approach to Trauma and Resilience. In F. J. Wertz, K. Charmaz, L. M. McMullen, R. Josselson, R. Anderson, and E. McSpadden (Eds.), Five Ways of Doing Qualitative Analysis: Phenomenological Psychology, Grounded Theory, Discourse Analysis, Narrative Research, and Intuitive Inquiry (pp.139-179). New York: *The Guilford Press.*

In: Organ Donation and Transplantation
Editor: Mary Anne Lauri

ISBN: 978-1-62948-257-6

Chapter 3

MOTIVATIONS FOR BEING A LIVING KIDNEY DONOR: A SOCIAL PSYCHOLOGICAL PERSPECTIVE OF ALTRUISM

Amy Camilleri-Zahra[*]
University of Malta, Malta

ABSTRACT

Altruism has often been cited as a motivation for organ donation. However, only a few studies have specifically investigated the experience of the living donor from this perspective. The aim of this study is to understand what motivates Maltese living donors to donate one of their kidneys whilst still alive. This study was conducted within the social psychological framework of prosocial behaviour. Participants for this study were recruited through the Transplant Support Group (Malta). Semi-structured interviews were used as a means of data collection, which were then analysed using thematic analysis. The three main themes that emerged from the study were: i) being in the world of the suffering other, ii) the bond with the patient suffering from kidney failure, and iii) the donor's disposition. Findings revealed that the primary aim of the act of organ donation for these donors was to relieve the other person from suffering. All the participants also had their own personal motivations. The outcome of this study can be useful in guiding the process of consent for live donors.

INTRODUCTION

It was William McDougall, who in the 1900s, first asked the question as to why people act or do not act prosocially (Clarke, 2003). However, it was not until the 1960s, after the "Kitty Genevose" incident that social psychologists really started to recognise the importance of prosocial behaviour (Clarke, 2003; Dovidio at al., 2006).

[*] E-mail: azah001@um.edu.mt.

Prosocial behaviour is an action, which is defined as being generally beneficial to other people and to the ongoing political system (Piliavin, Dovidio, Gaertner, & Clark, 1981, p.4). Dovidio et al. (2006) divide prosocial behaviour into three sub-categories: altruism, helping and cooperation. For the purpose of this study the focus is going to be solely on altruism.

According to Bar-Tal (1985-1986), altruistic behaviour is defined as the kind of behaviour which, "(a) must benefit another person, (b) must be performed voluntarily, (c) must be performed intentionally, (d) the benefit must be the goal by itself and (e) must be performed without expecting any external reward" (p.5). Theorists like Krebs (1982), and even more recently Aronson, Wilson, and Akert (2004), further limit the definition of altruism, by claiming that an altruistic act can only be defined as such when the act itself incurs a cost to the benefactor. This has lead to a discussion about altruism from different psychological perspectives.

In general, there is a fair amount of literature linking altruism to organ donation. The discussion on what motivates persons to donate an organ whilst still alive or several organs after death, as well as the decision by a donor's family to donate the organs of a deceased loved one, draws upon the above theories of pro-social behaviour and altruism. In my chapter, I will also be making reference to the debate between Cialdini and Batson about whether pure altruism exists, in order to understand the motivations of live donors.

The most common organ that is donated from a living donor is the kidney. One can live healthily with one kidney and can, therefore, donate the second one to someone suffering from kidney disease (Simmons, 1991). However, albeit this progress in medicine, in Malta, like in other countries, there still exists a great disparity between the number of people awaiting a kidney transplant and the number of donated kidneys (Eurobarometer, 2010).

Malta is a small island centrally located in the Mediterranean Sea, with an estimated population of 440,000 people. On average, in Malta there are approximately 130 patients on a waiting list for a kidney transplant at any given time (A. Bugeja, personal communication, November 4, 2012). Since 1992, the number of kidney transplantations amounted to 253, and of these, only 45 have been donated by living donors (E. Farrugia, personal communication, April 9, 2011).

Altruism from Different Perspectives

Altruism has been studied from various perspectives, including Freudian Psychoanalytic Perspective, Social Learning Theory, Sociobiological Theory, and Evolutionary Theory. In this chapter I will be focusing on sociobiological theory and evolutionary theory, since most studies on organ donation seem to point towards these two theories as their foundation.

Sociobiological Theory

Sociobiologists argue that altruism is innate and that therefore, altruism is genetically wired in the code of human being's behaviour (Hoffman, 1981). Wilson (1975, p. 578), a prominent sociobiologist, defines altruism as "self-destructive behaviour performed for the benefit of others". However, more generally, sociobiologists claim that behaviour is altruistic if it benefits the actor less than the recipient (Piliavin & Charng, 1990).

Wilson (1976, p. 371) refers to acts of altruism between kin, as "hard core" altruism. It is a kind of altruism that is depicted as irrational. They are, "spontaneous acts of bravery [which] are undertaken without any such conscious aim in view" (Hill, 1984, p. 24). This is because kin altruism requires less rational deliberation and self-persuasion (Vine, 1983). Notwithstanding, sociobiologists also claim that we are likely to act altruistically towards two other kinds of people, apart from next of kin: those whom we perceive as being similar to us, and those with whom we share "kin-like" ties (Piliavin & Charng, 1990).

Evolutionary Theory

Similarly to sociobiological theory, evolutionary theory, particularly the theory of kin altruism makes a specific reference to altruism between kin and shows how we are more inclined to act altruistically towards relatives than non-relatives. In 1964, Hamilton, a professor in evolutionary biology introduced the theory of Kin Altruism, also known as the inclusive fitness theory. Kin Altruism is a way of explaining self-sacrificing behaviour for the benefit of others. Hamilton argued that animals are likely to provide help to those with whom they shared genes through common descent. He also claimed that the amount of help given increases in a proportional manner to the amount of genes they shared (Workman & Reader, 2008).

Recently, after several studies, evolutionary psychologists have agreed that the theory of kin altruism can also be applied to humans. They argued that humans, through the years, have developed a mind set, which acts in ways that enables inclusive fitness (Workman & Reader, 2008). Kin selection theory explains how humans are more inclined to help and act altruistically towards their relatives than non-relatives, especially those with whom they shared more genes.

Empirical Studies on Organ Donation

Sociobiological theory, which refers to act of altruism as being "spontaneous acts of bravery" (Hill, 1984, p.24) is demonstrated in a study conducted in America by Simmons, Marine and Simmons (1987). Findings based on a multiple-choice questionnaire distributed amongst live kidney donors show that, 78% of the respondents claimed that they knew right away that they would be donating one of their kidneys and that they did not have to think it over. Furthermore, over 70% claimed that either the decision was not hard at all, or that there was actually no decision to make. Similarly, Wilms, Kiefer, Shanteau, and McIntyre (1987), also indicate that people who find themselves in the situation of donating a kidney whilst living actually think very little about their behaviour, but they automatically feel that it was the right thing to do.

Similarly, the theory of kin altruism as explained by evolutionary theorists is also shown in a study conducted by Borgida, Conner, and Manteufel (1992). Through this study with living kidney donors it resulted that donors were about three times as likely to donate an organ to a relative than to a nonrelative (73% vs. 27%). Similarly, a study carried out amongst

137 undergraduates at Kansas State University revealed that the students were more willing to donate an organ to their own child or a sibling, and less willing to donate to a friend or stranger (Shanteau & Skowronski, 1992). This clearly shows that the relatedness of the donor to the recipient is of great importance. However, Dovidio et al. (2006) give another possible explanation to this result, where they argue that people may help their kin more than they would help unrelated strangers, due to social pressure coming from one's own family. It is also important to point out that kin selection theory does not maintain that we will always help our kin but that we are more likely to do so (Workman & Reader, 2008).

Does Altruism Really Exist?

Whilst evolutionary psychologists and sociobiologists tend to define altruism purely by the act executed, social psychologists are primarily concerned with the intention behind the act (Workman & Reader, 2008). However, although most social psychologists tend to agree on the definition of altruism, there has been a long theoretical debate as to whether altruism really exists or not. The concrete issue is, whether people are really capable of performing an altruistic act sometimes at a cost through which they themselves gain nothing, or whether all prosocial acts are in fact done for some level or form of egoism.

On one side of this theoretical debate, there is Cialdini, who firmly believes that all actions, which appear altruistic, are in fact, hiding egoistical motives (Cialdini et al., 1987). Cialdini proposes various egoistical reasons for which a benefactor may offer to help someone else in need. One of the first reasons proposed, is the desire to produce a sense of well-being within oneself. Making use of learning theory, Cialdini, together with others, posited the idea that from an early age, we learn that through the act of helping others, we create a sense of well-being for ourselves (Manucia, Baumann, & Cialdini, 1984). According to Cialdini this can be done in two ways, either by offering to help to maintain a positive feeling, or by offering to help so as to relieve a negative feeling (Cialdini et al., 1987; Manucia et al., 1984). In addition, Cialdini proposes other rewards, which can motivate altruism. These include, the desire to increase one's own self-esteem, acquiring praise from other people, or even the projection of a positive image. Ultimately, one can also offer to help so as to avoid punishment (Piliavin & Charng, 1990; Simmons, 1991).

On the opposing side of this debate stands Batson (1987, 1991), who argues that there exists altruism, which is entirely focused on the other and is genuinely meant to provide aid. Batson further suggested that some circumstances elicit a specific kind of emotion, which he identifies as "empathic concern" (Batson & Oleson, 1991). He claims that it is this empathic concern that motivates the benefactor to perform an action with the sole aim of reducing the other person's distress. Nonetheless, Batson (1987, 1991) does not insist that egoistical motives are entirely absent, since he does acknowledge that in some cases egoistically motivated helping does occur. However, he claims, that for the most part, the primary motive is to help the other. The difference between Batson's and Cialdini's arguments is that Batson terms the motives posited by Cialdini as "subtle forms of self-benefit". Thus, according to Batson, these motives are only a by-product of the act of helping and not as Cialdini states, the primary aim (Batson, 1987).

According to Piliavin and Charng (1990), a present consensus has been reached, whereby it suggests that both types of helping, egoistical and altruistic, exist (Piliavin & Charng, 1990; Simmons, 1991). In addition, in her research, Simmons (1991) argues that as opposed to the laboratory, it is very difficult to disentangle altruistic and egoistical motives in real-life experiences. Her studies show that many organ donors are in fact motivated to act by concern for the sick person, but are at the same time happy that they could help.

ALTRUISM AND ORGAN DONATION

This chapter aims to understand what motivates Maltese donors to donate one of their kidneys whilst still alive, and whether they are motivated by altruism. The sample size was dictated by the inescapable fact that Malta is a small country, thus leading to a very small number of live donors. Furthermore, since a qualitative approach was adopted for this study, the sample size required is also small. Five participants were willing to take part in this study. Participants were recruited through the Transplant Support Group (Malta). Table 1 below portrays the pseudonym and characteristics of the five participants.

Table 1. Pseudonym and Demographic Characteristics of the Participants

Pseudonym	Age	Recipient	Time Since Transplant
Lara	54	Brother – Blood related	5 years
Mark	22	Male friend – Unrelated	3 months
Noel	50	Brother-in-law – Unrelated	7 years
Nina	63	Mother – Blood Related	5 years
Sarah	35	Daughter – Blood related	3 years

The following questions were put forward to the participants of this study, so as to assist the researcher in understanding the motivations of the act of kidney donation by live donors:

1. How did the participants get to know that their relative/friend needed a kidney transplant?
2. What was the participant's initial reaction to the knowledge that their relative/friend needed a kidney transplant?
3. What made the participants decide to become donors?
4. How was the kidney donation and transplantation experienced by the participants?

Data was collected by the means of semi-structured interviews. All 5 participants were given an information sheet and a consent form prior to each interview. The scheduled interviews were conducted on one-to-one basis. This gave the researcher and the participant the possibility to engage in deeper conversations, as well as the possibility to elaborate further on certain issues. The interviews were recorded with the permission of the participants and then transcribed by the researcher. Data was analysed using thematic analysis as described by Braun and Clarke (2006).

Results and Discussion

In this section each super-ordinate theme together with its subordinate themes will be discussed. Similarities to other results or theories as found in the literature review will be outlined. The classification of themes derived from the data is given in Table 2.

Table 2. Themes Derived from the Data

Superordinate Themes	Subordinate themes	Key Phrases
1. BEING IN THE WORLD OF THE SUFFERING OTHER	Witnessing the trials of dialysis	Complex procedure Associated problems (repeated infections, CADP – haemodialysis, fistula, adherence to prescribed regimes) Failing Health
	Deterioration in the quality of life	Limited choice of foods Restricted hobbies and activities
2. BOND WITH THE PATIENT	Familial Moral Obligation	Responsibility towards family members Responsibility towards the family of the recipient
	Deep friendships	Long friendships A sense of comradeship
3. DONOR'S DISPOSITION	Personality traits	Upbringing Influences
	Personal interest	Heavenly investment Redemption A better life
	Supported decision	Family's Support "Evidence-based"

Theme 1: Being in the World of the Suffering Other

Witnessing the Trials of Dialysis

During the interviews, most of the participants revealed that they were very much disturbed by the sight of the complexity of the dialysis procedure. They claimed that the sight of their friend or loved one being attached to a machine stirred a range of emotions within them. Nina claimed that she could not bear to see her daughter suffer and that the sight of the Vas Cath[1] coming out of her daughter's neck actually drove her to distraction.

[1] Vas Cath: a specialised central venous catheter used in dialysis. It is usually inserted in the sub-clavian or jugular vessels.

"When I saw it [Vas Cath], I was distraught. I just could not accept the sight of my daughter in that situation" (Nina)

Noel also claimed that the sight of his brother-in-law's blood flowing in and out of the dialysis machine "jolted" him.

"As soon as I went in and saw him there, to be honest, my first reaction, I was jolted, I was jolted . . . In that environment, hooked to a machine, pipes and tubes passing [through] and blood, coming out and going in and coming out of the tubes. It is not a happy scene! It is a scene, for those that are not used to it, like me at that time, it jolts you a bit!" (Noel)

All the participants also mentioned that the condition of kidney failure in conjunction with the dialysis procedure brought about a lot of other associated problems for the person needing a kidney. Such problems included repeated infections, intolerance to the dialysis procedure by the body, and problems with adherence to the demanding medical regimes. This created further suffering for the patient as well as for the participants, who were constantly being reminded of the fragility of the patient receiving the treatment.

"He'd been a while, and my brother had tried the home dialysis and that didn't work, he got a lot of infections, so he'd been through a lot of difficulties" (Lara)

"She started getting a lot of infections . . . her body could not tolerate [dialysis] anymore. She was very, very, very, weak, so that was the moment where, either death, she had come to the end my mother, she was a disaster . . . once she was, I don't know what happened and froth coming out of her mouth and that kind of thing, she was almost dying" (Sarah)

"Sometimes pain here and sometimes pain there. He used to come form dialysis with a big bump (referring to fistula), like this" (Mark)

It can be argued that these negative emotions that were stirred within the participants at the sight of the other's suffering was what initially drove them to think about donating one of their kidneys. Cialdini (Cialdini et al., 1987; Manucia et al., 1984) claims that humans may offer to help, either to create a positive feeling within oneself or else to relieve a negative feeling. It could be posited that for these living donors, apart from wanting to help so as to relieve the suffering of the other, the participants may have also wanted to donate one of their kidneys to relieve some of the suffering they were experiencing themselves. This reason would also be in adherence to Batson's (1987) claims where he says that the primary motive is always to help the victim, but that "subtle forms of self-benefit" may also exist. In this case the "self-benefit" would be the participants' own relief of the emotional pain they were feeling at the sight of their loved one's tribulations due to dialysis.

Deterioration in the Quality of Life

Apart from the complexity of the dialysis procedure, all five participants claimed that they also witnessed the patient's quality of life deteriorating before their very own eyes. This tormented each of them to various degrees. Nina made it very clear that her daughter's limited choice of foods and the fact that the daughter's appetite was always decreasing worried her significantly. Furthermore, she felt that her daughter was not being able to fulfill her role as a mother due to the effects of dialysis.

> "And that used to upset me. . . I didn't eat fruit in front of her. It used to get stuck here (referring to her throat). I used to say, I am eating fruit and she cannot . . . She ate nothing, nothing. . . That was my worry, I didn't see her eat, I didn't, God she was deteriorating rapidly" (Nina)

> "The machine (referring to the dialysis procedure) does not leave you with much strength to do the housework, and [her] son needs to be taken care of. He had enough tension as it was, poor boy" (Nina)

Similarly, Noel and Mark claimed that they had found it very hard to make sense of the change in their respective friend's lifestyle, considering that they had once led a very active life.

> "At one point I knew him like that and now seeing him, hooked to a machine, his life dependent so to say on a machine, I wanted to do something to see him back to leading a regular life, how I was used to seeing him" (Noel)

> "I remember him better, he used to go abroad and spend months abroad. He used to go to Peru, he went to Mexico to see the birds . . . He did not go abroad anymore" (Mark)

In this regard, it could be argued, that all participants were driven to act altruistically, by what Batson (Batson and Oleson, 1991) claims to be "empathic concern" for the patient's suffering. This "empathic concern" could have motivated the participants to donate one of their kidneys with the specific aim of reducing the other person's distress, or in this case, with the aim of restoring the original active lifestyle the patients had enjoyed, prior to kidney failure.

Theme 2: Bond with the Patient

Familial Moral Obligation

Three of the participants were related by blood to the recipients. The data analysis of the interviews with these participants revealed that they felt a sense of familial moral obligation towards their blood-relative who needed a kidney. However, these participants also claimed that they did not perform the act of donation solely out of a sense of duty.

> "Obviously, apart from all these, it is love. She is my mother . . . so for that respect, love, I don't know what I can call it" (Sarah)

> "Because, I say, if I don't help my daughter myself, who is going to help her? It's true she had her sister. . . but if I can give, I, her mother . . . for your children, you do everything" (Nina)

This sense of familial moral obligation could be highly linked to Hamilton's (1964) theory of kin altruism. All three participants were willing to perform self-sacrificing behaviour for the benefit of their family member. According to evolutionary psychologists, humans have developed this type of mindset as a way of enabling inclusive fitness (Workman and Reader, 2008).

Nina took this sense of familial moral obligation even further, and was not only feeling a sense of responsibility towards her own daughter but also towards her grandson.

> "I did not look at the fact that I might lose my life . . . I looked at her son. . . He was still young, 6 years old. I told him [the consultant], 'I am only looking at that child, she is still raising him'" (Nina)

Nevertheless, during the interview Nina also made it very clear that she would not donate a kidney to an "outsider" – someone other than an immediate family member.

> "I don't think I would do it for an outsider, but for my children I do it" (Nina).

This is in line with Hamilton's claim that humans are more inclined to help their relatives rather than non-relatives, due to inclusive fitness. The claims by these participants are also similar to the findings of a study carried out by Borgida, Conner, and Manteufel (1992), where they found that living donors are more likely to donate an organ to a relative than to a non-relative. Similarly, in a study conducted amongst university undergraduates, Shanteau and Skowronski (1992) found that students were more willing to donate to their own child or a sibling and less willing to donate to a friend or stranger.

Deep Friendships

The other two participants were not related by blood to the recipients, however, they made it very clear that the deep level of friendship they shared with the recipient was one of the motivators for their donation. Noel had known the recipient, Jake, for more than thirty years. Moreover, Jake had married his sister. Nevertheless, during the interview, Noel made it very clear that his donation was not specifically out of duty to his sister, but more to honour his friendship with Jake.

> "I have known Jake for the past 35 years . . . obviously there was a bond, there was a bond not because he was married to my sister . . . other than that we were friends. We used to share a lot of good times together and there was this sense of camaraderie . . . that sense of friendship" (Noel)

Similarly, Mark claimed that he had known Paul for a very long time and that a deep level of friendship had developed between them.

> "I have known him for 8 years, yes, that's how much, 8 years . . . Then you get to know the person more, personally, the things he has, secrets, friendships, women. The things we used to generally speak about" (Mark)

This altruistic act towards friends could be explained from the sociobiological perspective of altruism. Sociobiologists claim that humans are more likely to act altruistically towards two kinds of people, other than blood related relatives, those people whom we perceive as being similar to us, and those with whom we share “kin-like” ties (Pilliavin and Charng, 1990). For Noel and Mark it seems that the friendships they shared with their respective recipients fall into both of these categories. It is very highly probable that friends are chosen due to shared similarities, in line with the first category as suggested by sociobiologists. From the interviews, it also transpires that the level of friendship that both participants shared with the respective recipient was very much on the same level as one would share with kin relatives and this is in line with the second category.

Theme 3: The Donor’s Disposition

Personality Traits

A common feature amongst the participant’s motivations for donating a kidney was their personality and their upbringing. Lara claimed that the fact that she was a doctor’s daughter might have influenced her decision.

> “I think it’s very much to do with my personality . . . I think I was also influenced a bit by being a doctor’s daughter, I’d seen people ill . . . I see it very much as a decision making process that was, that really doesn’t happen on the day you take the decision to do it. I see it as something that is a life process really . . . the sort of formation process I had gone through previously, like my education, my formation as a whole” (Lara)

Similarly, Sarah, Mark, and Noel also believed that their personality and upbringing played a part in their motivations in donating one of their kidneys. Almost as if to prove that they had always been the helping kind, they also gave examples of other helping behaviours they had carried out, prior to donating one of their kidneys.

> “I think it’s my character, as a person I am positive and I always think of the future” (Sarah)

> “Always, always, from when I was young . . . I help people in their homework at school . . .Nowadays at Christmas, we go to a toyshop, I spend €200, €300, however much I have, and we buy toys, and we give them to an orphanage. At least we would have bought them a new toy” (Mark)

Literature is still very much inconsistent in its findings regarding specific personality characteristics, which are in correlation to an altruistic personality. According to Pilliavin and Charng (1990) to conduct such a study is indeed futile. For these participants it could be that they are merely repeating the behaviour, albeit on a higher level, which they would have learnt through experience and social modeling, since such behaviour would have left positive effects within them (Dovidio et al., 2006; Simmons, 1991).

Personal Interest

Another common theme was that most of the participants gave the impression that the act of donating one of their kidneys was not carried out solely and entirely for the other person’s benefit. Four participants out of the five that were interviewed spoke about some personal interest. Their reasons will be categorised under the heading of 'personal interest'.

The most outspoken of them all regarding his personal interest was Mark, who donated his kidney to a friend. During his interview, he explained quite bluntly that, in part, the donation was made as a way of atoning for his past sins. He also saw his donation as a way of achieving something in his life. In his eyes, it was a way of becoming at par with all the missed opportunities he had had in his life.

> "I am a person who did not have an easy life. From the beginning, I did not have an easy life . . . until I was 15 years old, I did not have much of a smooth life...Not at home, not outside . . . I became badly behaved and I did a lot of things . . . I, I never forgave myself and for me . . . For me, that is a form, a form of [seeking] redemption . . . That's how I felt it, like I gave back something . . . From the wrongdoing, and from the things I did not do in life, I gave something back . . . I felt relieved after the operation. Like, like . . . I'd achieved something" (Mark)

Similarly, during the interview, Sarah mentioned several times that she was seeing the transplant operation not only as a way of giving her mother a better life, but also as a way of giving herself, a better life. Sarah, repeated quite a few times that ever since she could remember, her mother had always been sick. She is the only daughter and was responsible for taking care of the house, her brother, her father, as well as her mother. This could be a further reason as to why Sarah felt that the responsibility to restore the family's stability was very much in her hands.

> "I said, 'if this succeeds, our lives would be normal'. We could have normality, because, I do not know for how long, after work I'd keep going to see her [the mother] at hospital. So, for me it was something, not fearful, but even something, 'positive' . . . So, for me it was the turning point of our lives, of my mum's life, of my life too because nowadays, thanks to the decision I took . . . that we took, I'm living a normal life" (Sarah)

Unlike Mark and Sarah, Noel's reason was not as straightforward. However, he still mentioned a personal reason. Noel saw the donation as an investment for an eternal life. He said that after this act, God would surely repay him. This might very well stem from the strong Maltese religious tradition, whereby we live in a culture where from a very early age, individuals are taught that, by giving, one will receive many more good graces in return.

> "However in life, without sounding as if I am some saint, however, I do have a lot of faith. I have enough faith to sell, and believe that when you give a present, God is going to repay many times over. I believe in that" (Noel)

During the interview, both Noel and Nina referred to the act of donation as if it were a calling or a vocation. Noel made it sound as if the donation was a mission bestowed upon him. Later in the interview, Noel also claimed that he would have still gone through the donation, even if it had resulted that Jake was not going to be a good match. Apart from showing his determination, this also shows that his motivation was not solely based on Jake's suffering or his obligation towards him, but almost as if it were his special mission.

> "A person that has many goals in my life, a person who lives to achieve those objectives . . . and this I wanted to do. Today I say, my dream came true" (Noel)

Similarly, Nina did not want anyone else to donate a kidney to her daughter and she felt that only her kidney would be the best. From the interview, one could realise that Nina was also very religious. The fact that she felt that it was her calling to donate the kidney, could be stemming from her religious background. Both Noel and Nina managed to convey the message that this was what God would have wanted them to do.

> "Because, I did not want anyone else to give it to her, I wanted to be the one to give it to her . . . Because I had something within, it told me, you. I told them, don't say anything, because I am going to give it to her" (Nina)

These revelations are very much in concordance with Batson's (1987) claims. Unlike Cialdini (Cialdini et al., 1987), Batson (1987) did believe in real altruism, however he also declared that egoistical motives for altruism are not entirely absent. It would be wrong to say that the participant's interests are entirely egoistical, as Cialdini proposed, since they all mentioned that the other person's suffering was the initial motivator. Nonetheless, this personal interest can be seen as a "subtle form of self-benefit" of their act of organ donation (Batson, 1987). It is interesting to note that these personal interests are also similar to Simmons' (1991) findings, who argued that as opposed to the laboratory, in real circumstances it is very hard to separate the altruistic motives from the egoistical motives.

Supported Decision

During the interviews, each of the five participants mentioned that the support they received from their family and friends had played an important role in increasing their motivations further. Nevertheless, they all maintained that this support did not in any way have any influence on their initial thought of being donors, but that it only consolidated their decision further.

> "I think that was also an important factor, that you know that you have the full support of the people around you and even at work" (Lara)

> "The people surrounding me, especially the friends that are the closest to me and more than that the relatives, you can say that they were a very important element, not of my decision, because my decision I took it myself and on my own and then I shared that wish with them. But they continued to consolidate that" (Noel)

It could be argued, that the fact that the participant's decision was met with support and maybe even with praise from friends and family, could have given rise to the creation of a sense of well-being within themselves. This could be linked to Cialdini's claims (as cited in Simmons, 1991), whereby he proposes that people might act altruistically, specifically for this purpose. Acquiring praise and support from other people could also in itself motivate altruism, which is in further accordance with Cialdini's claims (as cited in Simmons, 1991; Pilliavin and Charng, 1990). These claims are also in line with social learning theory, whereby it is claimed that praise is highly effective in reinforcing behaviour (Dovidio et al., 2006). However, in this case, it did not transpire that the major motive was to receive praise or support, but that the support that the participants received from their family and friends only made the decision seem more right.

Another common theme, which was revealed from the data of all the participants, was that they all carried out their own research regarding organ donation.

> "I started on my own, at home, seeing on the internet, about kidney donors . . . I downloaded some information from the internet, percentages that people with one kidney tend to live longer" (Mark)

> "Before the operation I used to do a lot of research . . . I used to keep contact with living donors" (Noel)

> "I like to read and find out so I was sort of going on the internet and checking . . . a lot of positive experiences of people who had given a kidney and saying how it had made them better people" (Lara)

This might not be directly linked to their motivations, however it discloses the fact that their final decision was based on "evidence". This goes to show that they were taking the act of organ donation very seriously and not as irrational and impulsive as Wilson (1976) claims altruism between relatives to be. This is with the exception of Nina, who conformed to Wilson's claims since she kept declaring that her decision was highly spontaneous.

CONCLUSION

Findings revealed that the primary aim of the act of organ donation for these donors was altruism. They wanted to relieve the other person from suffering, stemming from either a familial moral obligation or a deep friendship. Nevertheless, all the participants also had in addition their own personal motivations.

A significant strength of this study is the fact that this was the first time that the concept of altruism was applied to organ donation in Malta. Furthermore, this is also the first study in Malta, which aimed at shedding some light on the experience of the live organ donor. In addition to these strengths, it is also appropriate to refer to the various limitations of this study and suggestions for future research.

The small number of participants that were selected for this study was a possible limitation to the study. If more participants were selected it would have provided a better representative sample of Maltese donors. Although the relationships between donor and recipient, for this study, were all different, a bigger sample would have also provided other different relationships, thus giving rise to other different motivations. Further understanding of motivations could have also been achieved if other participants who were from different socio-economic backgrounds were included.

This study could also be used by policy makers in Malta during the writing of a national policy on organ donation, which to date, Malta still lacks. Further research would also benefit the guiding process that is required before consenting to donating one's own organ or those of a family member once departed. Rodrigue and Gunther (2006) claim that through such research, variables that can place donors at higher risks for negative outcomes or variables that provide a protective role, can be identified. In turn psychological interventions may be developed and put into practice so as to provide help to candidates whose risk factors may be modified. This kind of research along with this particular study would also be beneficial for The Transplant Support Group (Malta), who already offer support to donors before and after the transplant operation.

A suggestion for future research would be to study the experience of the donor before the transplantation operation. This will provide information to the professionals so as to provide the needed guidance to the donors before undergoing the operation. It would also enable the authorities to provide the donors with any adequate psychosocial assistance they might need.

It is hoped that the findings from this study will encourage further research and in turn provide the information needed for other donors to donate the "Gift of Life". Furthermore, it is hoped that this research gives a better understanding of altruism in relation to organ donation in Malta.

REFERENCES

Aronson, E., Wilson, T. D., & Akert, R. M. (2004). *Social psychology*. Upper Saddle River, NJ: Pearson Prentice Hall.

Bar-Tal, D. (1985-1986). Altruistic motivation to help: Definition, utility and operationalization. *Humboldt Journal of Social Relations, 13*(1-2), 3-14.

Batson, C. D. (1987). Pro-social motivation: Is it ever truly altruistic? In L. Berkowitz (Ed.), Advances in experimental social psychology (Vol. 20, pp. 65-122). New York: *Academic Press*.

Batson, C. D. (1991). *The altruism question: Toward a social-psychological answer*. Hillsdale, NJ: Lawrence Erlbaum Associates.

Batson, C. D., & Oleson, K. C. (1991). Current status of the empathy-altruism hypothesis. In M. S. Clark (Ed.), *Review of personality and social psychology: pro-social behavior* (Vol. 12, pp. 62-85). Newbury Park, CA: Sage.

Biller-Andorno, N. (2002). Gender imbalance in living organ donation. *Medicine Health Care and Philosophy*, *5*, 199-204. doi: 10.1023/A:1016053024671

Borgida, E., Conner, C., & Manteufel, L. (1992). Understanding living kidney donation: A behavioral decision-making perspective. In S. Spacapan & S. Oskamp (Eds.), Helping and being helped (pp. 183-212). Newbury Park, CA: *Sage*.

Braun V., & Clarke V. (2006). Using thematic analysis in psychology. *Qualitative Research in Psychology, 3*(2), 77-101.

Brug, J., Vugt, M. V., Borne, B. V. D., Brouwers, A., & Hooff, H. V. (2000). Predictors of willingness to register as an organ donor among Dutch adolescents. *Psychology & Health*, *15*(3), 357-368. doi: 10.1080/08870440008401998

Cialdini, R. B., Schaller, M., Houlihan, D., Arps, K., Fultz, J., & Beaman, A. L. (1987). Empathy based helping: Is it selflessly or selfishly motivated? *Journal of Personality and Social Psychology*, *52*(4), 749-758. doi:10.1037/0022-3514.52.4.749

Clarke, D. (2003). *Pro-Social and anti-social behaviour*. East Sussex: Routledge.

Dovidio, J. F., Pilliavin, J. A., Schroeder D. A., & Penner, L. A. (2006). The social psychology of prosocial behaviour. New Jersey: *Lawrence Erlbaum Associates*.

Eurobarometer (2010). *Organ donation and transplantation.* Retrieved from http://ec.europa.eu/public_opinion/archives/ebs/ebs_333a_en.pdf

Hill, J. (1984). Human altruism and sociocultural fitness. *Journal of Social and Biological Structures, 7*(1), 17-35. doi: 10.1016/S0140-1750(84)90062-9

Hoffman, M. L. (1981). Is Altruism part of human nature? *Journal of Personality and Social Psychology*, *40*(1), 121-137. doi: 10.1037/0022-3514.40.1.121

Hogg, M. A., & Cooper, J. (Eds.). (2007). The SAGE handbook of social psychology. London*: SAGE.*

Johnson, D. P. (2008). Contemporary sociological theory: an integrated multilevel approach. New York: *Springer.*

Krebs, D. (1982). Psychological approaches to altruism: an evaluation*. Ethics*, *92*(3), 447-458.

Manucia, G., Baumann, D. J., & Cialdini, R. B. (1984). Mood influences on helping: Direct effects or side effects? *Journal of Personality and Social Psycholgoy*, *46*(2), 357-364. doi: 10.1037/0022-3514.46.2.357

Piliavin, J. A., & Charng, H. (1990). Altruism: A review of recent theory and research. *Annual Review of Sociology*, *16*, 27-65.

Piliavin, J. A., Dovidio, J. F., Gaertner, S. L., & Clark, R. D. III. (1981). Emergency intervention. New York*: Academic Press.*

Rodrigue, J. R., & Gunther, R. T. (2006). Psychosocial evaluation of live donors. *Current Opinion in Organ Transplantation*, *11*(3), 234-240.

Romer, D., Gruder, C. L., & Lizzadro, T. (1986). A person-situation approach to altruistic behavior. *Journal of Personality and Social Psychology*, *51*(5), 1001-1012.

Rushton, J.P. (1982). Social learning theory and the development of prosocial behavior. In N. Eisenberg (Ed.), The development of prosocial behaviour (pp. 77-105). New York: *Academic Press.*

Schwartz, S. H. (1970). Elicitation of moral obligation and self-sacrificing behaviour: An experimental study of volunteering to be a bone marrow donor. *Journal of Personality and Social Psychology*, *15*, 283-293.

Schwartz, S. H., & Howard, A. (1984). Internalized values as motivators of altruism. In E. Staub, D. Bar-Tal, J. Karylowski & J. Reykowski (Eds.), Development and maintenance of prosocial behavior (pp.229-256). New York*: Plenum.*

Seelig, B., & Rosof, L. (2009). Altruism. In S. Akhtar (Ed.), Good feelings: psychoanalytic reflections on positive emotions and attitudes (pp. 63-94). London: *Karnac Books Ltd.*

Shanteau, J., & Skowronski, J. J. (1992). The decision to donate organs: An information-integration analysis. In J. Shanteau & R. J. Harris (Eds.), Organ donation and transplantation: Psychological and behavioral factors (pp. 59-67). Washington: *American Psychological Association.*

Simmons, R. G. (1991). Presidential address on altruism and sociology. *The Sociological Quarterly, 32*(1), 1-22.

Simmons, R. G., Marine, S. K., & Simmons, R. L. (1987). The Gift of Life: The Social and Psychological Impact of Organ Transplantation (2nd ed.). New York: *Wiley.*

Steinberg, D. (2003). Kidney and the kindness of strangers. *Health Affairs*, *22*, 184.

Vaillant, G. (1977). Adaptation to Life. Boston*: Little Brown.*

Vine, I. (1983). Sociobiology and social psychology – Rivalry or symbiosis? *British Journal of Social Psychology*, *22*, 1-11.

Wilms, G., Kiefer, S. W., Shanteau, J., & McIntyre, P. (1987). Knowledge and image of body organs: Impact on willingness to donate. In M. Wallendorf & P. Anderson (Eds.), Advances in consumer research (Vol. 14, pp. 338-341). Pruvo, UT: *Association for Consumer Research.*

Wilson, E. O. (1975). Sociobiology: a new synthesis. Boston: *Harvard University Press.*

Wilson, E. O. (1976). The war between the words: biological versus social evolution and some related issues (Section 2). Genetic basis of behavior – especially of altruism. *American Psychology*, *31*, 370-371.

Workman, L., & Reader, W. (2008). Evolutionary psychology: An introduction (2nd ed.). Cambridge, UK*: University Press.*

In: Organ Donation and Transplantation
Editor: Mary Anne Lauri
ISBN: 978-1-62948-257-6

Chapter 4

UNDERSTANDING DECISIONS TO COMMUNICATE ORGAN DONATION WISHES: A NARRATIVE REVIEW

Melissa K. Hyde*
Griffith Health Institute, Griffith University,
Queensland, Australia

ABSTRACT

Prior communication of organ donation wishes to family increases the likelihood of family consent for donation. However, many people have not shared their wishes. This chapter provides a narrative review of the psychosocial factors used to understand people's decisions to communicate their donation wishes via donor registries/cards and in conversation with family. Traditional (e.g., using demographic characteristics to create donor profiles) and more recent (e.g., using social-cognitive theory to predict communication intentions and behaviour) approaches applied to understand decisions to communicate donation wishes, and their associated limitations, are reviewed. Four key areas where there is scope for consideration are identified: consistency and compatibility in measurement; the assumption that decisions to communicate donation wishes are reasoned and rational, the intention-behaviour relationship, and the potential for other variables not tested to impact on communication decisions. Based on the review, recommendations are proposed that offer a way forward for research to increase communication of organ donation wishes. These include: increased focus on behaviour; further examination of emotional and affective variables; greater attention to family discussion as an extension to the research about joining donor registries; re-examining the conceptualisation of family discussion (conversation vs. notification); and including both individual and family perspectives in efforts to understand communication of donation wishes.

* Corresponding author: melissa.hyde@griffith.edu.au.

INTRODUCTION

Despite advances in transplantation surgery and post-transplant survival rates, the worldwide organ shortage continues to present as a major barrier for organ transplantation to those in need. At present there are 117,869 US (United Network for Organ Sharing, 2013), 7,288 UK (National Health Service Blood and Transplant, 2013), and approximately 1600 Australian (DonateLife, 2012) citizens on waiting lists to receive the therapeutic benefits of transplantation. Parallel to this, 95% of Americans and 94% of Australians surveyed indicated support for donation with approximately half indicating they had registered a preference for donation (Campbell Research & Consulting, 2006; The Gallup Organization Inc., 2005). Hence there appears to be a discrepancy between public majority support for and positive attitudes towards donating organs and organ donation rates which do not meet community demand (Simpkin, Robertson, Barber, & Young, 2009). In response at least in part, researchers have investigated demographic characteristics, beliefs, and attitudes that may explain a person's general preference for donating organs (for reviews see Nijkamp, Hollestelle, Zeegers, van den Borne, & Reubsaet, 2008; Radecki & Jaccard, 1997). However, a further research focus centers on family communication about organ donation. Specifically, it has been proposed that family conversations about organ donation need to increase so that next-of-kin have prior knowledge of their loved one's positive attitudes or wishes for donation in the event they are ever asked to authorise donation of their loved one's organs (i.e. consent). Family who are aware of their loved one's donation wishes are more likely to support them when a request for donation is made (Siminoff, Arnold, & Hewlett, 2001).

The importance of family in the consent process is underscored by a recent review of 54 nations with deceased donation programs in either a presumed consent or explicit consent legislative framework (Rosenblum et al., 2012). Presumed consent (opt-out) is a system where everyone is assumed to be a donor unless an objection is made by the individual prior to their death. An explicit consent system (opt-in or 'first person consent') requires people who wish to donate to designate their preference for donation on a donor registry or other official means. Family is then consulted for permission when donation wishes are unknown or family may be asked to confirm donation wishes when they are known. Regardless of the consent system in place, in practice next-of-kin were consulted in most nations to authorise donation of their loved one's organs and could veto donation even if the deceased's donation preference had been recorded previously (Rosenblum, et al., 2012). This is a critically important finding given international estimates show that approximately 30-60% of families refuse consent when approached for donation of their loved one's organs (DonateLife, 2012; Rosenblum, et al., 2012; Siminoff, et al., 2001; Simpkin, et al., 2009) and that family members who are unsure of their loved one's donation wishes are more likely to decline donation (Siminoff, et al., 2001). Many individuals have yet to communicate their donation wishes to family. Approximately 40% of Europeans surveyed had talked about organ donation with family (Opinion & Social, 2010), compared to 70% of Australians (DonateLife, 2012) and Americans (The Gallup Organization Inc., 2005) who had made their wishes known to family. Further, 43% of Australians did not know or were not sure about their loved one's donation wishes and 60% had not had a conversation about organ donation in the past year (DonateLife, 2012). Less than half of Americans had a family member share their donation preference (The Gallup Organization Inc., 2005). Hence, two key issues for organ donation practice and research are the extent to which people communicate their wishes for donation prior to death via a donor register, driver license, or donor card (i.e. *registering*) and advise family/next-of-kin of their donation wishes (i.e. *discussing*).

This chapter takes the form of a narrative review (Dixon-Woods, Agarwal, Jones, Young, & Sutton, 2005) which draws on empirically-based research and common social-cognitive decision-making theories from social and health psychology domains (see Conner & Norman, 2005) to understand family communication about organ donation wishes. It addresses three objectives. First, the socio-demographic characteristics (e.g., gender, age, donation experience) and beliefs associated with communicating organ donation wishes are described (Section 1). Second, the common social-cognitive decision-making theories (or constructs from these theories e.g., attitudes, norms, efficacy) applied to understand communication of donation wishes are reviewed (Section 2). Third, limitations of the research presented are discussed (Section 3) and future research recommendations to support efforts to increase communication of donation wishes are proposed (Section 4).

METHOD

Medline and PsycINFO databases were searched for peer-reviewed qualitative and quantitative journal articles published in English between January 1970 and October 2012. The following search string and keywords were used: (organ donat$.mp OR organ donor.mp OR transpl$.mp) AND (communicat$.mp OR consent.mp OR discuss.mp OR talk.mp OR convers$.mp OR licen$.mp OR register.mp OR registration.mp OR registry.mp OR sign.mp OR donor card.mp). The narrative review draws from articles that met the following criteria: conducted in countries with opt-in or explicit consent systems; AND included individuals eligible to record their donation preference via a donor register/card/driver license or family discussion; AND focused on communicating donation wishes for deceased organ/tissue donation for transplantation; AND included individual characteristics or beliefs related to communicating donation wishes AND/OR applied social-cognitive models (or their constructs) to understand individual decisions to communicate donation wishes.

RESULTS

Socio-Demographic Characteristics, Beliefs/Attitudes, and Communicating Organ Donation Wishes

Socio-demographic Characteristics Associated with Communicating Donation Wishes

Socio-demographic characteristics such as gender, age, ethnicity, education, income, religious affiliation, altruism, knowledge and experience with donation have been explored in relation to joining a donor registry/signing a donor card and family discussion and are reviewed below briefly.

Gender, age, and ethnicity. Females compared to males are more likely to have a donor card/designation on their driver license or to have joined a donor registry (e.g., Weber,

Martin, & Members of Comm401., 2006) and engaged in family discussion (e.g., Alvaro, Jones, Robles, & Siegel, 2005). Other studies suggest that males not females report greater readiness to discuss their organ donation preference (Guadagnoli et al., 1999), and some have found no relationship between donor card signing and gender (e.g., Besser, Amir, & Barkan, 2004). Being younger has been associated with higher rates of registering/donor card signing (e.g., Perkins, 1987), and in contrast, being middle aged has been related to donor card signing (Amir & Haskell, 1997), with older people more likely to have had family discussion (Newton, Burney, Hay, & Ewing, 2010). Some studies have found no relationship between gender, age, and registration status (Rodrigue et al., 2004). More consistently, being Caucasian compared to other ethnicities (e.g., African-American or Asian-American) has been associated with increased registering (e.g., Perkins, 1987) and family discussion (e.g., Guadagnoli, et al., 1999).

Education, income, and religious affiliation. Higher education levels and increased socioeconomic status or income are associated with donor card signing (e.g., Ashkenazi, Guttman, & Hornik, 2005) and family discussion (e.g., Sirois, Sears, & Marhefka, 2005). Religious affiliation has also been related to donor card signing (Amir & Haskell, 1997) and family discussion (Newton, et al., 2010); however, other studies have found that being less religious was associated with donor card signing (e.g., Ashkenazi, et al., 2005) or showed no evidence for a relationship between religious affiliation and communicating donation wishes (e.g., Besser, et al., 2004).

Altruism, knowledge about, and experience with donation. A positive link between altruism, that is the desire to help others without expectation of reward or personal gain, and willingness for organ donation has been widely cited in the literature (Radecki & Jaccard, 1997). There is some evidence for a link between altruistic beliefs or an altruistic tendency and registering/donor card signing (e.g., Kopfman & Smith, 1996) and family discussion (e.g., Morgan, 2004). Altruism in these studies however is related to the act of donating organs, rather than communicating donation wishes. Family discussion or joining a registry may also be associated with altruistic motivations such as saving family or loved ones from making a difficult decision (Hyde & White, 2007) or helping family to cope with death (Hyde & White, 2010b). People who have higher levels of factual knowledge about organ donation are more likely to have designated their preference on a donor registry or card or driver license (e.g., Horton & Horton, 1990); although some studies have found no relationship between knowledge and registering (e.g., Hyde & White, 2007). As well, increased knowledge has been linked to more family discussion about donation (e.g., Guadagnoli, et al., 1999). Similarly, having prior experience with organ donation such as knowing other potential donors is associated with increased registering (e.g., Nolan & Spanos, 1989) and knowing a potential donor/recipient with family discussion (Alvaro, et al., 2005).

Constructing a profile of the socio-demographic characteristics of people who communicate their donation wishes can help to match targeted health promotion messages to specific subgroups in efforts to increase communication of donation wishes (Haustein & Sellers, 2004). However, there appears a disproportionate focus on registering compared to discussing. With this constraint in mind, based on the research reviewed a preliminary communicator profile is offered (Table 1).

Beliefs and attitudes associated with communicating donation wishes

Beliefs and attitudes about organ donation generally may impact on willingness to communicate donation wishes (e.g., Besser, et al., 2004). For instance, beliefs shown to impact negatively on donation willingness generally such as fear that death will be declared prematurely for the purposes of recovering organs and fear of mutilation and the body not being whole after death (e.g., Parisi & Katz, 1986) may prevent communication of donation wishes. Conversely positive beliefs such as helping others, and saving or improving the quality of another person's life (e.g., Hyde & White, 2010b) may motivate discussion. People who have registered or signed a donor card or license, or have expressed their willingness or intention to do so, report more positive attitudes toward organ donation (e.g., Nijkamp, et al., 2008) and those who have not registered report more negative attitudes (Sirois, et al., 2005). Similarly, people who have talked with family demonstrate more positive attitudes (e.g., Morgan, 2004). However, other studies have found no relationship between attitude and donor card signing or that the correlation between attitude and behaviour is weak (Baluch, Randhawa, Holmes, & Duffy, 2001; Morgan, Stephenson, Harrison, Afifi, & Long, 2008). A recent trend in the research has been to consider cognitive (i.e. evaluations of a behaviour – e.g., good/bad) and affective (i.e. emotion or more visceral reactions – e.g., disgust) components of attitudes (e.g., Morgan, et al., 2008; O'Carroll, Foster, McGeechan, Sandford, & Ferguson, 2011). From this perspective, negative affective attitudes have been found to better discriminate between those who have and have not registered/signed donor cards (e.g., Morgan, et al., 2008; O'Carroll, Foster, et al., 2011).

Communicating donation wishes on a register or in family discussion is a different behaviour to being generally willing to donate (Hyde & White, 2009c) and may involve beliefs and attitudes that are not captured entirely by measures of general attitudes towards organ donation. An understanding of these specific beliefs, along with potential similarities and differences in beliefs for registering and discussing, is needed to develop effective strategies to promote communication of donation wishes.

Table 1. Preliminary communicator profile of the characteristics of people who register/sign a donor card or license and discuss donation wishes

Register/sign donor card	Discuss with family
• Female (1-7) • Younger (6,8-10) • Caucasian (1,6,10-13) • Higher education level (10,14) • Altruistic tendency (15-16) • No/less religious affiliation (1,14) • More donation knowledge (3,6,10,15,17-24) • Know other potential donors (6,17,19,22,25)	• Female (26-29) • Older (28) • Caucasian (5,27,30-31) • Higher education level (5) • Altruistic tendency (12,28,32-33) • More donation knowledge (28,30,32-33) • Know a potential donor/recipient (26)

1. Baughn et al., 2006; 2. Breitkopf, 2006; 3. Reubsaet, et al., 2001; 4. Sanner, 1998; 5. Sirois, et al., 2005; 6. Wakefield et al., 2011; 7. Weber, et al., 2006; 8. Downing & Jones, 2008; 9. Horton & Horton, 1991; 10. Perkins, 1987; 11. Afifi et al., 2006; 12. Morgan, et al., 2003; 13. Yuen et al., 1998; 14. Ashkenazi, et al., 2005; 15. Kopfman & Smith, 1996; 16. Morgan & Miller, 2002; 17. Besser, et al., 2004; 18. Horton & Horton, 1990; 19. Nolan & Spanos, 1989; 20. Pham & Spigner, 2004; 21. Radecki & Jaccard, 1999; 22. Rubens et al., 1998; 23. Ryckman et al., 2005; 24. Sander & Miller, 2005; 25. Amir & Haskell, 1997; 26. Alvaro, et al., 2005; 27. Minniefield et al., 2001; 28. Newton, et al., 2010; 29. Thompson et al., 2003; 30. Guadagnoli, et al., 1999; 31. Spigner et al., 2002; 32. Morgan, 2004; 33. Morgan & Miller, 2001.

Table 2. Summary of the perceived barriers to (-) and benefits of (+) communicating donation wishes

Theme	Registering/signing donor card or driver's license	Family discussion
Knowledge about the process of organ donation or communicating donation wishes	- Unsure how to register (Hyde & White, 2007; Saub et al., 1998) - Lack of general knowledge about organ donation (Hyde & White, 2007; 2009a; Siegel, et al., 2010) - Difficult to register (Reubsaet, et al., 2001) + Learn more about organ donation (Reubsaet, et al., 2001)	- Unsure how or when to raise the topic (Hyde & White, 2007; 2009a; Vincent, 2006; Waldrop et al., 2004) - Lack of general knowledge about organ donation (Hyde &. White, 2009a)
Decision confidence and motivation to communicate donation wishes	- Uncertainty about the donation decision (Breitkopf, 2006; Feeley & Servoss, 2005; Hyde & White, 2007; 2009a; Reubsaet, et al., 2001) - Lack of motivation to register (Feeley & Servoss, 2005; Hyde & White, 2007; 2009a; Saub, et al., 1998) - Have not thought about it (Feeley & Servoss, 2005) - Lack of opportunity to register (Feeley & Servoss, 2005; Siegel, et al., 2010) + Registering will strengthen belief in donation (Breitkopf, 2006) + Registering/signing as a good thing to do (Yuen, et al., 1998)	- Uncertainty about the donation decision (Hyde & White, 2009a) - Lack of motivation to discuss decision (Hyde & White, 2007; 2009a) - Have not thought about it (Yeung et al., 2000) - Not feeling ready to talk about it (Vincent, 2006; Yeung, et al., 2000)
Fear and (mis)trust in the organ donation and communicating process	- If registered, being unsure if life-saving measures would be taken (Baughn, et al., 2006; Brug, et al., 2000; Feeley & Servoss, 2005; Hyde & White, 2007; 2009a; Reubsaet, et al., 2001; Siegel, et al., 2010; Spigner, et al., 2002) - Being scared of or anxious about registering/signing (Brug, et al., 2000; Feeley & Servoss, 2005; Kopfman & Smith, 1996) + Registering as increasing the efficiency of the donation process (Hyde & White, 2007; 2009a)	- If registered, being unsure if life-saving measures would be taken (Alvaro, et al., 2005; Morgan, 2004) - Uncomfortable talking about death of self or others (Hyde & White, 2009a; Vincent, 2006; Waldrop, et al., 2004)

Theme	Registering/signing donor card or driver's license	Family discussion
Body integrity and control of organs	- Feeling the body will be mutilated or the need to preserve the body as whole after death (Baughn, et al., 2006; Brug, et al., 2000; Hardie et al.t, 1992; Hyde & White, 2007; Reubsaet, et al., 2001) - Organs traded (Brug, et al., 2000; Reubsaet, et al., 2001) + Body or organs survive after death (Reubsaet, et al., 2001) + Avoid waste of healthy organs (Hyde & White, 2007) + Can decide what happens to my organs after death (Brug, et al., 2000; Reubsaet, et al., 2001)	
Concern about family	- Create distress/conflict if family disagree (Feeley & Servoss, 2005; Hyde & White, 2007; 2009a; Rubens, et al., 1998) - Have to defend or justify decision to family (Breitkopf, 2006; Radecki & Jaccard, 1999)	- Create distress/conflict if family disagree (Hyde & White, 2009a) - Have to defend or justify decision to family (Hyde & White, 2009a) - Feel pressure from family to change decision (Hyde & White, 2009a)
Benefits to self or others	+ Make the decision/process easier for family (Brug, et al., 2000; Hyde & White, 2009a; Reubsaet, et al., 2001) + Help/save another person (Brug, et al., 2000) + Death positive for someone else (Brug, et al., 2000; Reubsaet, et al., 2001) + Better chance to receive a transplant (Brug, et al., 2000; Reubsaet, et al., 2001) + Make a good impression on others (Reubsaet, et al., 2001)	+ Make family aware of decision (Hyde & White, 2009a) + Gain approval from family for decision (Hyde & White, 2009a) + Be aware of important other's donation wishes (Hyde & White, 2009a)

Beliefs. Beliefs related to registering and family discussion identified in the review were grouped using six themes (Table 2): (1) knowledge about the process of organ donation and communicating donation wishes, (2) decision confidence and motivation to communicate donation wishes, (3) fear and (mis)trust in the organ donation and communication process, (4) body integrity and control of organs, (5) concern about family, and (6) benefits to self and others. While some of these themes reflect prior classifications of beliefs for organ donation generally such as knowledge (see Radecki & Jaccard, 1997), they also highlight beliefs related specifically to communicating donation wishes, such as decision confidence and concern about family (see also Breitkopf, 2006; Radecki & Jaccard, 1999). Within these themes, beliefs common to registering or signing and family discussion were: uncertainty about how to register or start family discussion, not feeling informed enough about organ donation generally, uncertainty about the actual donation preference, lack of motivation to communicate, not receiving adequate life-saving treatment if a positive donor status was communicated, and negative consequences associated with communicating donation wishes.

Differences in beliefs included registering but not family discussion elicited concerns about body integrity or control over organs. Benefits for others for discussion related solely to family, but for registering, benefits were predominantly for unknown others. Beliefs reflecting what could conceivably happen as a consequence of registering (e.g., helping or saving another person, organs being traded) suggest that registering is a behaviour clearly associated with organ donation. In contrast for family discussion, the potential for receiving inadequate life-saving medical care if donor status was known was the only belief related to donation. Family authorisation is needed in most cases for donation of a loved one's organs to occur, and it suggests the need to establish a clear link between sharing donation wishes with family and family carrying out these wishes.

Attitude. Specific attitudes toward communicating donation wishes (e.g., Breitkopf, 2006; Godin, Belanger-Gravel, Gagne, & Blondeau, 2008; Hyde & White, 2009b, 2009c), as opposed to more general attitudes about organ donation, are consistently and positively related to behaviour (and intention) (Table 3); the average correlation for attitudes and either registering or discussing behaviour being $r = 0.31$. This finding suggests a stronger relationship between corresponding attitudes and behaviour (consistent with meta-analyses of the attitude-behaviour relationship Kraus, 1995), compared to other studies linking general organ donation attitudes to registering/signing ($r = 0.23$, Morgan, et al., 2008; $r = -.01$, Feeley & Servoss, 2005) and discussing ($r = .11$, Wu, 2008; $r = .18$, Wu & Tang, 2009) behaviour.

Decision-Making Theories for Understanding Communication of Organ Donation Wishes

Organ donation models which include socio-demographic characteristics, beliefs, and attitudes (e.g., Organ Donor Willingness Model; Kopfman & Smith, 1996), Organ Donation Model; Morgan, 2004), as well as established social-cognitive theories (e.g., Theory of Reasoned Action; Weber, Martin, Corrigan, & 160, 2007; Theory of Planned Behaviour; Hyde & White, 2009c) and their extensions, have been applied to understand decisions to communicate donation wishes. These theories provide a framework from which to identify similarities and differences in predictors, and to develop interventions to increase communication about organ donation. These models are summarised below briefly and in Table 4.

Development of Specific Organ Donation Models

Horton and Horton's model. One of the first organ donation models developed was Horton and Horton's (1991) model which specified five variables proposed to positively influence the decision to sign or possess a donor card. In the original model, values (Rokeach's seven instrumental values, e.g., broadminded, helpful, honest), factual knowledge about organ donation, attitudes, and willingness to donate were directly or indirectly associated with signing or carrying a donor card. Revisions of this model included three additional variables: attitude towards death, age, and prior blood donation experience. Tests of this model showed that prior blood donation and attitude towards donation were associated with willingness to donate; and knowledge, prior blood donation and willingness to donate were directly linked to card signing or possession (Horton & Horton, 1991).

Organ Donation Willingness Model (ODWM). Using a variant of the theory of reasoned action (Fishbein & Ajzen, 1975), Kopfman and Smith (1996) extended Horton and Horton's model to create the Organ Donation Willingness Model. This model includes subjective norm (perceived support/approval from others in their social network), and replaces age, values, attitudes towards death, and prior blood donation with the variables of altruism and fear. Hypothesised relationships in this model were supported in discriminant analysis. Together, altruism, knowledge, fear, attitude, and subjective norm explained 60% of variance in level of intention to sign and reliably distinguished between people with weak intentions to donate, people with strong intentions who planned to sign a donor card, and committed donors who had signed (Kopfman & Smith, 1996).

Organ Donation Model (ODM). Morgan and colleagues (Morgan, 2004; Morgan & Miller, 2002; Morgan, Miller, & Arasaratnam, 2002, 2003) further extended these models to form the Organ Donation Model. This model specifies similar pathways to its Organ Donation Willingness Model predecessor with the exception that the variable fear is removed based on the argument that the measure of fear originally formed part of the knowledge measure used in Horton and Horton's model (Morgan & Miller, 2002). The Organ Donation Model differs further from prior models because it considers a person's willingness for family discussion to be a function of their willingness or intent and subsequent signing of a donor card (Morgan, 2004). Although links between intention and willingness to sign a donor card and actual signing behaviour, as well as between donor card signing and willingness to talk have been proposed in the Organ Donation Model, these relationships are rarely tested (for an exception see Morgan, et al., 2002). Intention to sign, willingness to talk, and actual donor card signing have all been predicted by attitude, subjective norm, and knowledge (Morgan & Miller, 2002; Morgan, et al., 2002); however, in other studies, knowledge was a significant contributor to intention to sign and willingness to talk only (Morgan, et al., 2003). Altruism was a direct predictor of willingness to talk (Morgan, et al., 2002, 2003) and donor card signing (Morgan & Miller, 2002).

Table 3. Specific attitude measures for communicating donation wishes

Author/s	Intentions/Behaviour	Measure	Scale	α	Attitude-behaviour or Attitude-intention relationship
(Breitkopf, 2006)	Intention to communicate wishes to family by signing a donation letter and signing behaviour	How favourable do you, personally, feel towards signing the donation letter at this time?	Extremely unfavourable/extremely favourable	-	Attitude correlated significantly with intention ($r = 0.45$) and behaviour ($r = 0.33$)
(Godin, et al., 2008)	Intentions and behaviour for signing the organ donor consent sticker	Would signing the organ donor consent sticker… Be a generous act? Be a rewarding act? Be a useful act? Be a stressful act? Be a source of anxiety? Make you nervous?	Very improbable/very probable	.74	Attitude predicted intention but did not predict behaviour
(Hubner & Kaiser, 2006)	Intention to sign an organ donor card	Signing an organ donor card is a good thing to do. Signing an organ donor card is sensible.	How strongly agreed or disagreed with the statements	.92	Attitude correlated significantly with intention ($r = .62$)
(Hyde & White, 2009c)	Intention to join the national organ donor registry and intention to discuss donation wishes with family	For me to register/continue to be registered as an organ donor would be… For me to talk to my family, partner, or close friend about my donation decision would be…	Good/bad Negative/positive Worthless/valuable Favourable/unfavourable	.88 for both behaviours	Attitude correlated significantly with intention ($r = .67$) for both registering and discussing
(Hyde & White, 2009b)	Intention to join the national organ donor registry and intention to discuss donation wishes with family	For me to register my consent to donate my organs upon death would be…	Good/bad Negative/ positive Worthless/valuable Favourable/unfavourable	.91 for both behaviours	Attitude correlated significantly with intention for registering ($r = .61$) and discussing ($r = .54$)

Author/s	**Intentions/Behaviour**	**Measure**	**Scale**	**α**	**Attitude-behaviour or Attitude-intention relationship**
		For me to discuss my organ donation decision with my partner or family members would be…			
(Hyde & White, 2010a)	Intention and behaviour for joining the national donor registry and discussing organ donation wishes with family	For me to register my consent in the next month to donate my organs upon death would be… For me to discuss my organ donation decision with my partner or family members in the next month would be…	Bad/good Valuable/worthless Negative/positive Favourable/unfavourable	.90 for registering .93 for discussing	Attitude correlated significantly with intention (r = .68) and behaviour (r = .31) for registering. Attitude correlated significantly with intention (r = .55) and behaviour (r = .28) for discussing.
(Park & Smith, 2007)	Intention to sign the donor registry and intention to talk with family about organ donation	Signing the state organ-donor registry is… Talking with my family about organ donation is…	Good/bad Unwise/wise Favourable/unfavourable Beneficial/not beneficial	.83 for signing and .87 for family discussion	Attitude correlated significantly with intention for signing (r = .56) and attitude correlated significantly with intention for family discussion (r = .42)
(Yun & Park, 2010)	Intention to sign an organ donor registry and intention to talk with family about organ donation	Signing an organ donor registry is… Talking with family about organ donation is…	Good/bad Unwise/wise Favourable/unfavourable Beneficial/not beneficial	.80 for signing a registry and .87 for family discussion	Attitudes to sign the registry were correlated significantly with intention (r = .53) and attitudes about family discussion were correlated significantly with intention (r = .49)

Table 4. Summary of theoretical approaches to understand communicating donation wishes

Author	Communication behaviour	Model/Theory	DV	R^2	INT	WILL	ATT	SN	PBC	MN	ID	PAST	KNOW	ALTR	OTHER
(Horton & Horton, 1991)	Sign donor card	Created model	Willingness				✓								✓ Prior blood donation
			Behaviour			✓							✓		✓ Prior blood donation
(Kopfman & Smith, 1996)	Sign donor card	ODWM	Willingness (discriminate between groups)	60%			✓	✓					✓	✓	✓ Fear (includes knowledge)
			Behaviour			✓									
(Morgan, et al., 2008)	Sign donor card	Extended ODM	Behaviour	15%			✓	✓					✓		✓ Non-cognitive beliefs (e.g. bodily integrity, ick factor)
(Morgan, et al., 2002)	Sign donor card	ODM	Intention				✓	✓						×	
			Behaviour				✓	×					✓		
(Morgan, et al., 2003)	Sign donor card	ODM	Intention	42%			✓	✓					✓	×	
			Behaviour				✓	✓					×	×	
(Feeley & Servoss, 2005)	Sign donor card	ODM	Behaviour			✓							✓		✓ Donation experience
(Brug, et al., 2000)	Register	Extended SCT*	Intention	62%			✓	✓	×			✓			
(Reubsaet, et al., 2001)	Register	Extended SCT	Intention	55%			✓	✓				✓	✓		✓ Gender ✓ Involvement ✓ Anxiety
(Breitkopf, 2006)	Signing donation letter	TRA	Intention	79%			✓	×							
			Behaviour		✓										
(Weber, et al., 2007)	Signed donor card	TRA	Behaviour	23%	✓										
(Bresnahan et al.,2007)	Register	Modified TPB	Intention				✓	✓	×				×		✓Communicate wishes to family

Author	Communication behaviour	Model/Theory	DV	R^2	INT	WILL	ATT	SN	PBC	MN	ID	PAST	KNOW	ALTR	OTHER
			Behaviour		✓										
(Hubner & Kaiser, 2006)	Sign donor card	TPB	Intention	69%			✓	✓	✓						
		Extended TPB	Intention	72%			✓	✓	✓	✓					
(Godin, et al., 2008)	Sign donor card	TPB	Intention				✓	×	✓						
		Extended TPB	Intention				✓	×	✓	✓		✓			✓Perceived barriers × Anticipated regret
		TPB	Behaviour		✓				✓						
		Extended TPB	Behaviour		✓				✓	✓		✓			
(Park & Smith, 2007)	Sign donor card	TPB	Intention	39%			✓	✓	×						
(Hyde & White, 2009c)	Continue to be registered	TPB	Intention	52%			✓	✓	✓						
		Extended TPB	Intention	57%			✓	✓	✓	✓	✓				
	Register	TPB	Intention	55%			✓	✓	✓						
		Extended TPB	Intention	79%			✓	×	✓	✓	✓				
(Hyde & White, 2009b)	Register	Extended TPB	Intention	74%			✓	✓	✓	✓	✓	✓			
(Hyde & White, 2010a)	Register	Augmented TPB and PWM	Intention	72%			×	✓	✓	✓	✓	✓			
			Willingness	50%			✓	×	×	✓	✓	×			
			Behaviour	44%	✓	×			✓			×			
(Yun & Park, 2010)	Register	TPB	Intention	47%			✓	✓	✓						✓ Culture
(Morgan, et al., 2002)	Talk	ODM	Willingness				✓	✓						✓	
(Morgan, et al., 2003)	Talk	ODM	Willingness	36%			✓	✓					✓	✓	

Table 4. (Continued)

Author	Communication behaviour	Model/Theory	DV	R^2	INT	WILL	ATT	SN	PBC	MN	ID	PAST	KNOW	ALTR	OTHER
(Wu, 2008)	Discuss	Extended TRA	Behaviour		✓		×	✓							✓ Death anxiety
(Wu & Tang, 2009)	Discuss	Extended TRA	Behaviour	15%			✓	✓							×Misconceptions ✓ Gender ✓ Ethnicity
(Park & Smith, 2007)	Talk	TPB	Intention	36%			✓	✓	×						
(Hyde & White, 2009c)	Discuss (Continue to be registered)	TPB	Intention	61%			✓	✓	✓						
		Extended TPB	Intention	68%			✓	✓	✓	✓	×				
	Discuss (Not registered)	TPB	Intention	60%			✓	✓	×						
		Extended TPB	Intention	69%			✓	✓	×	✓	×				
(Hyde & White, 2009b)	Discuss	Extended TPB	Intention	76%			×	×	✓	✓	✓	✓			
		TPB	Behaviour	11%	✓				×						
(Hyde & White, 2010a)	Discuss	Augmented TPB and PWM	Intention	69%			✓	✓	✓	✓	✓	×			
			Willingness	33%			✓	×	×	✓	×	✓			
			Behaviour	32%	✓	×			×			×			
(Yun & Park, 2010)	Discuss	TPB	Intention	56%			✓	✓	✓						× Culture

✓ = significant predictor; × = non-significant predictor.

Abbreviations: ALTR = Altruism; ATT = Attitude; DV = Dependent variable; ID = Identity (self); INT = Intention; KNOW = Knowledge; MN = Moral norm; ODM = Organ Donation Model; ODWM = Organ Donor Willingness Model; OTHER = Other variables including background characteristics; PAST = Past communication behaviour; PBC = Perceived Behavioural Control; PWM = Prototype/Willingness Model; SCT = Social Cognitive Theory; SN = Subjective norm; TPB = Theory of Planned Behaviour; TRA = Theory of Reasoned Action; WILL = Willingness

Note. * In Social Cognitive Theory, attitude is represented by positive and negative outcome beliefs and subjective norms are represented by social outcome expectancies

Revisions of the Organ Donation Model include additional variables such as perceived benefits (e.g., donors as heroes because they save lives) and 'non-cognitive' beliefs (e.g., body integrity, 'jinx' factor – making plans for death by signing a donor card will bring it about, 'ick' factor – organ donation as disgusting, and medical mistrust) proposed as either directly or indirectly contributing to donor card signing (Morgan, et al., 2008). A test of this revised Organ Donation Model showed knowledge, attitude, subjective norm, and 'non-cognitive' variables were direct and significant predictors of, and explained 15% of variance in, donor card signing (Morgan, et al., 2008).

Brug and colleagues' model. As a further extension to this research, Brug and colleagues (Brug, Van Vugt, van den Borne, Brouwers, & van Hooff, 2000; Reubsaet, van den Borne, Brug, Pruyn, & van Hooff, 2001) proposed a model grounded in social-cognitive theory to explain willingness to register as an organ donor. In this model, a person's motivation to register was proposed as a function of their positive and negative outcome expectancies (similar to attitudes), social outcome expectancies (similar to subjective norm), self-efficacy, past behaviour, and knowledge. Two tests of the model incorporating refinements explained 62% and 55% of variance in registering intentions. Consistent, direct and significant pathways were between intentions and negative outcome expectancies, positive outcome expectancies, past behaviour, and social outcome expectancies.

Overall, across these specific organ donation models, consistent predictors associated with intentions/willingness to communicate donation wishes and communication behaviour were: attitude, subjective norm, and knowledge (Table 4).

Theories of Reasoned Action and Planned Behaviour and their Extensions

Theory of reasoned action (TRA). The theory of reasoned action (Fishbein & Ajzen, 1975) proposes that behaviour is informed directly by a person's intention (i.e. readiness to act). Intention, in turn, is guided by a person's attitude (positive/negative evaluation of behaviour) and subjective norm (perceived approval/pressure from others in their social network). For example, Breitkopf (2006) used standard measures (i.e. conforming to the specifications of the model) to predict intention to sign an organ donation letter and signing behaviour. Intention to sign was the only significant predictor of signing behaviour, and attitude toward signing predicted signing intention. Similarly, Wu (2008) applied an extended theory of reasoned action, incorporating death anxiety and demographic factors, and found that subjective norm, death anxiety, and intention were associated significantly with past family discussion.

Theory of planned behaviour (TPB). The theory of planned behaviour extends the theory of reasoned action to explain behaviours that may not be entirely within an individual's control (Ajzen, 1991). For example, family discussion is contingent on family cooperation and, therefore, is not entirely a volitional behaviour. Further, some people may feel incapable of registering or discussing their wishes with family because they lack the necessary facts, skills, or resources to do so (e.g., Breitkopf, 2006). As with the theory of reasoned action, the main tenets of the theory of planned behaviour are that intention is the most proximal predictor of behaviour. Intention is a function of a person's attitude, subjective norm, and perceived behavioural control (or efficacy; perceived ease or difficulty of behavioural performance and whether behaviour is within a person's control). Also, perceived behavioural control is proposed to predict behaviour directly. Collectively, the assumptions of the theory of planned behaviour are supported in predicting people's communication of their donation wishes; attitude, and less so subjective norm and perceived behavioural control (e.g., Hyde & White, 2009c) contribute significantly to intentions to communicate, and intention is a significant predictor of communication behaviour (e.g., Godin, et al., 2008) (Table 4).

A further advantage of the theory of planned behaviour is the capacity to include as part of the model variables that may be relevant to the context studied and may explain a unique proportion of additional variance (Ajzen, 1991). In this respect, moral norm (i.e. perceived moral obligation or responsibility to act) and self-identity (i.e. being the type of person to perform a behaviour and importance of this role to one's self-concept) appear promising (e.g., Godin, et al., 2008; Hyde & White, 2009c). For instance, although being an organ donor is not a repeated behaviour like blood donation (Piliavin, 1992), it is possible that people have an organ donor identity and communicating donation wishes can confirm and strengthen this identity (Hyde & White, 2009c). In turn having a donor identity may encourage open communication about donation.

DISCUSSION

Limitations of the Research

The approaches to understand communication of donation wishes reviewed thus far have done much to encourage rigour and consistency in the research. These approaches, however, are not without their limitations. Two broader limitations are worth noting. First, there is a need for the consistent application of social-cognitive theories in studies which measure all core constructs and observe specifications of social-cognitive models, and use measures that are standard and empirically validated. Without this consistency it is difficult to make comparisons across studies and identify key predictors that could be used to develop interventions to increase communication of donation wishes. Second, in the literature there is a disproportionate focus on registering or signing as opposed to family discussion. Discussed below are four key aspects where there is scope for consideration: consistency and compatibility in measurement; the assumption that decisions to communicate donation wishes are reasoned or rational, the intention-behaviour relationship, and the potential for other variables not tested to impact on communication decisions.

Consistency and Compatibility in Measurement

Two main measurement limitations were identified. First, definitions of communicators and non-communicators lack consistency. For instance, some studies use the designation of 'donor' to refer to people who have previously registered or signed a donor card. Others use 'donor' to represent a person's willingness for or positive attitude towards donating upon death. Further, due to low rates of behaviour in some studies, people who are willing to register or sign have been combined in a single category with those who have actually registered or signed. Conceptually, willingness or intention and behaviour are different and although a person may be willing to communicate donation wishes, this does not mean that their willingness will translate to communication behaviour (Radecki & Jaccard, 1997, 1999).

Second, there is wide variation in measurement of attitudes and the weak correspondence in attitude-behaviour measures is problematic. Meta-analyses (Kraus, 1995) and extensive social and health psychology research demonstrate the importance of increasing the compatibility between attitude and behaviour measures. When both measures conform to the same level of specificity in terms of an identified target, a given action, a specific context, and a particular time (Ajzen, 1991), a stronger correlation results. Despite this research, most studies use measures of people's general attitudes towards organ donation, rather than attitudes toward communicating donation wishes specifically, to predict communication intentions and behaviour. It follows then that a weak attitude-behaviour relationship would result; a limitation which has only recently begun to receive attention.

Decisions to Communicate Donation Wishes – Reasoned or Reactive?

One assumption common to social-cognitive theories is that individuals adopt a rational, reasoned, or planned approach (e.g., by weighting up costs and benefits) to decision-making based on their attitudes, perceived normative pressure, control perceptions (theory of planned behaviour only), and intentions to communicate donation wishes (Conner & Norman, 2005). This reasoned decision-making process may be accurate for some people who make deliberate plans to communicate donation wishes; however, other people's decisions may be more reactive in nature and dependent on external cues (e.g., a family member sharing their donation wishes, a TV program with an organ donation segment) or circumstances (e.g., renewing the driver's license, knowing a friend or family member needs an organ transplant) (Hyde & White, 2010a). Furthermore, if a person feels uncertain about how others will react or does not feel equipped to answer questions or defend their decision (Breitkopf, 2006), they may wait to share their donation wishes until another person initiates a conversation or expresses a favourable opinion about organ donation. On this basis, there is the potential for communicating donation wishes to involve a more reactive decision-making process.

Hyde and White (2010a) tested this possibility using an augmented theory of planned behaviour and Prototype/Willingness Model (Gibbons, Gerrard, Blanton, & Russell, 1998) to represent the reasoned and reactive elements of decision-making. In the reactive pathway, rather than forming an intention for behaviour, a person may instead be willing to consider behaviour. In other words, they are open to the possibility of behavioural performance if the opportunity arises although they have formed no concrete plans to do so. Results showed that although people's decisions to communicate donation wishes may be better explained via a reasoned pathway based on model fit indices (especially registering), family discussion involved more reactive elements based on adequate model fit for the prototype/willingness model. A test of three interventions (a motivational intervention based on the theory of planned behaviour, a volitional intervention based on the Health Action Process Approach [Schwarzer, 2008], and a combined motivational and volitional intervention) to increase communication of donation wishes provided further support for this finding (Hyde & White, 2013). Participants exposed to the combined motivational and volitional intervention registered at significantly higher rates than participants in other conditions. There was no effect for any intervention on family discussion, indicating an approach that is something other than reasoned or rational is needed. In particular, almost half of the participants who engaged in family discussion used an external cue (e.g., TV advertisement) instead of their own internal resources as a way to start conversation. Recognising and exploring the reactive elements of communicating donation wishes warrants further research attention (Hyde & White, 2013).

Translating Intentions to Communicate Donation Wishes into Behaviour

Another assumption of social-cognitive and organ donation models is that a person's intention or willingness precedes their behaviour (Ajzen, 1991). In reviewing existing empirically-based studies using a social-cognitive theoretical framework (Table 4) it is evident there are few tests of the relationship between intention and behaviour for registering or family discussion. Of these studies, intention explains less than half the total variance in behaviour suggesting that, although important, intentions are not sufficient to explain behaviour. This may particularly be the case in situations where barriers such as anticipating (e.g., having to justify donation wishes) or encountering difficulty (e.g., a difference in opinion or being unable to answer a question), forgetfulness, or a lack of motivation (Hyde & White, 2007) prevent an individual from communicating donation wishes. In addition to further tests of the intention-behaviour relationship, an examination of variables which create links in memory between the behaviour and specific contextual cues to ensure a person recognises and responds to an opportunity to act is needed (Schwarzer, 2008). These post-volitional variables, such as implementation intentions or planning, can be included within predictive social-cognitive models or as part of interventions to increase communication of donation wishes.

For example, encouraging individuals to form action and coping plans detailing when, where, and how they will communicate donation wishes, in combination with a motivational intervention based on the theory of planned behaviour, may be effective in translating intentions to register into registration behaviour (Hyde & White, 2013). To further strengthen the likelihood that once prompted to do so people will communicate donation wishes, Siegel and colleagues highlight the importance of providing an immediate opportunity for the individual to act on their plans or intentions (Alvaro, Siegel, & Jones, 2011; Siegel et al., 2010). They demonstrated that those individuals given an immediate and complete registration opportunity and who were also aware of this opportunity registered at significantly higher rates (Alvaro, et al., 2011; see also Siegel and colleagues' chapter on the 'immediate opportunity, information, focused engagement, and favorable activation' model in this volume).

Other Influences Contributing to Communication of Donation Wishes

As with behaviour, there remains a large proportion of the total variance in intentions left unexplained by the constructs of social-cognitive models (Table 4), suggesting that other personal or social variables may inform decisions to communicate donation wishes. These influences, many of which are beyond the scope of this chapter, include but are not limited to: anticipated affect (van den Berg, Manstead, van der Pligt, & Wigboldus, 2005), death anxiety

(Wu, 2008), personality traits (Baluch, et al., 2001), descriptive or group norm (Park & Smith, 2007), attitudes towards organ donors and transplant recipients (Hyde & White, 2009; 2010b), 'non-cognitive' variables (Morgan, et al., 2008), and anticipated regret (O'Carroll, Foster, et al., 2011). With the exception of the latter two variables, there has been little inclusion of these potential influences in social-cognitive models to date.

'Non-cognitive' variables as conceptualised by the authors of the organ donation model (Morgan, et al., 2008) reflect visceral or emotional influences that may not be represented in more cognitive assessments of the benefits or barriers of donation and communication of donation wishes. Non-cognitive variables comprise the 'ick' factor (e.g., organ donation as disgusting), 'jinx' factor (e.g., tempting fate if donation wishes are communicated), body integrity (e.g., needing a whole body for burial), and medical mistrust (e.g., medical procedures performed without consent). One study has shown these 'non-cognitive' variables to have a direct impact on donor card signing; however, these variables are more often represented in the literature as misconceptions or myths about organ donation (Hyde, Wihardjo, & White, 2012) rather than as direct influences on decisions to communicate donation wishes.

Similarly, in response to criticisms of some social-cognitive theories (e.g., theory of planned behaviour) as less able to explain emotional or affective reactions in decision-making, some researchers (e.g., Godin, et al., 2008; O'Carroll, Dryden, Hamilton-Barclay, & Ferguson, 2011; O'Carroll, Foster, et al., 2011) have tested the impact of anticipated regret (i.e. feelings of regret due to action or inaction in a real or imagined situation) on decisions to register donation wishes. Anticipated regret toward not providing signed consent for donation moderated the relationship between intentions to sign and signing behaviour. This relationship, however, was in the opposite direction to that expected with people reporting higher levels of anticipated regret less likely to sign (although this finding was determined to be due to the behaviour of low intenders who were less likely to sign) (Godin, et al., 2008). Asking people whether they would regret not registering has also increased registering intentions (O'Carroll, Foster, et al., 2011) and behaviour (O'Carroll, Dryden, et al., 2011). More systematic exploration and further clarification of the impact of 'non-cognitive' variables and anticipated regret on registering and family discussion is one possible avenue for future research.

Recommendations - Where to From Here?

In reviewing the literature on communicating donation wishes published in the last 40 years, it is clear that there has been continuous development in the field. The research has progressed from an examination of individual characteristics associated with communicating donation wishes, to the development of organ donation models and adaptations of social-cognitive theories to understand decision-making about communicating donation wishes, and more recently the creation of interventions and communication campaigns (e.g., Feeley & Moon, 2009). At the same time, there has been a shift from a sole focus on signing donor registries or cards to one that increasingly includes family discussion about donation; likely corresponding to recognition of the importance of sharing donation wishes with family to increase consent for donation. Together, with limitations of the research in mind, the accumulated evidence across socio-demographics, beliefs, and social-cognitive factors shows several consistent predictors for both registering and discussing intentions (e.g., attitudes towards communicating donation wishes) and behaviour (e.g., intention) as well as some differences (e.g., knowledge as a predictor for registering behaviour only). These consistencies and differences in findings are displayed in Figure 1. Further to this, and to conclude, some key recommendations for future research avenues based on this overview are offered below.

CONCLUSION

First, the most critical need in the research is to focus on behaviour. This focus should include systematic tests of the relationship between intentions or willingness and behaviour as well as the capacity for post-volitional variables identified in other health domains (e.g., planning, implementation intentions, and anticipated regret) to support conversion of strong intentions to behaviour. Further, a more concerted effort is needed to develop interventions and experimental paradigms to increase understanding and actual communication of donation wishes if registering and discussing are to become behaviours that people routinely perform.

Second, a greater exploration of the emotional or affective reactions to communicating donation wishes is needed to understand how these variables operate within established social-cognitive models when all constructs are measured. Also, the non-reasoned aspects of decision-making (e.g., behaviour that is not planned but occurs in response to external cues), especially for family discussion, warrants further examination. Decision-making models that include both reasoned and reactive decision-making pathways (e.g., an augmented theory of planned behaviour and prototype/willingness model) may be useful in this respect.

Third, currently there is a greater focus on decisions to register or sign donor cards as compared to family discussion. Also, few studies consider both behaviours together to compare similarities and differences in decision-making pathways. Since both behaviours are recommended to maximise family consent, and in some models such as the organ donation model, donor card signing is proposed to inform discussion, it is crucial that future research addresses this gap.

A fourth and related point regards the conceptualisation of family discussion. If family discussion is conceptualised as a conversation, then in addition to acknowledging the spontaneous nature of conversations, people may also need greater encouragement to prepare for a conversation, practice it beforehand, and identify strategies to cope with conflict once a discussion has started or to overcome barriers to beginning an actual conversation. Including concrete strategies to start and maintain a conversation about donation wishes in persuasive message appeals or interventions may be useful options to explore. In some studies, participants simply told family their wishes and did not engage in discussion; a viable alternative may instead be to conceptualise family discussion as family notification. Specifically, letting family know by whatever means comfortable (e.g., social media, phone) may help reduce fear and pressure which prevent family discussion. Without empirical tests of these propositions, however, they remain purely speculative.

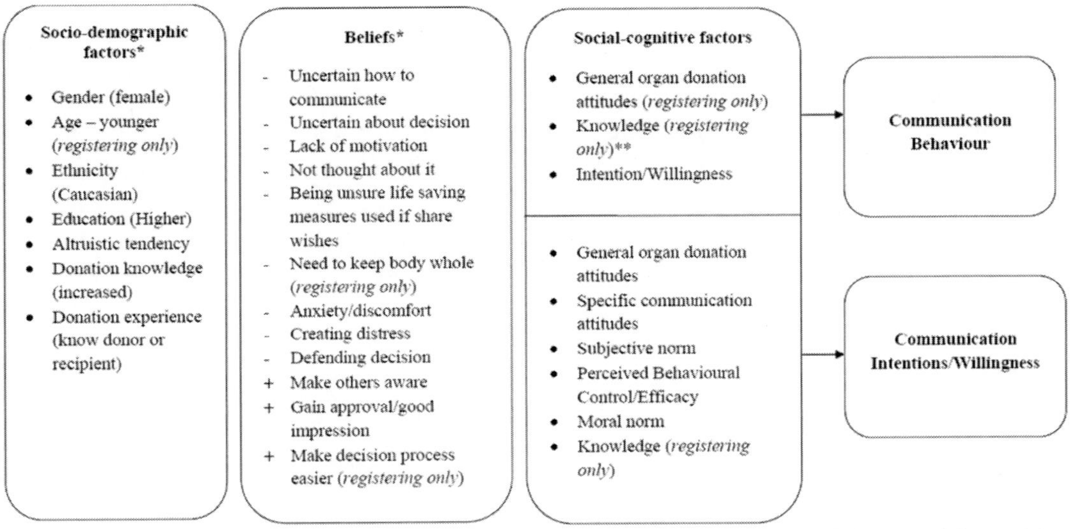

- denotes a barrier or negative belief, + denotes a motivator or positive belief; * In social-cognitive models such as the TRA/TPB, socio-demographic factors are proposed to be background factors captured by social-cognitive variables; beliefs are proposed to inform attitude, subjective norm, and perceived behavioural control. ** Knowledge is considered to be a background factor in the TRA/TPB.

Figure 1. Socio-demographics, beliefs, and social-cognitive factors consistently associated with communicating donation wishes.

Finally, and most importantly, the emphasis in the field has been on individual decision-making to communicate donation wishes when in reality consent for donation is not solely an individual decision. Regardless of the consent system in place, family more often than not have the final say or are involved in the process. Also, much of the research on family discussion identifies family objection to donation, family reaction to discussing death or donation, or fear of having to justify or defend donation wishes as barriers to donation conversations. Consistent with a family systems perspective, these findings suggest that family beliefs and values as well as prescriptions about the way in which particular family members act and the roles they fulfil can contribute to individual behaviour (Fingerman & Bermann, 2000). Recent work in communicating cancer risk also points to the usefulness of a family systems approach in exploring the relationship between family organisation and structure, shared family beliefs and values, and family communication (e.g., Harris et al., 2010). It follows that a critical next step and key future research focus is to bring family back into the decision-making equation so that we may understand how family and individual factors work together to inform decisions to communicate organ donation wishes.

ACKNOWLEDGMENTS

A sincere thank you to Suzanne Chambers for the support, encouragement, and helpful feedback. I also thank the editor for the opportunity and colleagues who provided suggestions and comments.

References

Afifi, W. A., Morgan, S. E., Stephenson, M. T., Morse, C., Harrison, T. R., Reichert, T. & Long, S. D. (2006). Examining the decision to talk with family about organ donation: Applying the theory of motivated information management. *Communication Monographs*, *73*(2), 188-215.

Ajzen, I. (1991). Theory of planned behavior. *Organizational Behavior and Human Decision Processes*, *50*, 179-211.

Alvaro, E. M., Jones, S. P., Robles, A. S. M. & Siegel, J. T. (2005). Predictors of organ donation behavior among Hispanic Americans. *Progress in Transplantation*, *15*(2), 149-156.

Alvaro, E. M., Siegel, J. T. & Jones, S. P. (2011). Increasing organ donor registration rates by providing an immediate and complete registration opportunity: An experimental assessment of the IFF model. *Psychology, Health & Medicine*, *16*(6), 686-694.

Amir, M. & Haskell, E. (1997). Organ donation: Who is not willing to commit? Psychological factors influencing the individual's decision to commit to organ donation after death. *International Journal of Behavioral Medicine*, *4*(3), 215-229.

Ashkenazi, T., Guttman, N. & Hornik, J. (2005). Signing on the dotted line. *Marketing Health Services*, *Summer*, 19-24.

Baluch, B., Randhawa, G., Holmes, S. L. & Duffy, L. J. (2001). Signing the organ donor card: The relationship between expressed attitude, the actual behavior, and personality traits. *The Journal of Social Psychology*, *141*(1), 124-126.

Baughn, D., Rodrigue, J. R. & Cornell, D. L. (2006). Intention to register as organ donors: A survey of adolescents. *Progress in Transplantation*, *16*(3), 260-267.

Besser, A., Amir, M. & Barkan, S. (2004). Who signs an organ transplant donor card? A study of personality and individual differences in a sample of Israeli university students. *Personality and Individual Differences*, *36*, 1709-1723.

Breitkopf, C. R. (2006). Perceived consequences of communicating organ donation wishes: An analysis of beliefs about defending one's decision. *Psychology and Health*, *21*(4), 481-497.

Bresnahan, M., Lee, S. Y., Smith, S. W., Shearman, S., Nebashi, R., Park, C. Y. & Yoo, J. (2007). A theory of planned behavior study of college students' intention to register as organ donors in Japan, Korea, and the United States. *Health Communication*, *21*(3), 201-211.

Brug, J., Van Vugt, M., van den Borne, B., Brouwers, A. & van Hooff, H. (2000). Predictors of willingness to register as an organ donor among dutch adolescents. *Psychology and Health*, *15*, 357-368.

Campbell Research & Consulting. (2006). Community perceptions on organ and tissue donation for transplantation. Victoria, Australia.

Conner, M. & Norman, P. (2005). *Predicting health behaviour: Research and practice with social cognition models.* (2nd ed.). Maidenhead, Berkshire: Open University Press.

Dixon-Woods, M., Agarwal, S., Jones, D., Young, B. & Sutton, A. (2005). Synthesising qualitative and quantitative evidence: a review of possible methods. *Journal of Health Services Research & Policy*, *10*, 45-53.

DonateLife. (2012). Facts and Statistics. Retrieved 16th March, 2012, from http://www.donatelife.gov.au/Discover/Facts-and-Statistics.html

Downing, K. & Jones, L. L. (2008). Designing an educational strategy for increasing organ donor registration among older adults. *Progress in Transplantation*, *18*(4), 290-296.

Feeley, T. H. & Moon, S. I. (2009). A meta-analytic review of communication campaigns to promote organ donation. *Communication Reports*, *22*(2), 63-73. doi: 10.1080/08934210903258852

Feeley, T. H. & Servoss, T. J. (2005). Examining college students' intentions to become organ donors. *Journal of Health Communication*, *10*, 237-249.

Fingerman, K. L. & Bermann, E. (2000). Applications of family systems theory to the study of adulthood. *International Journal of Aging and Human Development*, *51*, 5-29.

Fishbein, M. & Ajzen, I. (1975). *Belief, attitude, intention and behavior: An introduction to theory and research*. Reading, MA.: Addison-Wesley.

Gibbons, F. X., Gerrard, M., Blanton, H. & Russell, D. W. (1998). Reasoned action and social reaction: Willingness and intention as independent predictors of health risk. *Journal of Personality and Social Psychology*, *74*, 1164-1180.

Godin, G., Belanger-Gravel, A., Gagne, C. & Blondeau, D. (2008). Factors predictive of signed consent for posthumous organ donation. *Progress in Transplantation*, *18*(2), 109-117.

Guadagnoli, E., Christiansen, C. L., DeJong, W., McNamara, P., Beasley, C., Christiansen, E. & Evanisko, M. (1999). The public's willingness to discuss their preference for organ donation with family members. *Clinical Transplantation*, *13*, 342-348.

Hardie, I., Conomos, M., Higgins, C. & Smithurst, B. (1992). Attitudes of drivers towards organ donation. *Transplantation Proceedings*, *24*(1), 180.

Harris, J. N., Hay, J., Kuniyuki, A., Asgari, M. M., Press, N. & Bowen, D. J. (2010). Using a family systems approach to investigate cancer risk communication within melanoma families. *Psycho-Oncology*, *19*, 1102-1111.

Haustein, S. V. & Sellers, M. T. (2004). Factors associated with (un)willingness to be an organ donor: Importance of public exposure and knowledge. *Clinical Transplantation*, *18*, 193-200.

Horton, R. L. & Horton, P. J. (1990). Knowledge regarding organ donation: Identifying and overcoming barriers to organ donation. *Social Science & Medicine*, *31*, 791-800.

Horton, R. L. & Horton, P. J. (1991). A model of willingness to become a potential organ donor. *Social Science & Medicine*, *33*(9), 1037-1051.

Hubner, G. & Kaiser, F. G. (2006). The moderating role of subjective norms conflict on the link between moral norms and intention. *European Psychologist*, *11*(2), 99-109.

Hyde, M. K. & White, K. M. (2007). Young Australian adults' knowledge and beliefs about organ donation. *Progress in Transplantation*, *17*(3), 220-227.

Hyde, M. K. & White, K. M. (2009a). Communication prompts donation: Exploring the beliefs underlying registration and discussion of the organ donation decision. *British Journal of Health Psychology*, *14*, 423-435.

Hyde, M. K. & White, K. M. (2009b). Disclosing donation decisions: the role of organ donor prototypes in an extended theory of planned behaviour. *Health Education Research*, *24*(6), 1080-1092.

Hyde, M. K. & White, K. M. (2009). Student and community perceptions about organ donors, non-donors, and transplant recipients. *Journal of Community and Applied Social Psychology*, *19*, 125-141.

Hyde, M. K. & White, K. M. (2009c). To be a donor or not to be? Applying an extended theory of planned behavior to predict posthumous organ donation intentions. *Journal of Applied Social Psychology*, *39*(4), 880-900.

Hyde, M. K. & White, K. M. (2010a). Are organ donation communication decisions reasoned or reactive? A test of the utility of an augmented theory of planned behaviour with the prototype/willingness model. *British Journal of Health Psychology*, *15*, 435-442.

Hyde, M. K. & White, K. M. (2010b). Exploring donation decisions: Beliefs and preferences for organ donation in Australia. *Death Studies*, *34*(2), 172-185.

Hyde, M. K. & White, K. M. (2013). A test of three interventions to promote people's communication of their consent for organ donation. *Psychology & Health*, *28*(4), 399-417.

Hyde, M. K., Wihardjo, K. R. & White, K. M. (2012). Do the myths still exist? Revisiting people's negative beliefs about organ donation upon death. *Psychology, Health & Medicine*, *17*(5), 530-541.

Kopfman, J. E. & Smith, S. W. (1996). Understanding the audiences of a health communication campaign: A discriminant analysis of potential organ donors based on intent to donate. *Journal of Applied Communication Research*, *24*, 33-49.

Kraus, S. J. (1995). Attitudes and the prediction of behavior: A meta-analysis of the empirical literature. *Personality and Social Psychology Bulletin*, *21*(1), 58-75.

Minniefield, W. J., Yang, J. & Muti, P. (2001). Differences in attitudes towards organ donation among African Americans and whites in the United States. *Journal of the National Medical Association*, *93*(10), 372-379.

Morgan, S. E. (2004). The power of talk: African Americans' communication with family members about organ donation and its impact on the willingness to donate organs. *Journal of Social and Personal Relationships*, *21*(1), 112-124.

Morgan, S. E. & Miller, J. K. (2001). Beyond the organ donor card: The effect of knowledge, attitudes, and values on willingness to communicate about organ donation to family members. *Health Communication*, *14*(1), 121-134.

Morgan, S. E. & Miller, J. K. (2002). Communicating about gifts of life: The effect of knowledge, attitudes, and altruism on behavior and behavioural intentions regarding organ donation. *Journal of Applied Communication Research*, *30*, 163-178.

Morgan, S. E., Miller, J. K. & Arasaratnam, L. A. (2002). Signing cards, saving lives: An evaluation of the worksite organ donation promotion project. *Communication Monographs*, *69*(3), 253-273.

Morgan, S. E., Miller, J. K. & Arasaratnam, L. A. (2003). Similarities and differences between African Americans' and European Americans' attitudes, knowledge, and willingness to communicate about organ donation. *Journal of Applied Social Psychology*, *33*(4), 639-715.

Morgan, S. E., Stephenson, M. T., Harrison, T. R., Afifi, W. A. & Long, S. D. (2008). Facts versus feelings: How rational is the decision to become an organ donor? *Journal of Health Psychology*, *16*, 644-658.

National Health Service Blood and transplant. Available at: http://www.organdonation.nhs.uk/Last accessed 15th April, 2013.

Newton, J. D., Burney, S., Hay, M. & Ewing, M. T. (2010). A profile of Australian adults who have discussed their posthumous organ donation wishes with family members. *Journal of Health Communication*, *15*, 470-486.

Nijkamp, M. D., Hollestelle, M. L., Zeegers, M. P., van den Borne, B. & Reubsaet, A. (2008). To be(come) or not to be(come) an organ donor, that's the question: A meta-analysis of determinant and intervention studies. *Health Psychology Review*, *2*, 20-40.

Nolan, B. E. & Spanos, N. P. (1989). Psychosocial variables associated with willingness to donate organs. *CMAJ*, *141*(July 1), 27-32.

O'Carroll, R. E., Dryden, J., Hamilton-Barclay, T. & Ferguson, E. (2011). Anticipated regret and organ donor registration: A pilot study. *Health Psychology*, *30*(5), 661-664.

O'Carroll, R. E., Foster, C., McGeechan, G., Sandford, K. & Ferguson, E. (2011). The "ick" factor, anticipated regret, and willingness to become an organ donor. *Health Psychology*, *30*(2), 236-245.

Parisi, N. & Katz, I. (1986). Attitudes toward posthumous organ donation and commitment to donate. *Health Psychology*, *5*(6), 565-580.

Park, H. S. & Smith, S. W. (2007). Distinctiveness and influences of subjective norms, personal descriptive and injunctive norms, and societal descriptive and injunctive norms on behavioral intent: A case of two behaviors critical to organ donation. *Human Communication Research*, *33*, 194-218.

Perkins, K. A. (1987). The shortage of cadaver donor organs for transplantation: Can psychology help? *American Psychologist*, *42*(10), 921-930.

Pham, H. & Spigner, C. (2004). Knowledge and opinions about organ donation and transplantation among Vietnamese Americans in Seattle, Washington: A pilot study. *Clinical Transplantation*, *18*, 707-715.

Piliavin, J. A. (1992). Role identity and organ donation: Some suggestions based on blood-donation research. In J. Shanteau & R. J. Harris (Eds.), *Organ donation and transplantation: Psychological and behavioral factors* (pp. 150-158). Washington, DC.: American Psychological Association.

Radecki, C. M. & Jaccard, J. (1997). Psychological aspects of organ donation: A critical review and synthesis of individual and next-of-kin donation decisions. *Health Psychology*, *16*(2), 183-195.

Radecki, C. M. & Jaccard, J. (1999). Signing an organ donation letter: The prediction of behavior from behavioral intentions. *Journal of Applied Social Psychology*, *29*(9), 1833-1853.

Reubsaet, A., van den Borne, B., Brug, J., Pruyn, J. & van Hooff, H. (2001). Determinants of the intention of Dutch adolescents to register as organ donors. *Social Science & Medicine*, *53*, 383-392.

Rodrigue, J. R., Cornell, D. L., Jackson, S. I., Kanasky, W., Marhefka, S. & Reed, A. I. (2004). Are organ donation atittudes and beliefs, empathy, and life orientation related to donor registration status? *Progress in Transplantation*, *14*(1), 56-60.

Rosenblum, A. M., Horvat, L. D., Siminoff, L. A., Prakash, V., Beitel, J. & Garg, A. X. (2012). The authority of next-of-kin in explicit and presumed consent systems for deceased organ donation: An analysis of 54 nations. *Nephrology Dialysis Transplantation*, *27*(6), 2533-2546.

Rubens, A. J., Oleckno, W. A. & Ciesla, J. R. (1998). Knowledge, attitudes, and behaviors of college students regarding organ/tissue donation and implications for increasing organ/tissue donors. *College Student Journal*, *32*(2), 167-178.

Ryckman, R. M., van den Borne, B., Thornton, B. & Gold, J. A. (2005). Value priorities and organ donation in young adults. *Journal of Applied Social Psychology*, *35*(11), 2421-2435.

Sander, S. L. & Miller, B. K. (2005). Public knowledge and attitudes regarding organ and tissue donation: An analysis of the northwest Ohio community. *Patient Education and Counselling*, *58*, 154-163.

Sanner, M. A. (1998). Giving and taking - to whom and from whom? People's attitudes toward transplantation of organs and tissue from different sources. *Clinical Transplantation*, *12*, 530-537.

Saub, E. J., Shapiro, J. & Radecki, S. (1998). Do patients want to talk to their physicians about organ donation? Attitudes and knowledge about organ donation: A study of orange county, California residents. *Journal of Community Health*, *23*, 407-417.

Schwarzer, R. (2008). Modeling health behavior change: How to predict and modify the adoption and maintenance of health behaviors. *Applied Psychology*, *57*(1), 1-29.

Siegel, J. T., Alvaro, E. M., Crano, W. D., Gonzalez, A. V., Tang, J. C. & Jones, S. P. (2010). Passive-positive organ donor registration behavior: A mixed method assessment of the IIFF model. *Psychology, Health & Medicine*, *15*(2), 198-209.

Siminoff, L. A., Arnold, R. M. & Hewlett, J. (2001). The process of organ donation and its effect on consent. *Clinical Transplantation*, *15*, 39-47.

Simpkin, A., Robertson, L. C., Barber, V. S. & Young, J. D. (2009). Modifiable factors influencing relatives' decision to offer organ donation: Systematic review. *BMJ*, *339*, b991.

Sirois, B. C., Sears, S. F. J. & Marhefka, S. (2005). Do new drivers equal new donors? An examination of factors influencing organ donation attitudes and behaviors in adolescents. *Journal of Behavioral Medicine*, *28*(2), 201-212.

Spigner, C., Weaver, M., Cardenas, V. & Allen, M. D. (2002). Organ donation and transplantation: Ethnic differences in knowledge and opinions among urban high school students. *Ethnicity & Health*, *7*, 87-101.

The Gallup Organization Inc. (2005). 2005 National Survey of Organ and Tissue Donation Attitudes and Behaviors. Washington, DC.: The Gallup Organization.

Thompson, T. L., Robinson, J. D. & Kenny, R. W. (2003). Gender differences in family communication about organ donation. *Sex Roles*, *49*(11/12), 587-596.

TNS Opinion & Social. (2010). *Eurobarometer 72.3: Organ donation and Transplantation*. Brussels, Belgium: TNS Opinion & Social.

United Network for Organ Sharing. Available at http://unos.org. Last accessed 15th April, 2013.

van den Berg, H., Manstead, A. S. R., van der Pligt, J. & Wigboldus, D. H. J. (2005). The role of affect in attitudes toward organ donation and donor-relevant decisions. *Psychology and Health*, *26*(6), 789-802.

Vincent, D. E. (2006). Exploring college students' family discussions about organ and tissue donation. *Communication Research Reports*, *23*(4), 299-308.

Wakefield, C. E., Reid, J. & Homewood, J. (2011). Religious and ethnic influences on willingness to donate organs and donor behaviour: An Australian perspective. *Progress in Transplantation*, *21*(2), 161-168.

Waldrop, D. P., Tamburlin, J. A., Thompson, S. J. & Simon, M. (2004). Life and death decisions: Using school-based health education to facilitate family discussion about organ and tissue donation. *Death Studies*, *2004*(28), 643-657.

Weber, K., Martin, M. M., Corrigan, M. & 160, M. o. C. (2007). Real donors, real consent: Testing the theory of reasoned action on organ donor consent. *Journal of Applied Social Psychology*, *37*(10), 2435-2450.

Weber, K., Martin, M. M. & Members of Comm401. (2006). Gender and consent to organ donation. *The Journal of Social Psychology*, *146*(2), 247-249.

Wu, A. M. S. (2008). Discussion of posthumous organ donation in Chinese families. *Psychology, Health & Medicine*, *13*(1), 48-54.

Wu, A. M. S. & Tang, C. S. (2009). Solving the dilemma: Family communication about organ donation among Chinese, Japanese, and Caucasian American college students. *Journal of Applied Social Psychology*, *39*(7), 1639-1659.

Yeung, I., Kong, S. H. & Lee, J. (2000). Attitudes towards organ donation in Hong Kong. *Social Science & Medicine*, *50*, 1643-1654.

Yuen, C. C., Burton, W., Chiraseveenuprapund, P., Elmore, E., et al. (1998). Attitudes and beliefs about organ donation among different racial groups. *Journal of the National Medical Association*, *90*(1), 13-18.

Yun, D. & Park, H. S. (2010). Culture and the theory of planned behaviour: Organ donation intentions in Americans and Koreans. *Journal of Pacific Rim Psychology*, *4*(2), 130-137. doi: 10.1375/prp.4.2.130

In: Organ Donation and Transplantation
Editor: Mary Anne Lauri
ISBN: 978-1-62948-257-6

Chapter 5

ORGAN DONATION BEHAVIOR: WHY THE SHORTAGE OF ORGANS?

James Shanteau*
Kansas State University, Kansas, US

ABSTRACT

The purpose of this chapter is to describe research conducted as part of a 30-year effort at Kansas State University to understand organ donation behavior. We have incorporated the following perspectives into our studies: Helping Behavior and Altruism, Health Psychology, Cognitive Psychology, Psychology of Religion, Judgment and Decision Making, Social Psychology of Attitude Change, Individual Differences, and Legal Psychology.

This chapter contains an overview of our various research efforts. In addition, one relevant study is presented that explores the impact of prior actions of signing or not-signing organ donor statements on willingness to be a donor. The results of this study revealed that those who are opposed to signing such statements nonetheless are willing to be donors if the organs will benefit immediate family members. Thus, these *"Anti-Donors"* are not so much anti-organ donation as they are anti-stranger.

INTRODUCTION

With one-year success rates approaching 90%, organ transplantation is one of the marvels of modern medicine. The life expectancy of recipients is steadily increasing, with heart and kidney transplant survival rates of over 20 years. Improvements in medical procedures have also increased the types of organs and tissues that can be transplanted. A wide range of diseases and conditions can now be "cured" by organ transplants. Besides heart and kidney, a variety of other organs and tissues can be transplanted, eg, pancreas, liver, bone marrow, corneas, lungs, skin, joints, and blood vessels.

---

* Corresponding author: shanteau@k-state.edu.

One donor can donate up to 30–40 organs and tissues, and potentially save up to a dozen lives. But, there is a major roadblock in the ability to deliver this technology to patients in need. The roadblock is not neither a lack of skilled surgeons nor of competent medical teams; it is not even due to a lack of money in most cases. The roadblock is caused simply by a lack of enough donated organs.

The purpose of this chapter is to describe research conducted as part of a 30-year effort at Kansas State University (K-State) to understand organ donation behavior. When our research program began in 1981, there were 10,000 waiting for kidney transplants in the USA. Today, this number has increased to over 93,000 (OPTN, 2013). "Unless there are significant changes in the number of kidney transplants performed each year, there will soon be over 100,000 people waiting for a kidney transplant and the wait for some will exceed 10 years." (UNOS, 2013). At the same time, over 20,000 die each year under conditions where organ donation is possible. But, less than 1/4 of potential donations actually take place.

Consequences

Potential transplant recipients may wait for years, if they survive, before a suitable donor organ can be found. In addition, the longer the delay, the greater the likelihood of medical complications. Delays also increase the chances of a rejection of a transplanted organ. The recipient must then wait for another organ. Moreover, the cost per transplant is increased because of inefficiencies in the delivery of medical care. Finally, the ability of surgeons and medical teams to improve procedures and survivability is limited because there are too few organs to transplant.

A Psychological Approach to Organ Shortage

Our research program at Kansas State University K-State began with the belief that the answer to the shortage lies in a better understanding of the psychological processes involved. We assumed the reluctance to donate is due not to lack of knowledge, but is due instead to psychological reasons such as unstated motivations, perceived risks, and unarticulated fears. Our research team took an eclectic, broad-based behavioral approach to the problem. We incorporated the following psychological domains into our studies: cognitive psychology, helping behavior and altruism, health psychology, individual differences, judgment and decision making, legal psychology, psychology of religion, and social psychology of attitude change.

The goal of our research was to find reasons for the shortage of donated organs. In our studies, we looked at examined the following possibilities to explain the shortage:

(1) Knowledge of Organ Donation
(2) Attitudes and Opinions
(3) Motivation
(4) Knowledge and Beliefs About "Mystery Organs"

(5) Language of Donation and Transplantation
(6) Confusions About Organ Donor Cards and Urban Legends
(7) Cross-Cultural Differences Between Donors and Recipients
(8) Beliefs of Doctors, Nurses, and Health-Care Workers
(9) Decision Making by Anti-Donors

This chapter will briefly review research from the first eight issues. This will be followed by an extensive discussion of the ninth, since it provided one of our most compelling new insights.

Lack of Knowledge

The reason for the shortage most cited in the medical literature is that lack of knowledge in the general population (Shanteau & Harris, 1990b). Accordingly, considerable effort has been made to increase awareness (and sympathy) of the plight of potential organ recipients (Cantarovich, 2002).

In contrast, surveys have consistently shown that almost everyone is aware of the need for donated organs. In our studies of over 800 residents of Kansas and Ohio, almost 99% reported being aware of the need of donated organs for transplantations (McIntyre et al., 1987; Skowronski, 1987). Our results confirmed the findings of other researchers' surveys across the USA (eg, Manninen & Evans, 1985). Even non-English residents of America are aware of the need, although they are resistant to donating to non-family members (McIntyre, 1990). These studies also revealed that most are sympathetic to the plight of potential recipients. Therefore, the shortage of organs does not appear due to a lack of knowledge or an absence of empathy (Barnett et al., 1987).

Studies conducted by the Midwest Organ Bank (Jane Warmbrodt, Personal Communication, 1986) have concluded that only about 3,000 out of an estimated 23,000 who planned for donation were in fact donatedactually became donors. Even a modest increase in this rate of actual donation would go a long way in solving the shortage, since a single donor can provide 10 or more organs and tissues for transplantation.

The central question, of course, is why are there so few positive decisions to actually donate? One common answer in the medical community is that the public lacks knowledge about the need for donors. Accordingly, effort has been extended repeatedly to increase sympathy for the plight of potential organ transplant recipients.

Recent articles in medical journals continue to cite "lack of knowledge" as a major reason for the shortage (eg, Bean, 2006). Moreover, a just-publishedrecent meta-analysis of 18 studies involving 1,019 participants concluded that "ignorance about the donation process" was a major reason behind the shortage (Irving, et al., 2011, p. 7). Most of the studies, however, were based on focus groups and/or face-to-face interviews; both methods can lead to confirmation bias (Wason, 1960; Klayman & Ha, 1987).

A few years ago, I testified before a legislative committee in Kansas about a proposed law to provide tax incentives to the families of deceased organ donors. Being the first witness, I anticipated that some of the following witnesses would testify against the law because the "real problem" was lack of knowledge of the public. So I refuted that argument by providing data from surveys we conducted in Kansas which showed that 95%+ of residents were aware of the need for donated organs. The very next witness (from the Kansas Red Cross) in her prepared testimony said that the shortage was due to "a lack of knowledge of the need in Kansas." (Afterwards, she admitted totold me that she had no empirical evidence to support her position, but instead presented the traditional medical argument.)

The problem, of course, is that as long as the medical community continues to argue that lack of knowledge is the underlying cause to the shortage, more fruitful lines of inquiry continue tomay be overlooked. Therefore, it is critical to keep reminding those in the transplant community that virtually everyone is already aware of the shortage. The solution to the donor shortage must lie elsewhere.

Attitudes and Opinions

Studies of the social psychology of attitudes and opinions have reported favorable attitudes toward organ donation, but a lower proportion of people who actually sign organ donor cards (Prottas, 1983), with even fewer actually becoming organ donors (Shanteau & Harris, 1990a). This inconsistency between attitudes and behavior suggests underlying psychological sources of resistance to organ donation.

Field studies and observational research have identified several factors as important in attitude change, such as the presence of supportive others (Fulton, Fulton, & Simmons, 1977). The most successful requests for donation tend to provide the needed information sensitively and tactfully, in addition to refuting misconceptions and misinformation about organ donation (Harris et al., 1991).

However, discomfort in thinking about one's own death and even to make plans to buy life insurance are common (Coy, 2005). Avoidance to thinking about our mortality can provide a tremendous strong psychological barrier to signing a donor card. Still, there is obviously a sizeable minority who are able to overcome this discomfort in a positive manner and become organ donors.

Motivation

Organ donation is a particularly interesting example from the perspective of motivation and helping behavior. On the one hand, becoming a living donor (say of a kidney) represents one of the greatest, but potentially risky, examples of helping behavior. On the other hand, signing an organ donor card involves little or no immediate cost/risk, but the donor also never experiences the ultimate benefit.

Other factors are relevant from a motivational perspective. Agreeing as a next-of-kin to donate a loved one's organs is a type of helping behavior necessarily carried out under extreme stress due to time pressure and emotional pain. This act, however, has been reported to be a part of the healing process for many (Harris et al., 1991). Thus, organ donation may provide an activea means for a family to deal with the grief of losing a loved one.

In terms of motivation, most studies report that people's expressed reasons for donating organs are primarily altruistic and other oriented. But we gathered evidence that people respond more positively to a persuasive communication emphasizing benefits to self (it helps you feel better about yourself) than benefits to others (Barnett et al., 1987). Apparently, altruistic motivations are easier to understand, but self-centered reasons are more convincing.

"Mystery Organs"

One curious finding has been the willingness to donate some organs over others. For instance, people likely to donate kidneys and blood remain hesitant to donate their heart and corneas (Fulton, Fulton, & Simmons, 1977). This hesitancy may reflect, at least in part, differences in the image and knowledge of various organs. It may also reflect the importance or meaning attached to these various organs.

To investigate this possibility, we conducted several studies of the relationship between knowledge/andimage of organs and the willingness to donate those organs (Wilms et al., 1987). Participants were asked to identify the location and function of various internal organs, and also to state their willingness to donate these same organs. Results revealed a marginal relationship between knowledge measures and donation willingness. These results did demonstrate, moreover, that many people have surprisingly little knowledge of either the location or the function of their own body parts.

To illustrate the point, several "catch organs" were included in the study. For instance, an Abomassum was listed, although it is actually one of the stomachs found in cows. Roughly one third identified one of their internal organs as being an abomasum and with roughly the same proportion willing to donate theirs. Indeed, participants were willing to donate their (nonexistent) abomasum at about the same level as their (quite real) pancreas.

One curious result was a sizable gender difference, with females much less willing to donate heart and cornea (40% and 42%, respectively) compared to males (80% and 59%, respectively). Yet both genders were equally accurate/inaccurate in identifying the location and function of these organs.

Related research suggests that self-image may be an important moderating variable. Belk and Austin (1986) reported a relation between willing to donate and measures of one's self; the greater an organ is identified with self, the less willing an individual is willing to donate. Similarly, Pessemier, Bemmaor, and Hanssens (1977) found that living donors who placed less importance on body image were more likely to donate.

Language

A major portion of the organ donation bottleneck may lie within in the language used by the medical community itself. Doctors and nurses who have yet to come to an understanding of their own feelings about death and organ donation are unlikely to be effective in dealing with grieving families. Starting a conversation with "I have to ask you about organ donation…" is not likely to be effective in obtaining approval for organ donation.

This discomfort of health-care professionals is reflected by their use of technical terminology and jargon, such as "harvesting for organs," that distances themselves from their own uncertainties (Shanteau & Linin, 1990). Referring to a loved one as being on "life support" likely can makes it more difficult for families to accept the finality of the medical condition.

Unfortunately, such terminology can lead to miscommunication with the families of potential donors. Shanteau and Linin found, for example, that “brain dead” implies a finality of for a patient, whereas “brain death” is suggestive of someone still alive (or perhaps in a coma). , with at least some potential to live. Because the understanding of “brain death” is a vital step in obtaining permission (Hessing & Elffers, 1986), use of the term “brain death” may encourage an incorrect impression and give a false hope of recovery. Our research suggests that “brain dead” should be used instead.

Confusions and Urban Legends

Snopes.com, a website for debunking urban legends, describes nine such legends involving organ donation (as of March, 2013). These range from “Doctors let die those patients who’ve indicated they’ll donate their organs” at number one, to “Children abducted from stores and amusement parks … to be used as unwilling organ donors” at number nine. Probably the most (in)famous urban legend is number four: “Unwary travellers drugged as unwilling kidney donors by bands of organ thieves.”

Most of these urban legends are outrageous at first glance, eg, Harvard Medical School “pays thousands of dollars for the donation of a testicle” (number seven). As such, they are likely to elicit a chuckle or two. However, some of these legends have had grave, even deadly consequences. One example, is “June Weinstock, 51, a journalist from Fairbanks, Alaska, (who) suffered extensive injuries when a mob beat her with machetes, clubs, and metal pipes…in northeastern Guatemala…. Rumors of Americans stealing children – either to adopt or, in the more fantastic versions, to harvest their organs for transplants – have long circulated in Guatemala and other Latin American nations” (Orlebar, 1994). Weinstock remains critically impaired (Emery, 2013). (As a gruesome footnote, Campion-Vincent (2005) reported that a videotape of the Weinstock attack was widely circulated in both Guatemala and Miami.)

The author was told about an urban rumor in Australia that circulated 10 years ago that a deceased donor moved his hand just as his heart was being removed, as if trying to stop the removal. This rumor dried upreduced organ donation in Australia for many months resulting in an inestimable number of deaths to those waiting for transplants (Alex Wearing, Personal Communication, 2003).

When we first began our research on organ donation 25 years ago, little attention was paid to these word-of-mouth rumors. But as the stories above illustrate, these urban legends can have had damaging consequences. As a result, written information supporting organ donation now routinely dispels rumors and legends (eg, see Mayo Clinic, 2010). What has yet to be investigated, however, is how effective these truth-telling efforts are, given that those most likely to believe these rumors are also unlikely to check out websites such as the Mayo Clinic (Emery, 2013).

Cross-Cultural Differences

Gaining cross-national and cross-cultural insights is obviously vital. Ways to facilitate organ donation are being explored by different societies. Unfortunately, there is not enough information being shared of experiences elsewhere. For example, legal changes in presumed consent laws, such as instituting required-request or opting-out procedures, have had uneven results in various European countries (Hessing, 1990). Others have argued that opt-in (explicit consent) countries have higher lower rates of donation than opt-out (presumed consent) countries (Johnson & Goldstein, 2004).

Similarly, cultural differences within the USA produce different views about donation, eg, Cleveland (1975) reported 20% of Blacks support organ donation compared to 67% of the general population. Moreover, Prottas (1983) found that the Black donation rate was negligible, not over 1%. But, there has been surprisingly little research on the sources of these ethnic differences (for an exception, see McIntyre's (1990) analysis of the views of Hispanics).

Beliefs of Health Care Workers

At a 1998 conference at Kansas State University, "Psychological Research on Organ Donation," 25 investigators with different academic and professional backgrounds concluded that a major portion of the donation bottleneck lies within the medical community (Harris & Shanteau, 1990). While the tendency of these professionals is to "blame the public" for lack of knowledge about the shortage (see the discussion above), these same professionals may, in fact, be distancing themselves from their own uncertainties regarding organ donation and transplantation.

Recent studies suggest that health professionals share many of the same views as the general public concerning, for example, the part that financial incentives might play in organ donation (Barnieh et al., 2012). Moreover, it appears that medical education has minimal impact on these views (Tontus, Karabey, & Gurdal, 2011). This study also found that medical students were more willing to donate their own organs than those of a deceased relative by a 10:1 ratio (40% to 4%). If that is representative of the personal views of medical professionals, there is little wonder that these same professionals are often unsuccessful in convincing families to approve donation of a loved-one's organs.

One issue that affects the general population and medical professionals alike is religious concernsbeliefs. As Oliver et al. (2010) note, few if any patient families come forward about their religious concerns. Consequently, "health professionals may wish to avoid this sensitive issue altogether (because of) lack knowledge of religious issues pertaining to transplantation (p. 1)." In our research efforts, we consulted with a minister/graduate student who after checking numerous written and personal sources concluded that no major world religion has a ban on organ donation, although many religions have specific concerns about handling of bodies after death (Rev. Michael Klassen, personal communication, 1987).

Research on Anti-Donors

It is rare that one figure or one table can tell a compelling story that can impact social policy. In our effort to evaluate those we called "anti donors," we had such an experience (Shanteau & Skowronski, 2013). The One purpose of this research effort was to investigate the decision strategies of those most opposed to donating organs. Information integration theory (IIT) developed by Anderson (1981) was used to determine how various pieces of information combine to form donation likelihood judgments. Using this paradigm, Skowronski and Shanteau (1990) evaluated willingness-to-donate organs as a function of:

- Whether the donor is living or deceased
- The relation of recipient to donor
- What organ /tissue is to be donated
- Prior commitment of subject participants to be a donor

Two studies were conducted which will be summarized before describing the key result.

Experiment 1

137 undergraduates at Kansas State University completed a questionnaire that contained an IIT analysis of willingness to donate under various conditions. (For a description of other results from this study, see McIntyre et al., 1987). Students were felt to be appropriate for donation research because (1) the age of their organs is ideal for transplantation, (2) they are more likely to engage in risky activities, and (3) they may called up on to make donation decisions for themselves, for parents, or for children.

Two factorial designs were used. The first was a 4 x 4, organ-to-donate x relationship, while-living design and the second was an 11 x 2, organ-to-donate x relationship, after-death design. These designs were used to describe possible organ donation under varying conditions, eg, . For instance, participants were asked to evaluate “Donate Kidney to Stranger, While Living.” The instructions read: “Indicate your willingness (to donate) by using the following scale:”

0	1	2	3	4	5	6	7	8	9	10
Highly unwilling to donate					Neutral					Highly willing to donate

In groups of 20 to 25, each participant judged every stimulus combination once. (Note: in most IIT studies, participants are run individually with several replications of the stimulus materials.)

Results. The results were quite orderly in that participants followed systematic decision strategies. Thus, the use of group data-collection procedures did not impact the ability to conduct IIT analyses of organ donation intentions.

The Living Donation results revealed: (a) relatively small differences across organ type, with (b) greater willingness to donate to relatives or friends as opposed to strangers. The Deceased Donation results showed: (c) about 20% higher rates for relative donation compared to stranger donation, and (d) greater willingness to donate organs listed separately compared to donating “All Organs.” The comparison of living and deceased donation showed: (e) increased likelihood of donating to relatives while living, but (f) greater willingness to donate to strangers after death.

Based on the success ofAs a follow-up to Experiment 1, a second study was conducted. In addition to the variables included in the first study, participants were asked how willing they were towhether they had signed their driver's license to give approval for organ donation.

Experiment 2

A larger and somewhat older sample of subjects was used; 243 night-school students at Ohio State University were separated into four groups: (1) Signed-Donors, who had already signed a donor card (n = 53, 22%); (2) Favorable-to-Sign, who are willing to signed if asked (n = 51, 21%); (3) Uncertain-About-Signing, whose minds are not yet made up (n = 113, 46%); and (4) Anti-Donors, who had decided not to sign (n = 26, 11%). The procedure and stimulus materials were identical to first experiment, except that a different experimenter conducted the study.

Results. Despite differences of when and where the two studies were conducted, the findings were quite similar. For instance, "willingness-to-donate kidneys to strangers while living" averaged just over 4 on the 10-point scale in Experiment 1 and just under 4 in Experiment 2. Similarly, "willingness-to-donate kidneys to relatives while living" was slightly greater than 9 in Experiment 1 and averaged a little less than 9 in Experiment 2.

Analysis of "willingness-to-donatedonation while living" across all groups indicates: (a) consistently high willingness-to-donate to family relatives (son/daughter or brother/sister), and (b) relatively little difference in donation rates across organ or tissue type. As shown in Figure 1, analysis of living donation for the 4 groups revealed: (c) clear differences between groups, especially for donating to strangers, and (d) high willingness across groups to donate organs/tissues to relatives.

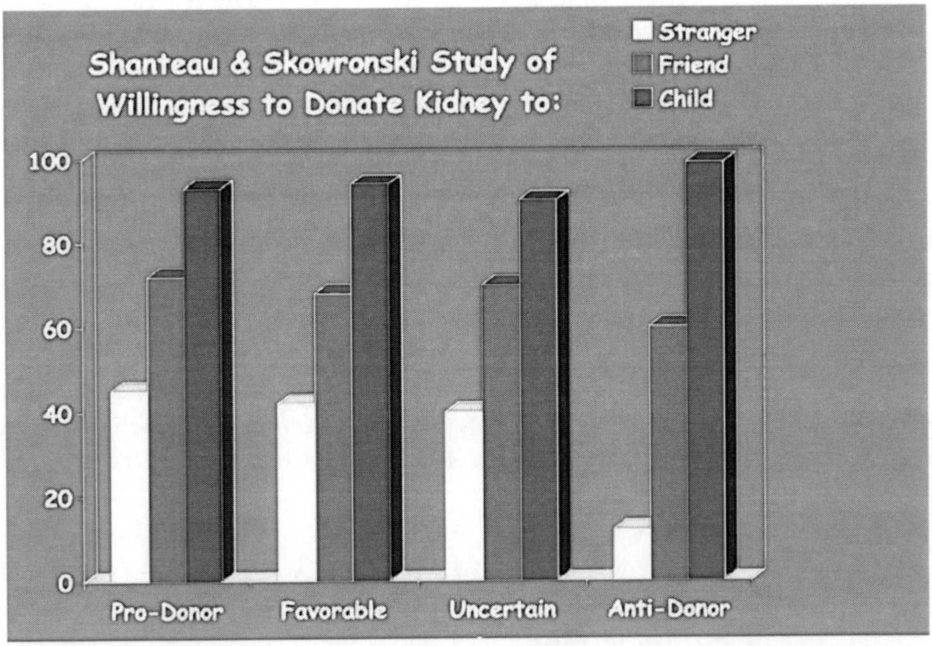

Figure 1. Chart of willingness to be a living kidney donor to stranger, friend, or child for 4 groups, where groups defined by views toward signing or not signing organ-donor card.

Discussion. The results revealed a *"cognitive algebra"* underlying organ donation, that is, there are were consistent, explainable patterns. One important result was a greater willingness to donate to relatives while living and to strangers after death. There are at least two possible explanations: (a) the benefits of living donation can be shared, or (b) living donors don't think, they just react.

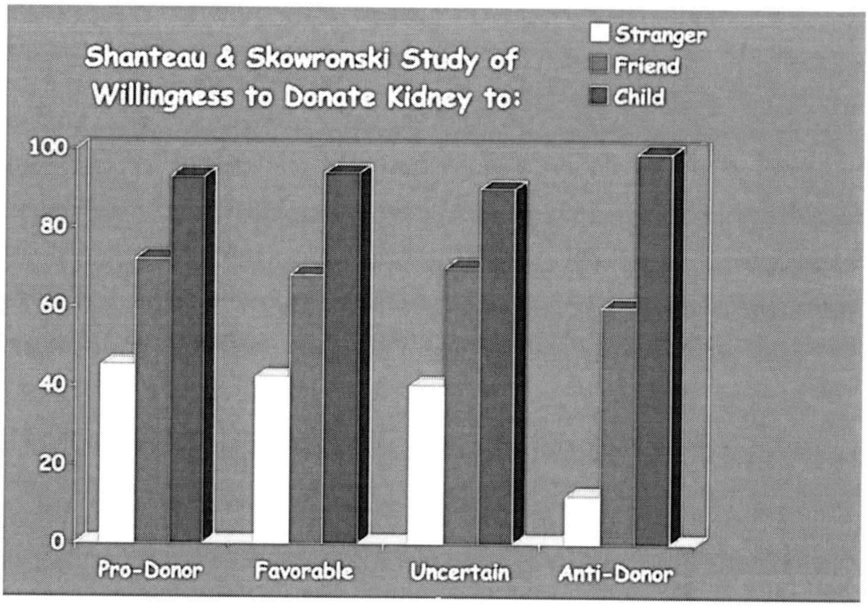

Figure 1.

Interestingly, request for All Organs was treated less favorably than a request for each organ individually. This may reflect either a lack of knowledge of what constitutes "All Organs," or a preference to have more control over the organ donation process.

Signed donors were quite likely to donate to relatives and fairly likely to donate to friends and strangers. Apparently, donors they are comfortable with death and the idea of donating body organsparts. Other groups were equally willing to donate to relatives, but less likely to donate to strangers.

The anti-donors group is that which is of most interest. Figure 1 reveals that they are probably misnamed. They are not anti-donation, but rather anti-stranger. Therefore, one approach to increasing donation rates would be to broaden the class of those considered to be *"family."* The goal would be to reduce the perceived distance between insiders and outsiders of one's family. Possible appeals might state that the lives saved through donation could be those of your friends and neighbors, i.e., . Specifically, *"organ donation can save the life of someone just like yourself."*

CONCLUSION

The studies summarized here have at least five implications for research on organ donation behavior. First, attempts to educate or persuade consumers to increase organ donation are unlikely to succeed, unless more is known about the psychological issues involved. Simply repeating the mantra of *"educate consumers"* is not going to change rates of donation until the psychological reasons for resistance are addressed. Second, despite all that is not known about organ donor behavior, people are not random or unpredictable in their decisions about organ donation. As can be seen in Figure 1, clear patterns of behavior emerge. Third, few people are opposed to donations under all circumstances; almost everyone is willing to donate…if the circumstances are right. Thus, fears of upsetting people by raising the topic of donation appear unfounded. Fourth, there are definable differences between people in their willingness to donate. These differences are analyzable and reveal systematic trends. This suggests that market segmentation might be a useful approach to increasing organ donation. Finally, fifth, the IIT approach (Anderson, 1981) provided useful new insights into organ donation decisions. Despite less than optimal data-collection methods, IIT revealed clear behavioral trends, especially in regards to the behavior of so-called anti-donors.

We can make several suggestions based on our other lines of research, as well as the work of others. At least three recommendations seem noteworthy:

(i) Because of continuing frustration by doctors and patients over the organ shortage, efforts have been made to change the laws regarding requests for donation. Most states in the USA, including Kansas, instituted *"required request"* laws; patients entering hospitals must be asked about donation. However, research by Prottas and Batten (1988) suggests that medical professionals are often reluctant to make requests for organs, despite the law.

(ii) A related finding is that doctors and nurses frequently have difficulty with their own personal feelings about death and how to deal with the family of the deceased (Carroll, 2005). Medical workers also have difficulty defining brain death, both to themselves and to others. Not surprisingly, therefore, there is considerable confusion among consumers about the terminology of organ donation/transplantation, for example, what is meant by "brain death" (Shanteau & Linin, 1991).

(iii) There are numerous rumors and urban legends surrounding organ donation and transplantation that raise doubts in people's minds about the appropriateness of being a donor. Rather than ignoring such rumors, we recommend addressing them directly in communications with consumers, eg, see the responses provided at Snopes.com.

ACKNOWLEDGMENTS

The research described in this chapter was supported, in part, by grants from the American Psychological Association, the U.S. Department of Health and Human Services, the Bureau of General Research at Kansas State University, and the Office of Research and Sponsored Programs at K-State. Preparation of this chapter was supported by an award from the Division of Organ Transplantation in DHHS.

I wish to thank Mark Barnett, Richard Harris, J. D. Jasper, Stephen Kiefer, Jim Springer, Jane Warmbrodt, and especially Patricia McIntyre and John Skowronski for their insightful comments and helpful suggestions. I should also recognize the inspiration provided by Vinod Thukral to start the Kansas State University Organ Donation Laboratory.

Further information on the research described here can be obtained by contacting: James Shanteau, Department of Psychology, Bluemont Hall 492, Kansas State University, Manhattan, Kansas, 66506-5302 USA.

REFERENCES

Anderson, N. H. (1981). *Foundations of information integration theory*. NY: Academic Press.

Barnieh, L., Klarenbach, S. Gill, J. S., Caulfield, T. & Mannis, B. (2012). Attitudes toward strategies to increase organ donation: Vies of the general public and health professionals. *Clinical Journal of the American Society of Nephrology*, 12(Dec), 1956-63.

Barnett, M. A., Klassen, M., McMinimy, V., & Schwarz, L. (1987). *The role of self- and other-oriented motivation in the organ donation decision*. In M. Wallendorf & P. Anderson (Eds.), Advances in Consumer Research. Provo, UT: Association for Consumer Research.

Bean, K. B. (2006). Crisis in American organ donation. *Gastroenterology Nursing*, *29*(2), 97-181.

Belk, R. W. & Austin, M. C. (1986). *Organ donation willingness as a function of extended self and materialism*. In M. Ven Venkatesen (Ed.), Association for Health Care Research.

Campion-Vincent, V. (2005). *Organ theft legends*. (Translated by J. Simpson). Jackson: University Press of Mississippi.

Cantarovich, F. (2002). Improvement in organ shortage through education. *Transplantation*, *73*, 1844.

Carroll, K. A. (2005). Does how we ask for organs determine whether people decide to donate? *American Medical Association Journal of Ethics*, *7*, Number 6.

Cleveland, S. (1975). Personality characteristics, body image and social attitudes of organ transplant donors versus non-donors. *Psychosomatic Medicine*, *37*(July-August), 313-319.

Cohen, E. L. (2007). *My loss is your gain: Examining the role of message frame, perceived risk, and ambivalence in the decision to become an organ donor*. Communication Theses, Paper 26.

Coy, P. (2005). Scared to death of life insurance. *Bloomberg Business Week Magazine,Magazine* posted February 20, 2005.

Emery, D. (2013). *The kidney thieves: An urban legend*. Retrieved March 2, 2013 from http://urbanlegends.about.com/od/horrors/a/kidney_thieves_2_htm.

Fulton, J., Fulton, R. & Simmons R. G. (1977). The cadaver donor and the gift of life (338-376). In R. G. Simmons. S. D. Klein, & R. L. Simmons (Eds.), *The gift of life: The social and psychological impact of organ transplantation*. NY: John Wiley & Sons.

Harris, R. J., Jasper, J. D., Shanteau, J. & Smith, S. A. (1990). *Organ donation consent decisions by the next of kin: An experimental simulation approach*. In J. Shanteau & R. J. Harris (Eds.), Organ donation and transplantation: Psychological and behavioral factors. Washington, DC: American Psychological Association Publications.

Harris, R. J. & Shanteau, J. (1990). *Conclusion: We've only just begun*. In J. Shanteau & R. J. Harris (Eds.), Organ donation & transplantation: Psychological & behavioral factors. Washington, DC: American Psychological Association Publications.

Harris, R. J., Jasper, J. D. & Lee, B. C. (1991). Consenting to donate organs: Whose wishes carry the most weight? *Journal of Applied Social Psychology*, *21*, 3-14.

Hessing, D. J. (1990). The social dilemma or organ donation: Opting in or opting out. In J. Shanteau & R. J. Harris (Eds.), *Organ donation and transplantation: Psychological and behavioral factors*. Washington, DC: American Psychological Association.

Hessing, D. J. & Elffers, H. (1986). Attitude toward death, fear of being declared dead too soon, and donation of organs after death. *Omega Journal of Death and Dying*, *17*, 115-126.

Irving, J. I., Tong, A., Jan, S., Cass, A., Rose, J., Chadban, S., Allen, R. D., Craig, J. C., Wong, G. & Howard, K. (2011). Factors that influence the decision to be an organ donor: A systematic review of the qualitative literature. *Nephrology Dialysis Transplantation*, *10*, 1-8.

Johnson, E. J. & Goldstein, D. G. (2004). Defaults and donation decisions. *Transplantation*, *78*(Dec), 1713-1716.

Klayman, J. & Ha, Y. W. (1987). Confirmation, disconfirmation, and information in hypothesis testing. *Psychological Review*, *94*, 211-228.

Manninen, D. & Evans, R. (1985). Public attitudes and behavior regarding organ donation. *Journal of the American Medical Association*, *253*(June), 3111-3115.

Mayo Clinic (2010). Retrieved March 21, 2013 from http://www.mayoclinic.com/health/organ-donation/FL00077/NSECTIONGROUP=2

McIntyre, P. (1990). Perceptions of Mexican-Americans and Anglo-Americans regarding organ donation advertisements. In J. Shanteau & R. J. Harris (Eds.), *Organ donation and transplantation: Psychological and behavioral factors*. Washington, DC: American Psychological Association.

McIntyre, P., Barnett, M. A., Harris, R. J., Shanteau, J., Skowronski, J. & Klassen, M. (1987). *Psychological factors influencing decisions to donate organs*. In M. Wallendorf & P. F. Anderson (Eds.), Advances in consumer research, Vol. XIV, Toronto: Association for Consumer Research.

Oliver, M., Woywodt, A., Ahmed, A. & Saif, I. (2010). Organ donation, transplantation and religion. *Nephrology Dialysis Transplantation*, *19*, 1-8.

Orlebar, E. (1994). *Child kidnaping rumors fuel attacks on Americans: Guatemala: Military may be fomenting fear of foreigners: Hysteria may invite hard-liner backlash*. Retrieved March 21, 2013 from http//articles.latimes.com/pring/1994-04-02/news/mn-41338_1_ military intelligence

Pessemier, E. A., Bemmaor, A. C. & Hanssens, D. M. (1977). Willingness to supply human body parts: Some empirical results. *Journal of Consumer Research*, *4*, 131-140.

Prottas, J. (1983). Encouraging altruism: Public attitudes and the marketing of organ donation. *Health and Society*, *61*(2), 278-306.

Prottas, J. & Batten, H. L. (1988). Health professionals and hospital administrators in organ procurement: Attitudes, reservations, and their resolutions. *American Journal of Public Health*, *78*, 642-645.

Shanteau, J. (1988). *The decision to donate organs. A consumer research perspective*. In V. L. Hampton (Ed.), American council on consumer interests. Austin, TX: American Council on Consumer Interests.

Shanteau, J. & Harris, R. J. (1990). *Why psychological research on organ donation*? In J. Shanteau & R. J. Harris (Eds.), Organ donation and transplantation: Psychological and behavioral factors. Washington, DC: American Psychological Association Publications.

Shanteau, J. & Harris, R. J. (Eds.). (1990). *Organ donation and transplantation: Psychological and behavioral factors*. Washington, DC: American Psychological Association.

Shanteau, J. & Linin, K. A. (1990). *Subjective meaning of terms used in organ donation: Analysis of word associations*. In J. Shanteau & R. J. Harris (Eds.), Organ donation and transplantation: Psychological and behavioral factors. Washington, DC: American Psychological Association.

Shanteau, J. & Skowronski, J. J. (1990). *The decision to donate organs: An information integration analysis*. In J. Shanteau & R. J. Harris (Eds.), Organ donation and transplantation: Psychological and behavioral factors. Washington, DC: American Psychological Association Publications.

Shanteau, J. & Skowronski, J. J. (2013, August*). Who Is Opposed to Organ Donation? A Judgment/Decision Making Analysis*. Paper presented at the Subjective Probability, Utility, and Decision Making Conference, Barcelona.

Skowronski, J. (1987, May). *Psychological factors influencing decisions to donate organs*. Paper presented at the meeting of the Midwest Psychological Association, Chicago, IL.

Snopes.com (2013). Retrieved March 2, 2013 from http://search.atomz.com/search/?sp-q=Organ+Donor&x=34&y=13&sp-a=00062d45-sp00000000&sp-advanced=1&sp-p=all&sp-w-control=1&sp-w=alike&sp-date-range=-1&sp-x=any&sp-c=100&sp-m=1&sp-s=0

Tontus, H. O., Karabey, M. & Gurdal, N. (2011). Survey of medical students' attitudes, religious beliefs, and knowledge of organ donation. *Organs, tissues & cells*, *14*, 203-206.

UNOS. (2013). *The kidney transplant waiting list*. Retrieved March 27, 2013 from www.unos.org

Wason, P. C. (1960). On the failure to eliminate hypotheses in a conceptual task. *Quarterly Journal of Experimental Psychology*, *12*, 129-140.

Wilms, G., Kiefer. S. W., Shanteau, J. & McIntyre, P. (1987). Knowledge and image of body organs: Impact on willingness to donate. In M. Wallendorf & P. F. Anderson (Eds.), *Advances in consumer research*, Vol. *XIV*, Toronto: Association for Consumer Research.

In: Organ Donation and Transplantation
Editor: Mary Anne Lauri
ISBN: 978-1-62948-257-6

Chapter 6

LOVE IS ALL YOU NEED: ORGAN DONATION IN THE TEACHINGS OF DIFFERENT RELIGIONS

Joseph Borg*
University of Malta, Malta

ABSTRACT

Research has shown that in many cultures, religious convictions are still an important factor that influence people's attitudes and actions. These religious convictions influence, amongst other things, the decision whether or not one could or should donate organs while living or after one's death.

This chapter analyses the position that major religions take on this issue. It is to be expected that a religion's theological anthropology, its concept of the afterlife and its theology of the body have particular relevance for the religious understanding of organ donation. However this paper argues that although the major religions of the world have different theological positions and perspectives on these subjects there is a general consensus – albeit with different emphasis - in favour of organ donation because all religions accept the basic rule – Do to others, what you would like them to do to you.

The chapter also discusses in some detail the position on organ donation of the world's three largest religions, namely Christianity, Islam and Hinduism.

INTRODUCTION

Religion is as old as humanity itself while organ donation is a far more recent phenomenon; the first successful living-related kidney transplant is as recent as 1954. Both religion and organ donation are very complex and multifaceted as both address complicated issues. Religion is one of those phenomena that are easy to describe but very difficult to define. In a simple way religion can be described as a system of beliefs, moral precepts and ritual celebrations. Literature on the subject provides more intricate descriptions and definitions. The sociologist Durkheim (1915) described religion as a unified system of beliefs

* Corresponding author: Email: joseph.borg@um.edu.mt.

and practices relative to the sacred. Anthropologist Geertz (1973) called religion a cultural system while the theologian Tillich (1959) described it as the substance, the ground, and the depth of man's spiritual life.

This chapter will not explore these definitions and the complexities they encompass. It will use the term religion as it is commonly used to refer to established religions. This paper will address the basic ethical principle adopted by different religions to support organ donation and will then focus on the position of the three largest world religions, that is, Christianity, Islam and Hinduism.

Even the words "organ donation" encompass many issues. There is a difference between the donation of renewable tissue such as blood or bone marrow and the reception of more vital organs such as kidneys, liver, heart and lungs. The donation of such non-renewable organs will be the subject of this chapter. Some organs can be donated while one is still alive, for example a kidney, but others can only be donated after one's death, for example the heart. Organs can be extracted even from animals, as in cases of transplanted heart valves from pigs. These interventions elicit a battery of ethical and religious questions. Does the donation of organs imply that humans exercise sovereignty over their bodies over and above that of God? Does it create any conflict with the belief in the resurrection? Does xenotransplantation contradict the concept of man as an image of God? Are we morally obliged to donate organs to those who need them? Who should decide how to fairly allocate organs? Can one give organs against payment? When is the point of death or when does the soul definitively leaves the body? The ethical and religious implications of these questions clearly manifest themselves in the discussion about organ donation.

Influence of Religion on Organ Donors

The 1960s brought with them several theories of secularisation all predicting a diminishing role for religion in the public sphere (Berger, 1969; Martin, 1978). Developments however showed the emergence of a situation which is more complex than predicted. Some churches, for example Christian mainline churches particularly in Europe, lost their former relevance (Donnelly & Inglis, 2010). Other Churches increased their political clout in several countries; for example the rise of Islamic fundamentalists (Hoover, 2008). The move for the establishment of Sharia law in a number of Arab countries is just one example of what can be described as secularisation in reverse.

Experience shows that the religious beliefs, even if divorced from institutional roots, have not lost their influence on the formation of attitudes adopted by individuals and the resultant actions. People's decisions for or against organ donation are certainly an area wherein religion still plays an important role. This applies to different countries and cultures. Davis and Randhawa (2006) studied the black Caribbean and black African population in the United Kingdom. They found that a common element present during all focus groups' discussions was the importance given to the influence of religion in the decision whether one should become an organ donor or not. Moreover religion was often viewed as a barrier to organ donation. Some participants in the focus groups were not certain whether or not their religion allowed them to become organ donors or whether their God considered such donations to be justified. Reubsaet, Brug and Van Den Borne (2001) studied the reactions of Dutch adolescents following the 1998 implementation of a new organ donor registration scheme in the Netherlands. They concluded that religion was a significant predictor of returning a completed registration form. The results of a study of Filipinos by Albright, Glanz and Wong (2005) also showed that religion was one of the major themes influencing their attitude to organ donation. Religious concerns play a role even among Muslim physicians. A 2005 survey in Turkey showed that as many as 21% of doctors cited religious concerns as a reason for not pushing for organ donation (Oliver, Woywodt, Ahmed, & Saif, 2011). Other studies showed that both the laity and some religious ministers are not well informed on the religious dimension of the subject and consequently object to organ donation on religious grounds. Such an objection is not justified as none of the world's main religions have a formal objection to the donation or reception of organs from living or dead donors (Bruzzone, 2008; Davis & Randhawa, 2006; Gallagher, 1996; Oliver et al., 2011).

A Unifying Ethical Principle

Vast theological differences separate the large number of world religions. These differences sometimes led to open warfare, for example the Christian Crusades against the Moslems, the Moslem originated jihads against Christians, the violent flare-ups between Moslems and Hindus in India and the fighting between different Christian groups in Ireland. The theological differences between the world religions are enormous. Islam's monotheism is radically different from Christianity's. There is disagreement whether Hinduism is polytheistic, pantheistic, or perhaps monotheistic. Classical Buddhism does not recognise the existence of a deity. The different concepts of deity lead to different anthropologies. The Judeo-Christian tradition looks at humans as created in the image of God. Islam's emphasis on God's transcendence makes it refute this doctrine. On the other hand, Hinduism and Buddhism believe in reincarnation but not in the resurrection.

Such fundamental theological and anthropological differences could make one conclude that religions would have dissimilar views about organ donation. However this is not the case as all religions agree on one very important ethical principle, that is, the Golden Rule. Different variations of the Rule describe it as either "do to others what you wish others do to you" or "love your neighbour as yourself". This Ethic of Reciprocity is common to all religions which also believe that it over-rides other principles such as the prohibition of mutilating the human body or touching the body after death. Consequently all religions agree that giving an organ to a person who needs it is morally acceptable if not also laudable. The general acceptance of this principle provides the ground for the campaigns of ethical publicity conducted in many countries in an attempt to keep organ donation as a voluntary activity and prevent it from sliding into the realm of markets and commodities (Cohen, 1999).

Judaism's and Christianity's acceptance of the Golden Rule is buttressed by quotations from their sacred books. "Love your neighbour as yourself" is mandated by the Old Testament book of Leviticus (19:18). The great Hebrew rabbi, Hillel the Elder, described the Golden Rule as the kernel of the Torah. When a heathen who wished to become a Jew asked him for a summary of the Jewish religion, Hillel said that what one finds to be hateful, one should not do to fellow humans (Hillel, n.d.). The same teaching is further developed in the New Testament so much so that the Golden Rule is "sometimes claimed by Christianity as its own" (Blackburn, 2001, p. 101). This could be because Jesus did not only ask his disciples to love others as they love themselves (Matthew 5:43; Luke 6:31) but he upped the ante by enjoining them to love others as He loves them (John 13:34-35). In the parable of the Good Samaritan, Jesus widened the definition of neighbour to include anyone in need of help. The Samaritan is praised for treating the wounded Jew as a neighbour and helping him even though the two ethnic groups were adversaries.

Even Islam's positive attitude towards organ donation is based on the importance that the Qur'an gives to altruism. It states that saving the life of one person is tantamount to saving all mankind (Qur'an 5:32). Although Islam prohibits any violation of the human body, whether living or dead, organ donation supersedes these prohibitions as it is considered that necessity overrides prohibition (Oliver et al., 2011). In the *Sunnah*, which included Muhammad's specific words and practices, the Prophet states that no one is to be considered as a believer until one desires for others what one desires for oneself (as cited in Yorkley, 2008). Such references in Islam give support to the practice of organ donation without however going so far as to consider it to be a mandatory act that has to be practised by all believers.

The Golden Rule is also accepted in the Hindu scriptures and such references come in handy to justify organ donation. According to the Hindu holy book, *Padmapuraana, shrushti* the entire *dharma* or spiritual and moral laws can be summarised thus: that which one finds to be unfavourable, one should not do that to others (Ramsukhdas, n.d.). Of particular importance to organ donation is the fact that giving without thought of reward referred to as *daan* in the Sankrist language, is listed as the third in the list of the ten *Niyamas* or virtuous acts (NHS, 2012).

The Buddha adopted the Golden Rule as one of the foundations of his ethical system. There are several sayings in the *Tripitaka* or the Buddhist scriptures which exhort believers not to behave towards others in ways that they themselves find hurtful; and to seek for others the happiness one desires for oneself (as cited in Yorkley, 2008). Consequently Buddhism gives great importance to charitable gifts. In the *Anguttara Nikaya*, another holy book, the Buddha says that "the noble disciple lives at home with a heart free from the taint of stinginess; he is open-handed, pure-handed, delighting in self-surrender, one to ask a favour of, one who delights in dispensing charitable gifts" (Anguttara Nikaya II 66 as cited in Harvey 2000, p. 63).

This universal acceptance of the Golden Rule brings with it an ethos of solidarity and mutual responsibility conducive to organ donation but no religion formally obliges one to donate organs or considers the donation of organs as a compulsory religious duty (Bruzzone, 2008). Religions' approval of the Golden Rule extends the practice of organ donation also to people one does not know personally. Only some Orthodox Jews and some Islamic Ulemas/Muftis depart from this attitude by proposing directed organ donation, that is, organ donation to specific groups only, for example members of the religion of the donor (Bruzzone, 2008). This attitude unfortunately betrays a very myopic vision of human solidarity and undermines the very rationale of the Golden Rule. How can one constrict the altruism proposed by the Golden Rule just to members of one's religion or ethnic grouping? It is understandable that this restrictive position is supported only by a very tiny minority among religious leaders.

Some may say that donation, at least in a number of cases, is not a selfless act of generosity. People donate organs during their lives for a number of reasons including the belief that they are buying a ticket to heaven or for enhancing their self-esteem (Lauri, 2009). Even in cadaveric donation there is some benefit for the families of the donors who believe that their departed dear ones will live on in the person receiving the organ donated. Some medical personnel do not discourage families from thinking that their relatives may live on in someone else's body although this belief does not hold ground medically. Religions do not in any way discourage this strategy of coping and comfort adopted by these relatives as the generosity shown by the act of giving even within such parameters is still laudable. No religion expects its adherents to be motivated only by the most pure selfless intentions in order for acts to considered as religiously positive ones.

CHRISTIANITY AND ORGAN DONATION

Christianity encompasses different churches and denominations, that is, Catholicism, Orthodoxy and Protestantism. For the purposes of this chapter they will be grouped together as all have the same position on the subject. The Catechism of the Catholic Church (Catholic Church, 1992) approves organ donation from living persons "if the physical and psychological dangers and risks to the donor are proportionate to the good sought for the recipient" (Para. 2296). In the same paragraph it also states that "organ donation after death is a noble and meritorious act and is to be encouraged as an expression of generous solidarity."

A similar position is taken by the Orthodox Church. Milton Efthimiou, a high official of the Greek Orthodox Church in the United States, says that the Greek Orthodox Church is not opposed to organ donation as long as the organs and tissue in questions are used to better human life, that is for transplantation or for research that will lead to improvements in the treatment and prevention of disease (Cooper and Taylor, 2000). There are, though some Orthodox hierarchs who have objected to heart transplants because they consider the heart to be the seat of the soul (Harakas, 2012). On the other hand, in 2005, the head of the Greek Orthodox Church, Archbishop of Athens and All Greece Christodoulos announced that he and the members of the Holy Synod had signed organ donor forms (RIA Novotsi, 2005).

The mainline Protestant denominations also support organ donation. Dr Morgan, Anglican Archbishop of Wales, described organ donation as "the most generous of self-giving imaginable" (NHS, 2012) and Lutheran congregations in the USA consider it to be an expression of sacrificial love for a neighbour (O'Connell, 2001). The United Methodist Church officially encourages organ donation considering it to be an example of *agape* or selfless love and self-sacrifice for others (O'Connell, 2001).

On more than one occasion Pope John Paul II praised the practice of organ donation, but Pope Benedict XVI seems to have gone a step beyond. When still a cardinal and Prefect of the Congregation for the Doctrine of the Faith he said that "I have agreed to give my organs to whoever might be in need. I registered years ago and I always carry this document with me. In addition to personal data, it states that I offer my organs to help whoever is in need; it is simply an act of love" (Bruzzone, 2008, p.1066).

But strangely enough the Pope has been banned from performing this act of love! Mgr. Georg Gaenswein, Benedict XVI's personal secretary wrote that the donation card was rendered "obsolete" when Benedict XVI was elected Pope (Catholic News Agency, 2011). While the Vatican's "health minister," Archbishop Zygmunt Zimowski, told Italy's *La*

Repubblica newspaper that the Pope's body must remain intact "because it belongs to and for the Church, in body and soul ... It is also understandable in view of possible future veneration," he said, referring to possible future declaration of sainthood (Catholic News Agency, 2011). This statement raises an obvious question. How could it be possible to prohibit the Pope from doing something he declares he wants to do as it is an act of love?

Some Christians fear that organ donation does not leave the body intact and thus in some way hinders the proper rendering of the final universal resurrection of all humanity. This writer encountered such fear while participating in the Organ Donation Campaign he helped organise in Malta in 2005/6. In an answer to this fear the Episcopalian theologian Simcox (1986) refers to Rousseau who claims that the only thing that a man clutches when he dies is what he has given away during his lifetime. Simcox (1986) describes as defective the Christianity of anyone who is more concerned about what happens to a liver after death than about what happens to somebody who needs a healthy liver while still alive!

The positive approach taken by Christian Churches to the practice of organ donation does not mean that they are not conscious of ethical issues connected with the practice. Pope John Paul II, while addressing the participants of the first International Congress on the Transplant of Organs, June 20, 1991, referred to shameful abuses committed such as when the body is treated as a merely physical or biological entity or when its organs and tissues are used as items for sale or exchange (Bruzzone, 2008). In his Encyclical Letter, *Evangelium Vitae* (The Gospel of Life), John Paul II (1995) condemned the practice "when, in order to increase the availability of organs for transplants, organs are removed without respecting objective and adequate criteria which verify the death of the donor" (Para.15). Other Christian denominations point towards other abuses that can occur. For example, some Baptists oppose the use of foetal tissues for transplantation, Lutherans object to the procurement of organs for anencephalic new-borns or human foetuses, if death were the result, and Presbyterians take a stand against abortion of foetuses solely to obtain parts for transplantation (O'Connell, 2001).

ISLAM AND ORGAN DONATION

Islam, like other religions, is not monolithic and therefore one is to expect that although it approves of organ donation, different scholars and religious currents may hold contrasting attitudes and positions towards the subject. Oliver et al. (2011), for example, noted that Indo-Asian scholars are less approving of organ donation than Arab Muslim ones. As a consequence Muslims are automatically exempt from the presumed consent system operative in Singapore. Bruzzone (2008) notes that the objection of some of these scholars is based on the belief that organ donation can be a desecration of the human body which is an *amanat* (trusteeship) from God. However, they approve of xenotransplantation as this danger of desecration does not apply. Concerns are also raised by Muslim burial customs which mandate burial within 24 hours and by the controversies about the concept and definition of brain death; both issues create obstacles for the acceptance of organ donation (Oliver et al., 2011). Similar reasons united British Jews and Muslims, to show concern about the proposed legislation in favour of presumed consent in Wales (BBC, 2012). Cadaveric donation is still looked at sceptically by some Muslims. Oliver et al. (2011) give the example of Iran where only 13% of renal transplants done in 2006 were cadaveric donations. While reporting similarly low figures in Turkey and Saudi Arabia, Oliver et al. (2011) propose that this could be in part explained because of logistical factors.

These objections notwithstanding, it can be said that Islam is generally in favour of organ donation (Ghaly, 2012). A review of 70 contemporary *fatwas* or religious laws confirmed some degree of heterogeneity, although all supported organ transplants (Oliver et al., 2011). An outstanding example is the decision of the 1998 Islamic Jurisprudence Assembly Council in Saudi Arabia approving cadaveric and live donation. As explained above the main justification of organ donation is based on the principle of altruism. This is given precedence over other considerations, for example the prohibition against violating the human body. The same principle was used to justify products originating from swine in the production of insulin and in performing bone grafts (Oliver et al., 2011).

Three *fatwas* originating from Muslim organisations based in Europe are of particular importance. These are the 1995 *fatwa* of the UK Muslim Shariah Council; the 2000 *fatwa* of the Ireland based European Council for Fatwa and Research (ECFR) which included three *fatwas* previously issued by notable Muslim academies; and the 2006 *fatwa* of Mustafa Ben Hamza decreed during a conference held in the Netherlands (Ghaly, 2012). These three *fatwas* have contributed greatly towards the nurturing of a positive attitude towards organ donation by Muslims. The following points from the fatwas show the wide ranging approval for organ donation (Ghaly, 2012):

- donation to third parties is permissible both while a person is alive and also after death;
- the definition of the moment of death is the responsibility of the medical profession;
- brain stem death is accepted as the end of life as this belief is based on the best current medical knowledge;
- organ transplantation is permissible when it is a means of assuaging pain or saving life in line with Sharia law;
- the donation of someone's testicle or ovum to another person is forbidden because such a donation would entail the transfer of the genetic characteristics of the donor;
- it is permissible for Muslims to carry donor cards;
- if the dead person was not a registered donor or had not clearly expressed his desire to donate organs after the death, his/her relatives may authorise the needed operation to obtain organs from the body to save other people's lives;
- organs must be donated freely. The donor should not be given rewards and trading in organs is prohibited;
- organs can be donated to non-Muslims and can be received from non-Muslims.

The imams, as can be said about other religious leaders, can play an important role in the advancement of an attitude in favour of organ donation as their advice is respected by the rest of the community. The targeting of such opinion leaders is essential for the successful adoption of organ donation by Muslims. Moreover, religious seasons such as Ramadan can be very fruitful in persuading the faithful to become organ donors as during these seasons emphasis is made on altruistic behaviour. Studies conducted in Iran show that the inscription for organ donation cards increases during Ramadan (Oliver et al., 2011).

Hinduism and Organ Donation

Hinduism, the world's third largest religion, is the least centralised of the religions discussed so far. It is a composite of various philosophies, without a universal authority and without a single founder (Osborne, 2005). Within such a scenario it is reasonable to expect the co-existence of diverse trends and positions although there is a generally accepted framework albeit not at all rigid. This holds true of Hinduism in general and of the Hindu position on organ donation.

The belief in life after death and the on-going process of re-incarnation are a basic tenet of Hinduism. The law of Karma determines which way the soul will go in the next life. The Bhagavad Gita, one of Hinduism's holy books, compares the relationship of the mortal body and the immortal soul to the relationship of clothes to a body. Hindus believe that whatever one does during one's life will have an effect on what will happen to that person after death, thus actions during this life have an effect on the process of re-incarnation. The donation of an organ can entail that some of the donor's karma will be carried on to the recipient. Even the donor can be influenced. Since parts of his or her physical body are still "alive", organ donation may somehow interfere with the moving on to the next incarnation. These dangers potentially could fade if the donor would finally move to the next incarnation, but some of the donor traits could have already been integrated into the recipient's personality (Rampazzo, Bassiri Gharb, & Siemionow, 2011).

This way of reasoning by some Hindu scholars explain their scepticism about organ donation. Gurudeva, Satguru Sivaya Subramuniyaswami, founder of Kauai's Hindu Monastery was asked whether donating organs at death would stop one's soul from going into higher realms (Kauai's Hindu Monastery, 2001). Gurudeva said that whoever donates organs will remain earthbound, attached to the person who received the organ. He explained that if the person who received the organs was an unhappy person, then the person who donated the organs will also be in an unhappy situation. The donor would remain earth bound until the recipient passed on.

Swami Satchidananda, one of the most revered Yoga masters of our time, said that the replacing of organs in a body which is clearly dying is tantamount to not allowing the soul to fulfil its karma in this life by dying at the proper time and getting a new body through re-incarnation. He added that it is not correct to keep the soul indefinitely in the same old body by changing the organs (Satchidananda as cited in Editors of Hinduism Today, 2007). On the other hand, there are many Hindu scholars who are supportive of organ donation. The Hindu Temple Society of North America says that Hindus can, if they do so wish, be organ donors (Cooper & Taylor, 2000). Swani Bua, the founder of the Indo-American Yoga-Vedanta Society, said that Hindus should support *bona fide* scientist working on organ donation but they should guard against the unscrupulous traders in human organs (Editors of Hinduism Today, 2007). Swami Chidanand Saraswati, the President and spiritual head of one of India's largest and most renowned spiritual institutions, feels that it is important to donate organs as this is in line with the Hindu spirit of giving and sacrifice. Dr. Sodhi, from the Ayurvedic and Naturopathic Medical Clinic, Washington USA, favours the donation of some organs but not of the heart as Ayurveda, the Hindu system of traditional medicine, considers it to be the seat of the soul (Editors of Hinduism Today, 2007). A leaflet published on the site of the department responsible for organ donation within the National Health Scheme of the United

Kingdom quotes several Hindu authorities in support of organ donation. These include, for example, Om Parkash Sharma MBE, President, National Council of Hindu Temples and Dr Bal Mukund Bhala, Co-ordinator Hindu International Medical Mission (NHS, 2012).

Hinduism's acceptance of the Golden Rule discussed in the introduction forms the basis of the acceptance of organ donation. Love of others is considered to be more important than other considerations. In fact the *Manusmruti*, a Hindi holy book, states that of all the things that it is possible to donate, to donate one's own body is infinitely more worthwhile (as cited in NHS, 2012). Moreover, Hindu mythology narrates several episodes in which different human organs are used for the benefit of other humans. For example it is said that Brahma, the creator, cut away part of his own body to bring into existence his wife, Saraswati. Hindu mythology also includes the legend of Ganesha the God who is part human and part elephant. Kahan (1989) says that this provides the basis of the support of xenotransplantation. In another myth a hunter plucks out his right and then his left eye to give it to Shiva, one of the Hindu deities. The God, Shiva, stretched his arms out in order to stop the hunter. Because the hunter received the grateful love of the god himself, Doniger (1996) says that these myths are evidence of the positive attitude of Hinduism towards organ donation among the living.

Conclusion

The foregoing review of the position of the world's main religions about organ donation clearly manifests a generally positive approach to the subject. However the debate is complex and a number of doubts are stated. These caveats or doubts should not be lightly dismissed by the scientific community or considered to be unwelcome obstacles in promoting organ donation. These difficulties perhaps reflect that there is something ingrained within the collective human psyche that hesitates at the idea of giving or receiving organs (Youngner, Fox. & O'Connell, 1996). The experience of those working with people faced by the possibility of donating the organs of their loved ones after their death attests the fact that religious and spiritual considerations play a very important part in the process of deciding (O'Connell, 2001). Religion, thus, should be considered as an ally to the efforts of the scientific community. Different religions present some of the fears that people feel unconsciously. At the same time religions also propose the way forward as they present organ donation as a generous act worthy of praise. This positive attitude has to be harnessed by the scientific community to help people overcome their fears and look forward enthusiastically to the possibility of donating organs.

References

Albright C. L., Glanz K. & Wong L. (2005). Knowledge and attitudes about deceased donor organ donation in Filipinos: A qualitative assessment. *Transplantation Proceedings*, *37*(10), 4153-4158.

BBC (2012, November 5). Organ donation: Jewish and Muslim presumed consent worries. *BBC news*. Retrieved from http://www.bbc.co.uk/news/uk-wales-20182517

Berger, P. L. (1969). *A rumor of angels. Modern society and the rediscovery of the supernatural*. New York: Doubleday.

Blackburn, S. (2001). *Ethics: A very short introduction*. Oxford: Oxford University Press.

Bruzzone, P. (2008). Religious aspects of organ transplantation. *Transplantation Proceedings*, *40*, 1064-1067.

Catholic Church (1992). *Catechism of the Catholic Church*. Citta del Vaticano: Libreria Editrice Vaticana.

Catholic News Agency. (2011, February 5). Pope's secretary puts papal organ donation discussion to rest. *Catholic News Agency*. Retrieved from http://www.catholicnewsagency.com/news/popes-secretary-puts-papal-organ-donation-discussion-to-rest/

Cohen, L. (1999). Where it hurts: Indian material for an ethics of organ transplantation. *Daedalus*, *128*(4), 135-66.

Cooper, M. L. & Taylor, G. J. (Eds.). *Organ and tissue donation: A reference guide for clergy* (4th ed.). Richmond, VA: SEOPF/UNOS.

Davis, C. & Randhawa, G. (2006). The influence of Religion on organ donation and transplantation among the Black Caribbean and Black African population – A pilot study in the United Kingdom. *Ethnicity & Disease*, *16*, 281– 285.

Doniger, W. (1996). Transplanting Myths of Organ transplants. In I. S. Youngner, R. Fox & L. J. O'Connell (Eds.), *Organ transplantation: Meanings and realities* (194-220). Madison, Wisconsin: University of Wisconsin Press.

Donnelly, S. & Inglis T. (2010). The media and the Catholic Church in Ireland: Reporting clerical child sex abuse. *Journal of Contemporary Religion*, *25*(1), 1- 19.

Durkheim, E. (1915). *The elementary forms of the religious life*. London: George Allen & Unwin.

Editors of Hinduism Today (2007). *What Is Hinduism? Modern Adventures into a Profound Global Faith*. Kapaa, HI USA: Himalayan Academy Publications.

Gallagher, C. (1996). Religious attitudes regarding organ donation. *Journal of Transplant Coordination*, *6*, 186-190.

Geertz, C. (1973). *The interpretation of culture*. New York: Basic Books.

Ghaly, M. (2012). Religio-ethical discussions on organ donation among Muslims in Europe: An example of transnational Islamic bioethics. *Medical Health Care and Philosophy*, *15*, 207–220.

Harakas, S. S. (2012). *For the health of body and soul: an Eastern Orthodox introduction to bioethics*. Retrieved from http://www.goarch.org/ourfaith/ ourfaith8076

Harvey, P. (2000). *An introduction to Buddhist ethics*. Cambridge: University Press.

Hoover, S. M. (2008). *Media and religion*. A White Paper from The Center for Media, Religion, and Culture. Colorado, USA: University of Colorado at Boulder.

Hillel. (n.d). Hillel. In the unedited full text of the *1906* Jewish *Encylopedia*. Retrieved from http://www.jewishencyclopedia.com/articles/7698-hillel

John Paul II (1995). *Encyclical Letter: Evangelium Vitae*. Retrieved from http://www.vatican.va/holy_father/john_paul_ii/encyclicals/documents/hf_jp-ii_enc_25031995_evangelium-vitae_en.html

Kahan, B. D. (1989). Ganesha: the principal Hindu xenograft. *Transplantation Proceedings*, *21*(3), 1 – 8.

Kauai's Hindu Monastery (2001). *Organ Donation at death*. Retrieved from http://www.himalayanacademy.com/view/gr_2001-04-05_organ-donation-at-death

Lauri, M. A. (2009). Metaphors of organ donation, social representations of the body and the opt-out system. *British Journal of Health Psychology, 14*, 647-666.

Martin D. (1978). *A general theory of secularization*. Oxford: Blackwell.

NHS (2012). *A guide to organ donation and Hindu beliefs*. Retrieved from http://www.organdonation.nhs.uk/ukt/newsroom/fact_sheets/religious_leaflets/hindu_dharma_and_organ_donation/hindu_dharma_and_organ_donation.pdf

O'Connell, L. J. (2001). The religious and spiritual perspective toward human organ donation and transplantation. In W. Shelton & J. Balint (Eds.), *The ethics of organ transplantation. Advances in Bioethics* (277-292). Bradford: Emerald Group Publishing.

Oliver, M., Woywodt, A., Ahmed, A. & Saif, I. (2011). Organ donation, transplantation and religion. *Nephrology Dialysis Transplantation, 26* (2), 437-444.

Osborne, E. (2005). *Accessing R.E. Founders & Leaders, Buddhism, Hinduism and Sikhism Teacher's Book Mainstream*. Dublin, Ireland: Folens Limited.

Rampazzo A., Bassiri Gharb B. & Siemionow M. Z. (2011). Addressing Religious and Cultural differences. In M. Z Siemionow (Ed.), *The know-how of face transplantation* (287-296). Berlin: Springer Verlag.

Ramsukhdas, S. (n.d.). *The essense of spiritual truths*. Retrieved from http://www.swamiramsukhdasji.net/eBooks/Essence-of-Dharma.htm

Reubsaet, A., Brug, J. & Van Den Borne, B. (2001). Predictors of organ donation registration among Dutch adolescents. *Transplantation, 72*(1), 51-56.

RIA Novosti (2005, July 1). *Head of Greek Orthodox Church intends to become organ donor*. Retrieved from http://en.rian.ru/society/20050701/40831584.html

Simcox, C. E. (1986). *The Case of the Missing Liver* (I Cor. 15:44). Retrieved from http://www.religion-online.org/showarticle.asp?title=1000

Tillich, P. (1959). *Theology of culture*. Oxford: Oxford University Press.

Yorkley, J.M. (2008). *Social responsibility therapy for adolescents and young adults. A multicultural treatment manual for harmful behaviour*. New York: Routledge.

Youngner, S. J., Fox, R.C. & O'Connell, L. J. (1996). *Organ transplantation: Meanings and realities*. Madison, Wisconsin: University of Wisconsin Press.

In: Organ Donation and Transplantation
Editor: Mary Anne Lauri
ISBN: 978-1-62948-257-6

Chapter 7

ILLUMINATING THE PSYCHOLOGICAL PROCESSES ASSOCIATED WITH RENAL FAILURE DIAGNOSIS AND LIVING DONATION CONSIDERATIONS: AN APPLICATION OF GOAL DISRUPTION THEORY

Jason T. Siegel*
Claremont Graduate University, US

ABSTRACT

Goal disruption theory offers a framework for understanding when goal expectancy violations (e.g., being diagnosed with renal disease) are most likely to cause a state of goal disruption (i.e., psychological disequilibrium caused by a goal expectancy violation), and the adaptive responses that are automatically catalyzed as a result (e.g., reduced cognitive complexity, increased impulsivity, decreased willingness to forgive). The current chapter gives an overview of the disruptive force of chronic disease, provides an introduction of goal disruption theory, identifies the relevance of goal disruption theory for renal patients and medical personnel, and offers insight into how the theoretical framework can be used to increase the health and wellness of patients with renal disease.

INTRODUCTION

A renal patient considering living donation (i.e., receiving an organ from a living donor) is making a decision that will have life-altering ramifications. Ideally, such a decision would be made with a clear mind. Unfortunately, given the manifold challenges faced by someone with renal disease (e.g., constant threat of death, frequent uncertainty, economic tension, dependency on others; Devins, Hunsley, Mandin, Taub, & Paul, 1997), a state of *goal disruption* is more likely. As described by goal disruption theory (GDT; see Siegel, 2004,

* Corresponding author: Email: Jason.Siegel@cgu.edu.

2011; Siegel et al., 2012 for initial theorizing), a goal disruption refers to a state of persistent psychological disequilibrium caused by having one's expectations violated (e.g., expectations of good health). When psychological disequilibrium occurs, the individual's sole purpose is to restore psychological balance as quickly as possible. This restoration ascends to the top of an individual's goal hierarchy, often at the expense of other, and sometimes more important, goals.

Equally problematic for the patient and medical practitioners is the array of additional adaptive changes that are catalyzed as a result of a goal disruption. These adaptive changes include, but are not limited to, reduced cognitive complexity (Fraunfelder, 1974; Ionescu, 2012; Pennell, 1996), impaired ability to take the perspective of others (Amici, Aurelli, Visalberghi, & Call, 2009), increased impulsivity (Nordgren & Chou, 2012), increased tendency to stereotype (Kugler, Cooper, & Nosek, 2010), and increased willingness to endure physical harm to reach a needed goal (Rosenberg, Lewandowski, & Siegel, in press; Siegel, 2011). To be sure, these adaptive responses are useful in some contexts (e.g., finding food when hungry), but not useful in others (e.g., when contemplating living donation).

Given patients with renal disease will likely experience a consistent barrage of expectancy violations (e.g., unexpected loss of health, freedom, vocation, friends), there is vast utility in knowing when these violations are most likely to cause a state of disruption, the intensity with which the disruption will be experienced, and the system-wide adaptive processes that will occur as a result.

The Disruptive Force of Chronic Illness

Being diagnosed with a severe chronic illness can wreak havoc on a patient's psychological functioning (e.g., Caress, Luker, & Ackrill, 1999). Feelings of strife can overwhelm a patient as a storm of expectancy violations are experienced. The patient feels vulnerable; survival comes into question. As noted by Becker (1999), "If an illness comes on or is discovered suddenly, people's sense of continuity may completely unravel. Illness necessitates the surrender of the cherished assumption of personal indestructability" (p. 40). Likewise, **Levealahti**, **Tishelman**, and Ohlen (2007) discuss how a diagnosis, "...could disrupt structures of everyday life, expectations, and normal rules of reciprocity and mutual support" (p. 470). Reactions to the diagnosis of a severe chronic illness have been considered as debilitating as the actual disease (Lewis, 1998); terms such as "traumatic surprise" are common in qualitative investigations of illness (Power, Brown, & Ritzo, 2008, p. 337).

Patients with end stage renal disease experience disequilibrium and upset in line with this profile. Being diagnosed with kidney disease can lead patients to question the predictability of the world, the utility of their body, and the security of their existence (Devins et al., 1997). When Dollard and colleagues (1939) needed an example of something that would likely cause a high level of goal frustration, kidney disease was tapped: "The interference may be slight, as when a mosquito hums near a person absorbed in a thought, or great, as when an individual suffers the effects of kidney disease" (p. 7). In addition to a loss of kidney function, patients with renal disease must respond to changes in their family role, work capabilities, personal freedom, and sexual function (e.g., Kimmel, 2001). Renal patients also must adjust to medication side effects, dietary constraints, dependency on treatment, and fears of death (e.g.,

Chilcot, Wellsted, Da Silve-Gana, & Farrington, 2008; Gonzalez, Siegel, Alvaro, & O'Brien, 2013).

Accordingly, once dialysis begins, the prevalence of depression among renal patients is approximately three times higher than that of the general population (Akman, Ozdemir, Sezer, Micozkadioglu, & Haberal, 2004; also see Chilcot, Wellsted, Da Silve-Gana, & Farrington, 2008). More than 80% of patients with renal disease agree that the *biggest problem* in their life is finding a new kidney, and 85% agree that some days they think they need a new kidney *more than anything else* (Siegel, Alvaro, Hohman, & Mauer, 2011). As described by Devins and colleagues (1997), "Affected individuals experience the continuing threat of death, decreased physical strength and stamina, dependencies on medical machinery and personnel, vocational and economic strains, stringent dietary and fluid-intake restrictions, and complex medical and pharmacologic regimens" (p. 325).

It is during this storm of expectancy violations (e.g., realizing one is not as healthy as expected) that myriad life-changing decisions have to be made (Alvaro et al., 2008), including whether to consider asking a loved one to donate his or her kidney (e.g., Rodrigue, Cornell, Kaplan, & Howard, 2008; Waterman, Rodrigue, Purnell, Ladin, & Boulware, 2010; also see Siegel & Alvaro, 2010; Siegel, Alvaro, Lac, Crano, & Alexander, 2008). Receiving a transplant from a living donor can increase the likelihood of long-term survival and quality of life beyond the benefits of a non-living donor transplant (e.g., Neipp et al., 2006). Living donor transplants can also reduce the length of time the patient has to be on dialysis, lower the likelihood of acute graft rejection, increase the likelihood of a high-quality kidney graft, and expand the donor eligibility criteria (Rodrigue, Cornell, Kaplan, & Howard, 2008; Tarantino, 2000). Further, if a patient finds a living donor, the patient will not have to wait an unknown period of time for an organ to become available (Meier-Kriesche & Kaplan, 2002).

On the flip side, living donation requires the patient to make numerous additional decisions, including asking someone to risk his or her life so the patient can be healthier (Glannon, 2008). As noted by Kleinman and Lowy (1992), "Nowhere else in medicine is a part of a healthy person removed without the procedure being of direct physical benefit to that individual" (p. 1484). Further, the patient must decide whether to directly ask family members or friends to donate or to wait until someone comes forward on their own (e.g., Kranenburg et al., 2009; Simmons & Klein, 1972). If the patient decides to be proactive, the patient must then determine how to relay the decision and the need for a donation to family members (e.g., Pradel, Suwannaprom, Mullins, Sadler, & Bartlett, 2008). If a family member comes forward, the potential recipient has to decide whether to accept the offer (e.g., Gordon, 2001). Fears about other people being hurt are commonplace among potential recipients (Franklin & Crombie, 2003). If no one comes forward, the patient has to decide how to respond, as familial relations may be negatively altered (e.g., Simmons, Hickey, Kjellstrand, & Simmons, 1971). As noted by Simmons and colleagues (1971), the end result can be bitterness on the part of the person in the greatest need.

Decisions such as whether to ask a family member to engage in a potentially life ending surgery, how to do so, and how to respond if acceptance or rejection occurs, would ideally be made with a clear and stable mind. Unfortunately, given that renal patients' worlds are turned upside by the diagnosis and ongoing goal frustrations, this will rarely be the case. By knowing when violations associated with living donation (e.g., no one volunteering to be a living donor) are most likely to cause disruption, and the adaptive changes to thought and action that will result if disruption occurs, medical practitioners can prepare patients to minimize the likelihood of a goal disruption occurring and minimize the damage that will be caused if a disruption takes place.

Goal Disruption Theory

Goal disruption theory (GDT; Siegel, 2004; 2011; Siegel et al., 2012; also see GDTheory.com; Lewandowski, Rosenberg, Parks, & Siegel, 2011) offers a framework for understanding the contexts in which a goal expectancy violation (e.g., being diagnosed with renal disease) is most likely to cause goal disruption (i.e., a state of psychological disequilibrium caused by a goal violation), and the adaptive processes that automatically engage as a result (e.g., tunnel vision, dichotomous thinking, no economy of action, increased false consensus).

Goal disruption theory is relatively unique in its focus on expectations and expectancy violations. As such, a discussion of each is provided. A discussion of the contexts in which goal expectancy violations are most likely to cause a state of disruption will follow. Next, the range of adaptive changes that will ensue as a result of the violation will be described. Lastly, the chapter will conclude with insight on the utility of GDT for assisting medical personnel working with renal disease patients.

Goal Expectations

Moskowitz and Grant (2009) eloquently refer to goals as "…the desired end state the individual reaches for; it is the ultimate aim of one's adopted action, the very cause of the action; it is the purpose toward which one is striving; it is the reason for doing and thinking" (p. 1). In the most general sense, expectations can be considered beliefs about a person's goals. Tolman (1925) first wrote about goal expectations nearly a century ago, and considered expectations to act as a foundation for guiding thought and action. He perceived expectations to be a combination of memories and perceptions, as "there are probably no actual cases of pure perceptions" (Tolman, 1932, p. 139). While Tolman's contemplations on outcome expectations (e.g., Bolles, 1972; Conklin, Dahling, & Garcia, 2013) and self-efficacy (Bandura, 1977) have historically garnered the most interest, Tolman's conceptualization of expectations included a far broader range of beliefs (e.g., expectations about the best path for reaching a goal, expectations of the distance remaining between the person and the goal). Scholars have recently shown increased appreciation for the range of expectations proposed by Tolman (e.g., Fuhrman, Flannagan, & Matamoros, 2009; Seidel, Franks, Stephens & Rook, 2012; Siegel & Burgoon, 2002).

In line with Tolman's (1932, 1933, 1959) expansive view of expectations, GDT defines goal expectations as the broad range of beliefs people hold about the goals they want to achieve. This range of beliefs includes, but is not limited to, expectations about the future (also see Thompson et al., 2012), expectations about the rewards associated with specific goals, the paths through which the goal can be achieved, the person's capabilities for achieving the goal, the skills that will be needed for achieving the goal, and the level of performance the person can expect to achieve (Cumming & Ramsey, 2011). Also included are expectations for resources and support that exist for achieving the goal (including social support; Kelly & Burgoon, 1991), the situations that will be encountered as a result of goal-related behavior (Gurland, Grolnick, & Friendly, 2012), and expectations about the knowledge that was used to form goal expectations (van Rompay, de Vries, Bontekoe, & Tanja-Dijkstra, 2012). Further, people hold expectations about the goals they have already accomplished and the distance remaining between the person and the goal. Tolman (1955) also noted that individual expectations could interact with each other and create new expectations.

Expectancy Violations

In addition to shining a light on the expectation construct, Tolman (1932) theorized about what occurs when an expectation is violated. A goal expectancy violation refers to any internal or external event that runs counter to the beliefs and expectations of the individual. Simply, a goal expectancy violation occurs when people's expectations and beliefs about their goals are deemed inaccurate (e.g., a patient believes their kidneys are healthy but are told they have kidney disease).

The unexpected nature of the violation was at the heart of Tolman's (1932) and Elliot-Smith's (1928) description of disruption. Tolman (1932) used the term disruption to describe the breakdown and upset in behavior that occurs when a goal expectation is violated. Other scholars have had a similar interest in the impact of unexpected occurrences (e.g., Erikson, 1968; Lipman-Bluman, 1973; Mendes, **Blascovich**, Lickel, & **Hunter, 2007**). The focus of these scholars is well placed—decades of research conducted since Tolman's theorizing empirically support his focus on cognitive expectations and the violations thereof (e.g., Pyszczynski & Greenberg, 1981; Skenderian, Siegel, Crano, Alvaro, & Lac, 2008).

Central to the experience of a goal disruption is the unexpected nature of the violation; the unexpected quality of the occurrence is particularly threatening to the person's sense of psychological equilibrium. Goal expectancy violations do not only impair the person's goal capabilities, but the person's world is revealed to be less predictable than believed. As noted by Lewin (1959), "Being in unstructured surroundings leads to uncertainty of behavior because it is not clear whether a certain action will lead to or away from the goal" (p. 255). The unexpected nature of the violation will influence the extent to which the violation will make people feel that their worlds are unpredictable, unstable, uncertain, and, most importantly, threatening (e.g., Mendes et al., 2007). As noted by Clary and Tesser (1983), "It may be that unexpected events represent a challenge to one's prior ideas, and explanatory activity is undertaken as a means of reestablishing a sense of control" (p. 617).

Decades of empirical research support the unique influence of unexpected violations (e.g., Bettencourt, Dill, Greathouse, Charlton, & Mulholland, 1997). For example, unexpected failure is associated with greater dissatisfaction and is more aversive than expected failure (Feather, 1969; House & Perney, 1974); unexpected events catalyze more aggression and hostility than expected events (e.g., Berkowitz, 1960; Kregarman & Worchel, 1961). Likewise, levels of performance often diminish as a result of an expectancy violation (Mendes et al.**, 2007), and** the same information can lead to vastly different interpretations and predictions based on whether the experienced event was unexpected or expected (Harvey, Harkins, & Kagehiro, 1976; Bettencourt et al., 1997).

Even though goal expectancy violations will likely be numerous for patients diagnosed with renal disease, not all patients will enter disruption. Goal disruption theory is useful to medical practitioners because the framework can be used to broadly consider whether psychological disequilibrium is likely to occur, as well as the intensity with which the patient might experience it. Goal disruption theory puts forth five categories of factors that influence the likelihood that a goal violation will become a goal disruption, and the intensity with which the disruption will be felt: 1) *violation severity*, 2) *violation imprint*, 3) *opinion of efficacy*, 4) *structural harmony (state of the system)*, and 5) *personality traits*. The first two, (i.e., severity and imprint) focus on the expectancy violation itself, while the latter three (i.e., opinion of efficacy, structural harmony, and personality traits) focus on the person who experiences the violation. All factors can be seen as offering insight into when a goal expectancy violation is most likely to lead a patient to psychological disequilibrium in a patient.

Violation Severity

Violation severity has two components. The first refers to the extent to which the violation was unexpected. To be sure, all expectancy violations are unexpected; however, some violations will be more unexpected than others. The second component of violation severity refers to the strength with which the violated expectations were held. Simply, not all expectations will be held with equal levels of strength.

Violation severity: Unexpectedness. All goal disruptions are caused by expectancy violations; however, not all expectancy violations will be of equal intensity. Put another way, the distance between what was expected and what occurred will vary. The more unexpected the occurrence, the greater the likelihood that psychological disequilibrium will result. For example, if no one comes forward to offer a kidney, but a patient did not expect anyone to come forward, disruption will be less likely. On the other hand, if the patient expected numerous family members to volunteer, but no one did, the likelihood of disruption amplifies.

Violation severity: Strength of violated expectations. Expectancy strength refers to the level of confidence the person had in the expectation that was violated. Borrowing heavily from the research on attitude strength (Crano & Prislin, 2008; Petty & Krosnick, 1995), all expectancy violations are not equally predictive of whether a disruption will occur. Expectations that are held with high certainty (Bizer, Larsen, & Petty, 2011), that are easily accessible (see Fazio, 1995), that are non-ambivalent, or non-conflicting (Henderson, de Liver, & Gollwitzer, 2008), and that are based on knowledge and experience (Prislin, 1996), will be most likely to cause disruption if violated.

Two patients can both expect to be given a clean bill of health, but their expectations may be held with different levels of strength. If one patient was confident (e.g., based on knowledge and experience) that a clean bill of health was forthcoming and another patient less so, the more confident patient, all else being equal, would be more likely to experience disruption. From a GDT perspective, violations of strongly held expectations (e.g., those that are based on knowledge, experience, held with high certainty, are non-conflicting) are more likely to arouse psychological equilibrium than weakly held expectations (e.g., expectations that are not certain). When a weakly held expectation is violated, it is less likely to threaten peoples' understanding of their worlds, or their ability to predict their world, because they were not very confident of the outcome to start with. On the other hand, if a strongly held expectation is violated, the person's perceived ability to predict and explain the world is more likely to be shattered. Feelings of safety and security are difficult to come by when the world cannot be predicted or understood (Lewin, 1959).

Violation Imprint

The violation imprint refers to the extent of the changes that occur as a result of the violation. At the most global level, the size of the imprint is impacted by the number of related expectations that become violated as a result of the initial violation (Tolman, 1932, 1959). If a person's expectations can be considered akin to a sheet of glass, violation imprint refers to how shattered the glass becomes as a result of the violation. Just as a small chip in someone's windshield can stay small or end up spreading across the entire windshield, a violation can impact only one goal or it can impact multiple goals; the integrity of the windshield could stay in place, or it can come completely shattered. If having renal failure damages numerous goals, disruption will be more likely than if the number of impaired goals is minimal.

Opinion of Efficacy

Another variable that will dictate whether an expectancy violation will become a goal disruption is whether the person feels capable of adjusting to the violation. Certainly, a person will feel more or less capable based on the severity and the imprint, but all else being equal, peoples' perceived capabilities of finding an alternative path to restore their feelings of safety will also moderate the likelihood of a goal expectancy violation becoming a disruption. As such, a person's knowledge (Frings, Hurst, Cleveland, Blascovich, & Abrams, 2012), skills (Tomaka, Blascovich, Kelsey, & Leitten, 1993), and experience (Lipman-Bluman, 1973) will play a role in whether psychological disequilibrium occurs as a result of the expectancy violation. Likewise, patients' perceptions of their social, financial, and interpersonal resources will influence whether a disruption occurs (e.g., MacGeorge et al., 2008). Accordingly, patients diagnosed with diabetes are less likely to report distress when they believe that their illness can be managed and when they feel capable of doing so (Polonsky et al., 2010).

Structural Harmony (State of the System)

The balance and coherence of the person's current psychological state and goal structure will also moderate whether a goal expectancy violation will cause a disruption. Borrowing from the work of Lipman-Bluman (1973), a person's goal structure is proposed to have varying degrees of structural soundness or integrity. This can also be considered in line with Lovinger's (1976) considerations of ego, Antonovsky's (1987) sense of coherence, as well as variables such as stability of self (Rosenberg, 1989). For example, if a violation occurs to a patient who is experiencing a general state of anxiety (Kohli, Batra, & Aggarwal, 2011), the patient's likelihood of entering a state of goal disruption will increase. Further, the flexibility/rigidity of the patient's goal structure (i.e., its ability to adjust to new situations), the level of goal organization (Lipman-Bluman, 1973), and the person's self-stability (Rosenthal & Zimmerman, 1976) will come into play. The length of time since the most recent violation, as well as past neglect or abuse, will also influence whether a disruption occurs (Harkness & Lumley, 2007).

Personality Traits

Two people could experience identical violations (e.g., renal disease, no one coming forward to donate), have identical environments, and yet one becomes disrupted and one does not. A list of every personality trait that will play a role in predicting disruption is beyond the scope of this chapter; however, GDT posits that specific personality traits will play a particularly large role in allowing a renal patient to retain psychological equilibrium when a goal expectancy violation occurs. If a renal patient tends to have highly stable self-esteem (Auerbach, Abela, Ho, Mcwhinnie, & Czajkowska, 2010), have an optimistic outlook (Carver, Lehman, & Michael, 2003)—whether it tends to be realistic or unrealistic optimism (Schneider, 2001)—and tends not to be bothered by uncertainty inducing events (Chen & Hong, 2010), a goal expectancy violation will be less likely to cause a disruption. A renal patient will also be less likely to enter a state of disruption if they have low levels of need for structure (e.g., Routledge & Juhl, 2012), a more internal locus of control (Rotter, 1954), and are not typically hypersensitive to threatening stimuli (McLaughlin & Hatzenbuehler, 2009).

Reducing the Likelihood of Disruption

This part of the framework, focusing on understanding when goal disruptions are most likely to occur, offers a potential means for reducing the likelihood of disruption. For the sake of illustration, and to show the depth of the utility of GDT, all examples used will focus on one specific type of expectancy violation. Please imagine a situation where a renal patient attempted to indirectly communicate the need for an organ donor to family members. The patient expected at least one person to come forward, yet no one did.

The patient could have been intensely confident that someone would come forward, or the patient could have also known that obstacles could have thwarted the possibility of an offer (e.g., kidney disease inflicting numerous family members). If the patient did not expect anyone to come forward, disruption will be less likely; if the patient expected numerous family members to volunteer, the likelihood of disruption amplifies. As such, medical personnel can work with renal patients to increase the likelihood that patient's expectations are as accurate as possible. Even better, the medical personnel can work to help the patient understand that anything is possible, including someone coming forward, but that it is also possible that someone will not. Openness to either occurrence will reduce the likelihood that the outcome will be unexpected.

The imprint of the violation is the next consideration. Due to concerns with the length of the waitlist for non-living donation (see Ganikos, 2010), the patient may perceive living donation as the only means for a desirable life. If so, a dearth of people volunteering to donate would be more likely to cause a disruption than if the patient perceived dialysis as acceptable. As such, medical personnel might put particular focus on the alternatives to living donation. If potential alternative paths are discussed with patients prior to moving forward with living donation, their opinion of efficacy will increase, and the expectancy violation will be less likely to cause disequilibrium.

Goal disruption theory would also suggest consideration of the state of the patient. For example, if the patient were having a particularly rough time adjusting to renal failure, a disruption would be more likely to occur. Since the state will impact how the violation is responded to, medical personnel could consider the right and wrong time to have a patient breach the topic of living donation. Also, while medical personnel can do little to change a patient's enduring personality traits, consideration of personality variables could inform medical personnel about the patients who are most susceptible to experiencing a disruption.

Psychological Disequilibrium

The extent to which the occurrence was unexpected, the strength of the violated expectations, the extent of the violation imprint, the state of the system, the perceived efficacy, and the personality of the patient are all considered with one goal: predicting whether psychological disequilibrium will occur. Psychological disequilibrium can best be defined as a disturbance of homeostasis (Britt & Janus, 1940), a state of imbalance in the person's psychological systems (see Cannon, 1932; Raup, 1925; Inhelder & Piaget, 1958). Goal disruption theory is one of numerous theories that places psychological equilibrium at its center. The notion of a balanced system has existed in psychological scholarship for nearly a century (e.g., Cannon, 1920; Festinger, 1957; Heider, 1958; Henning, 2011; Higgins, 1989; Selye, 1956; Young & Hollands, 2012). This line of thought can be traced back to Cannon's homeostasis theory (1920, 1926, 1932, 1941) in physiology, which held that the body self-organizes to strive for stability and balance. As recently noted by Moskowitz (2009), "humans have a natural tendency toward homeostasis, balance, and equilibrium. Imbalance, tension, and disequilibrium need to be reduced" (p. 331).

When a person is not in a state of psychological balance, discomfort will be experienced. As noted by Tolman, "The ultimate drive is for the removal of the driving physiological condition (or the prevention of the physiological injury or interference)" (1926, p. 354). Disequilibrium is an aversive state that causes adaptive processes to instinctively engage (Festinger, 1957; Richter, 1943). If psychological disequilibrium occurs, GDT suggests that this slew of adaptive process are enacted to attempt a return to equilibrium. This is in line with Tolman's (1932) theorizing of a heightened drive state, Barker, Dembo, and Lewin's (1941) conceptualization of regression, and recent studies on terror management theory (e.g., Ardnt & Solomon, 2003). A return to equilibrium will become the paramount focus as system-wide adaptive processes engage with the goal of maximizing the likelihood of a return to equilibrium (for similar conceptualization see Ardnt & Solomon, 2003; Lewin, 1946; Perls, Hefferline, & Goodman, 1951). All other goals beyond returning to equilibrium will become secondary. Psychological disequilibrium and the resulting discomfort will persist until psychological balance is restored (Kessen, 1971; Tolman, 1926).

The range of adaptive responses that is put forth by GDT, known as goal adaptation, is a culmination of over a century of scholarship looking at responses to disequilibrium within a variety of contexts. Tolman's consideration of behavior during a heightened drive state and Lewin's considerations of behavior during general frustration served as the foundation for the manifold adaptive adjustments to be presented. Adding to Tolman (1932, 1959) and Lewin's (1941) considerations are decades of contributions from scholars across numerous domains (e.g., Becker, 1999; Fredrickson & Branigan, 2005; Yaniv & Choshen-Hillel, 2012). Some streams of research tend to look at one adaptive response (e.g., aggression; Dollard et al., 1939), others consider many (e.g., terror-management theory; Greenberg, Pyszczynski, & Solomon, 1986). Goal disruption theory attempts to uncover the breadth of adaptive changes that might occur.

The range of automatic and adaptive responses that occur as a result of goal disruption (i.e., a state of psychological disequilibrium caused by an expectancy violation) are placed into five categories: 1) *ability*, 2) *disposition*, 3) *allocation of mental resources*, 4) *processing and perception*, and 5) *tactics*. These adaptive processes are interdependent; they constitute parts of a system. For example, changes in allocations of resources will cause changes in processing and disposition. Changes in processing will cause changes in ability and tactics. Changes in ability will influence the tactics used.

Automatic Changes in Ability

A patient's ability to learn about the goal expectancy violation, including ways of returning to equilibrium, can increase while in a state of disruption. However, a patient in disruption will be unable to think and behave on a higher level (Lewin, 1951). This reduction in cognitive complexity is associated with a variety of deficits. To begin, there is less fluidity with which to switch between goals (Lewin, 1941); also, a renal patient in a state of disruption will have a reduced ability to accomplish simultaneous goals at once (Lewin, 1941). There will also be a decrease in the variety of the behavior exhibited (Lewin, 1951). The disrupted patient will also be less creative (e.g., Isen, Daubman, & Nowicki, 1987) and will exhibit a reduced ability to come up with alternative solutions (e.g., Lewin, 1941; Plessow, Kiesel, Kirschbaum, & Fischer, 2012). Further, as will be mentioned in the discussion of resource allocation, solutions will be chosen without any consideration for economy of action (i.e., striving to obtain a maximum result with minimal effort; Lewin, 1941). The disrupted patient will also be less likely to control his or her impulses (Hofmann, Friese, & Wiers 2008) and less likely to pull him- or herself out of the situation (Marien, Aarts, & Custers, 2012). In other words, a patient in disruption will be unlikely to "rise above" the current situation because they are automatically committed to the most immediate return to equilibrium possible. Further impairing the disrupted patient's abilities, the patient will be fixated on resolving the disruption; put another way, the patient will not be able to shut out thoughts on the topic or focus on anything unrelated (Bryant & Harvey, 1995). The patient will only be able to focus on returning to equilibrium (Nissim et al., 2012).

Automatic Changes in Disposition

A patient in disruption will exhibit characteristics and temperament that are not common to the patient. These changes are not random, but purposive. The patient is in survival mode caused by the unexpected occurrence; focusing on the self and perceiving uncertainty and ambiguity as noxious is an adaptive response to the situation (Hogg, 2007, 2009).

For example, compared to the patient's norm, a lower tolerance for ambiguity (Smock, 1955), an increased desire for structure (Ardnt & Solomon, 2003), an increased need for certainty (Hogg, 2007), and an increased need for closure (Kruganski & Webster, 1996) will be exhibited. Further insight into dispositional changes can be gleaned from scholarship focused on the automatic responses that occur when a person is experiencing positive emotions. Specifically, given that positive emotions have been empirically revealed to be associated with increased concern for others (Thomson & Siegel, 2013), more openness to new experiences (Fredrickson & Branigan, 1998), more optimism (Froh, Kashdan, Ozmkowski, & Miller, 2009), and more trust (Dunn & Schweitzer, 2005), the opposite may also be true. Patients in a state of disruption should be less empathetic, more conservative regarding new experiences, less optimistic, and less trusting.

Because some renal patients will be hyper-focused on returning to equilibrium, such a patient will also likely be more irritable and hostile toward anything impeding a return to balance (Berkowitz, 1960, 1989; Dollard, Doob, Miller, Mower, & Sears, 1939; Erikson, 1959; Zander, 1944). The patient will be closed to feedback that is not specific to regaining goal integrity (Trope & Pomerantz, 1998) and egocentrism will be exhibited (Becker, 1999); the disrupted patient will also be less inclined to take the other person's perspective (Hale & Delia, 1976). The patient will be more defensive and less willing to forgive (DeShea, 2003), which can be particularly problematic if the patient is in disruption when a family member is unwilling to come forward as a donor. Again, these dispositional changes, such as egocentrism are not due to the patient becoming evil, but rather an automatic and adaptive response to the state of disequilibrium being experienced.

Automatic Changes in Allocation of Mental Resources

When in disruption, a patient's mental resources will automatically be distributed toward understanding the violation and restoring equilibrium (Moriya & Tanno, 2009; Tolman, 1932). Also, as all resources are allocated to restoring equilibrium, no resources are dedicated to other needs that the individual might possess—in the current moment, satiation is the only goal (Conway, Meares, & Standart, 2004; Cropanzano, Citera, Howes, 1995). As described by Lewin (1951), there will be little or no economy of action; all resources are applied regardless of whether all resources are actually needed. There will be little to no concern for the problems that might be caused as a result of shifting resources away from other goals.

Automatic Changes in Processing and Perception

Lewin (1941, 1951) and Tolman (1932, 1959) often noted that a person would see the world differently based on their state of mind. Tolman focused on variables such as attention bias and learning. Lewin theorized about changes in cognitive simplicity and the inability of someone experiencing frustration, insecurity, and emotional tension to think at a higher level. Changes in processing and perception posited by GDT are absconded from the thoughts of Tolman and Lewin, as well as the theoretical advances made since.

Tolman's (1932) discussion of processing and perception while in a heightened drive state posits the disrupted person will have an attention bias toward salient stimuli and a hyper bias toward anything perceived as relevant or threatening. A patient in disruption will also exhibit hyper-vigilance and oversensitivity to surroundings regarding violation-specific information (Weiss, 2004). Information perceived to be relevant to the disruption is processed with vigilance; information perceived irrelevant is relatively ignored (Zotter & Crowther, 1991). The importance of the goal is also exaggerated (Pinquart, Nixdorg-Hanchen, & Silbereisen, 2005), the fear of failure is exaggerated, the outcomes associated with failure are amplified, and a reduced likelihood of success is perceived (House & Perney, 1974; Nakhleh et al., 2011). Parts of the patient's memories, expectations, and beliefs will not be accessible, and commitment to one specific chosen course of action will increase (Wolff & Moser, 2008). These processes are not necessarily negative. It is useful for a hungry person to notice food more quickly than someone who is not hungry. However, not all adaptive processes are useful in every context.

Lewin's theorizing further elucidates changes in processing and perception that occur during what GDT refers to as a disruption. At the heart of Lewin's theorizing was that frustration would cause a change, "from an abstract to a more concrete type of thinking, from reasoning to learning, from flexible to stereotyped behavior" (p. 95, 1951). The patient becomes less cognitively complex (Lewin, 1951), the patient's processing becomes less flexible (Lewin, 1951), and the patient's thinking will be less organized (Lewin, 1951). The patient will be more likely to exhibit absolutistic, dichotomous thinking (Byrne, Dove, Watt, & Nathan, 2008), and will be more likely to believe that others see the world as they do (Koenig & King, 1964).

Goal disruption theory also proposes that even if the patient does not want to think about the topic, they will not be able to think about anything else. Scholars have described this specific phenomenon as intrusive thoughts, frequent reappraisals, and rumination (e.g., Lazarus, 1991; Nissim et al., 2012;). Rumination, which is known to instigate and maintain mental disorders (de Jong-Meyer, Beck, & Riede, 2009), will persist until there is a return to psychological equilibrium (Martin & Tesser, 1989). Ruminative response styles may act as a barrier to complex thinking and interpersonal problem solving (Lyubomirsky, Tucker, Cladwell, & Berg, 1999).

Automatic Changes in Tactics

Not only will the disrupted patient see the world differently and have different capabilities available to them, the disrupted patient will also take an altered approach to behavioral engagement. A patient in disruption will take the most direct approach toward achieving equilibrium (Shows, Gentry, & Wyrick, 1974). Indeed, people not receiving the expected reward have been reported to respond with increased vigor (Amsel & Hancock, 1957). As eloquently noted by Barker, Dembo, and Lewin (1941), "If the tension in frustrating situations is too high, the actions in the direction of the goal are likely to become emotional and more primitive" (p. 184). As further described by Barker, Dembo, and Lewin (1941), "instead of trying to find round-about routes in an organized systematic way, direct actions occur which are frequently vague and primitive in character" (p. 184). The direct or aggressive approach (Zander, 1944) can be considered the result of focusing only on the immediate, not having any cognitive flexibility, and not seeing nuances. Put differently, the patient will not have as many behavioral options available due to the intense focus on returning to equilibrium, which includes a narrowing of the psychological environment (Lewin, 1941). The direct approach is likely seen as the only approach. Further, as the disrupted patient is less open to feedback, it is unlikely that the disrupted patient will make good use of trial and error.

The patient will be highly likely to exhibit purposive aggression and purposive risk taking (Siegel, 2011; Siegel et al., 2012; see also Rosenberg et al., in press). In other words, the more intense the level of disruption, the more the individual will be willing to injure themselves, physically or otherwise, if it would lead to their desired goal. Collateral damage is likely irrelevant, and future ramifications of behavior are likely inaccessible to the disrupted individual (Lewin, 1951). They will be unlikely to consider the most efficient means of reaching their goal; instead, they will be focused on the quickest route to equilibrium.

Reducing Harms of Disruption in the Renal Context

Once again, please imagine a situation where a renal patient attempted to indirectly communicate their need for an organ donor to their family. The patient expected at least one person to come forward, yet no one did. Ideally, the renal patient would be able to think of the numerous reasons as to why no one came forward to donate an organ (e.g., no one realized that the renal patient was making an indirect request). The patient would ideally be able to consider other ways of finding a living donor (e.g., communicating more directly, indirectly asking more people). A patient who experiences goal disruption, however, will be unlikely to take other people's perspective or come up with creative solutions. Further, if the disrupted patient wants to lash out, he or she will have less than typical willpower to refrain. If the patient is too disrupted to be at his or her intellectual best, medical personnel can possibly offer basic cognitive coaching. Further, medical personnel can help the patient consider possible reasons as to why no one volunteered to donate while providing the patient assistance in discovering alternative approaches for finding a living donor (e.g., indirectly asking friends and extended family). Providing the patient tools for overcoming the inclination to engage in impulsive behavior can also be beneficial.

Regarding changes in disposition, the disrupted renal patient will exhibit characteristics different than what is typical. While trying to understand why no one volunteered to be a living donor, the patient will be more neurotic, less empathetic, more selfish, less forgiving, and more easily frustrated with uncertainty. Medical personnel can assist the disrupted patient by making them self-aware of the dispositional changes that are occurring. The patient can be provided with tools that will allow for increased self-monitoring. Alerting family members to the changes they might observe in their loved one could serve as another means of helping the disrupted renal patient. Family members might be able to be more sympathetic and more helpful if they are made aware that the renal patient is not fully to blame for the behavioral transgressions likely to be exhibited (Weiner, 1980).

Medical personnel might also be able to minimize harm caused by changes in the patient's allocation of resources. When disruption occurs, most of the patient's resources will be focused on orchestrating a return to psychological equilibrium. The renal patient would also benefit if medical practitioners were able to expand the patient's scope of consideration. If no one comes forward to donate, and this puts the patient in a state of disruption, encouraging the patient to focus on other aspects of their life and helping the patient do so could allow for the tunnel vision focus to subside. If other, more satiated, components of the patient's life are considered, there is a chance of reducing the persistent disequilibrium caused by the disruption. Further, medical personnel can inform family members of the patient's fixation on a goal and ask for assistance in helping the patient to broaden the range of the goals deemed important to the patient. With proper guidance, family can help the patient think of the other goals that he or she has accomplished or wants to accomplish.

The patient will also be processing and perceiving the world differently than he or she would have otherwise. For example, the patient will have a reduced time perspective, engage in biased processing, and will be more likely to make false consensus errors. The disrupted patient will also make more casual attributions, ruminate more, use increased stereotyping, and will be more likely to engage in dichotomous thinking. Medical personnel could be critical in the patient being able to accurately process their environment. For example, as perspective taking will be reduced, medical personnel could help the patient to be cognizant of the perspectives of others. The patient could be helped to understand why people might not have come forward to donate (e.g., concerns about their children, lack of information, lack of awareness of the indirect request). As the renal patient will be processing in an all-or-nothing manner, the patient might think, "Clearly my family does not care about me. If they did, they would have volunteered to donate." Medical personnel can help the patient see the range of possible reasons why family member might care deeply, but not be able to donate. Medical personnel can help reduce the tunnel vision, help the patient see things from a different perspective, let the patient know of expected changes in processing that are occurring (e.g., an increased belief that everyone else will share one's point of view), and expand the range of considerations contemplated by the patient.

The patient who expected someone to come forward, only to have that expectation violated, will also have to decide what to do next. Goal disruption theory explains that a disrupted patient will choose the most direct path, regardless of the collateral damage to the self, other people, and other goals. There will be a decrease in the variety of behaviors that are considered and the actions will be wrought with impulsivity. As with the other changes caused by goal disruption, medical personnel can inform the patient and family members of the changes that could occur. Working with renal patients to be cognizant of the changes they will experience can help them adjust their thoughts and actions accordingly. Convincing patients to get assistance in extensively weighing the costs and benefits, both short and long term, of each behavior being considered, can minimize the potentially harmful aspects of this adaptive change.

A final consideration: Knowing the goals that are most salient to the renal patient can maximize the utility of GDT. If a renal patient is fixated on the health and wellness of their family, the patient will engage in very different thoughts and actions than if the patient was fixated on his or her own survival. Patients concerned about their families above all else will impulsively refuse to accept a living donation from a loved one; a patient fixated on self-survival will impulsively accept. Knowing the goals that were most intensely violated by the renal disease diagnosis might be a crucial first step in assisting patients with renal disease. Fortunately, a simple question such as "What would make your life perfect?" could possibly help practitioners obtain a quick image of the goals activated in the mind of the renal patient (Rosenberg et al., in press; Siegel, 2004).

CONCLUSION

The goal of this chapter was to use GDT to elucidate changes in thoughts and actions that can occur as a result of a renal disease diagnosis, with a focus on the living donation process. Goal disruption theory was not created specifically for this context; however, it is clearly applicable. If medical practitioners contemplate the variables that are associated with an increased likelihood of goal disruption, steps might to be taken to prevent a goal disruption from occurring. Further, if a goal disruption appears inevitable, GDT can inform medical personnel as to the intensity with which the disruption will likely be experienced. Knowing the adaptive changes that goal disruption may cause can help minimize the impact that the adaptive changes have on the renal patient and the patient's family when disruption does occur. Simply, consideration and application of GDT can positively influence the course of treatment for patients with renal disease.

REFERENCES

Alvaro, E. A., Siegel, J. T., Turcotte, D., Lisha, N., Crano W. D. & Dominick, S. A. (2008). Hispanic living kidney donation: A qualitative examination of barriers and opportunities. *Progress in Transplantation*, *18*, 243-250.

Amici, F., Aureli, F., Visalberghi, E. & Call, J. (2009). Spider monkeys (Ateles geoffroyi) and capuchin monkeys (Cebus apella) follow gaze around barriers: evidence for perspective taking? *Journal of Comparative Psychology*, *123*, 368–74. doi:10.1037/a0017079.

Amsel, A. & Hancock, W. (1957). Motivational properties of frustration. III. Relation of frustration effect to antedating goal factors. *Journal of Experimental Psychology*, *53*, 126-131.

Antonovsky, A. (1987). *Unraveling the mystery of health: How people manage stress and stay well.* San-Francisco, CA: Jossey-Bass.

Ardnt, J. & Solomon, S. (2003). The control of death and the death of control: The effects of mortality salience, neuroticism, and worldview threat on the desire for control. *Journal of Research In Personality*, *37*, 1-22. doi:10.1016/S0092-6566(02)00530-5.

Auerbach, R. P., Abela, J. Z., Ho, M., McWhinnie, C. M. & Czaikowska, Z. (2010). A prospective examination of depressive symptomology: Understanding the relationship between negative events, self-esteem, and neuroticism. *Journal Of Social And Clinical Psychology*, *29*, 438-461. doi:10.1521/jscp.2010.29.4.438.

Bandura, A. (1977). Self-efficacy: Toward a unifying theory of behavioral change. *Psychological Review*, *84*, 191-215. doi:10.1037/0033-295X.84.2.191.

Barker, R. R., Dembo, T. T. & Lewin, K. K. (1941). Frustration and regression: an experiment with young children. *University Of Iowa Studies: Child Welfare*, *18,* xv-314. Becker, G. (1999). *Disrupted lives: How people create meaning in a chaotic world.* Berkley, California: University of California Press.

Berkowitz, L. L. (1960). Repeated frustrations and expectations in hostility arousal. *The Journal of Abnormal and Social Psychology*, *60*, 422-429. doi:10.1037/h0044601.

Berkowitz, L. (1989). Frustration-aggression hypothesis: Examination and reformulation. *Psychological Bulletin*, *106*, 59-73. doi:10.1037/0033-2909.106.1.59.

Bettencourt, B., Dill, K. E., Greathouse, S. A., Charlton, K., & Mulholland, A. (1997). Evaluations of ingroup and outgroup members: The role of category-based expectancy violation. *Journal of Experimental Social Psychology, 33,* 244-275.

Bizer, G. Y., Larsen, J. T. & Petty, R. E. (2011). Exploring the valence-framing effect: Negative framing enhances attitude strength. *Political Psychology*, *32*, 59-80. doi:10. 1111/j.1467- 9221.2010.00795.x.

Bolles, R. (1972). Reinforcement, expectancy, and learning. *Psychological Review*, *79*(5), 394-409.

Britt, S. H. & Janus, S. Q. (1940). Criteria of frustration. *Psychological Review*, *47*, 451-470. doi:10.1037/h0061381.

Bryant, R. A. & Harvey, A. G. (1995). Psychological impairment following motor vehicle accidents. *Australian journal of public health, 19*, 185-188.

Byrne, S., Allen, K., Dove, E., Watt, F. & Nathan, P. (2008). The reliability and validity of the dichotomous thinking in eating disorders scale. *Eating Behaviors, 9*, 154-162. doi:10.1016/j.eatbeh.2007.07.002.

Cannon, W. B. (1920). *Bodily changes in pain hunger fear and rage.* New York, NY: D. Appleton & Company.

Cannon, W. B. (1926). Physiological regulation of normal states: some tentative postulates concerning biological homeostatics. *Jubilee volume for Charles Richet*, 91-93.

Cannon, W. B. (1932). *Wisdom of the body.* New York, NY: WW Norton & Company.

Cannon, W. B. (1941). The body physiologic and the body politic. *Science, 93*, 1-10.

Caress, A., Luker, K. & Ackrill, P. (1999). Exploring the effect of renal disease and its treatment on patients' well-being: Across sectional study of anxiety and depression in a sample of renal patients. *Clinical Effectiveness in Nursing, 2*, 185-196.

Carver, C. S., Lehman, J. M. & Antoni, M. H. (2003). Dispositional pessimism predicts illness- related disruption of social and recreational activities among breast cancer patients. *Journal of Personality and Social Psychology, 84*, 813-821. doi:10.1037/0022-3514.84.4.813.

Chen, C. Y. & Hong, R. Y. (2010). Intolerance of uncertainty moderates the relation between negative life events and anxiety. *Personality and Individual Differences, 49*, 49-53.

Chilcot, J., Wellsted, D., Da Silve-Gane, M. & Farrington, K. (2008). Depression on dialysis. *Nephron Clinical Practice, 108*, 256-264.

Clary, E. & Tesser, A. (1983). Reactions to unexpected events: The naive scientist and interpretive activity. *Personality and Social Psychology Bulletin, 9*, 609-620. doi:10. 1177/0146167283094010.

Conklin, A. M., Dahling, J. J. & Garcia, P. A. (2013). Linking affective commitment, career self-efficacy, and outcome expectations A test of social cognitive career theory. *Journal of Career Development, 40*, 68-83.

Conway, M. A., Meares, K. & Standart, S. (2004). Images and goals. *Memory, 12*, 525-531. doi:10.1080/09658210444000151.

Crano, W. D. & Prislin, R. (2008). *Attitudes and attitude change.* Boca Raton, Florida: CRC Press.

Cropanzano, R., Citera, M. & Howes, J. (1995). Goal hierarchies and plan revision. *Motivation And Emotion, 19,* 77-98. doi:10.1007/BF02250564.

Cumming, J. & Ramsey, R. (2011). Investigating the effect of model type and practice format on performance expectations and actual physical performance. *International Journal Of Sport And Exercise Psychology, 9*, 267-283. doi:10.1080/1612197X.2011.614852.

de Jong-Meyer, R., Beck, B. & Riede, K. (2009). Relationships between rumination, worry, intolerance of uncertainty and metacognitive beliefs. *Personality & Individual Differences, 46*, 547-551. doi:10.1016/j.paid.2008.12.010.

DeShea, L. (2003). A Scenario-Based Scale of Willingness to Forgive. *Individual Differences Research, 1*, 201-217.

Devins, G. M., Binik, Y. M., Hollomby, D. J., Barre, P. E. & Guttmann, R. D. (1981). Helplessness and depression in end-stage renal disease. *Journal of Abnormal Psychology, 90*, 531.

Devins, G. M., Hunsley, J., Mandin, H., Taub, K. J. & Paul, L. C. (1997). The marital context of end-stage renal disease: Illness intrusiveness and perceived changes in family environment. *Annals of Behavioral Medicine*, *19*, 325-332.

Dollard, J., Doob, L., Miller, N.E., Mowrer, O.H. & Sears, R.R. (1939). *Frustration and aggression.* New Haven, CT: Yale University Press.

Dunn, J. R. & Schweitzer, M. E. (2005). Feeling and believing: the influence of emotion on trust. *Journal of personality and social psychology*, *88*, 736-748.

Elliot-Smith, G. G. (1928). *The evolution of man. (2nd ed.).* Oxford, England: Univ. Press.

Erikson, E. H. (1959). *Identity and the life cycle: selected papers.* Oxford, England: International Universities Press.

Erikson, E. H. (1968). *Identity: youth and crisis.* Oxford, England: Norton & Co.

Fazio, R. H. (1995). Attitudes as object-evaluation associations: Determinants, consequences, and correlates of attitude accessibility. In R. E. Petty, J. A. Krosnick (Eds.), *Attitude strength: Antecedents and consequences* (247-282). Hillsdale, NJ England: Lawrence Erlbaum Associates, Inc.

Feather, N. T. (1969). Cognitive differentiation attitude strength, and dogmatism. *Journal of Personality*, *37*, 111-126. doi:10.1111/j.1467-6494.1969.tb01734.x.

Festinger, L. (1957). *A theory of cognitive dissonance.* Evanston, IL: Row, Peterson.

Franklin, P. M. & Crombie, A. K. (2003). Live related renal transplantation: psychological, social, and cultural issues. *Transplantation*, *76*, 1247-1252.

Frauenfelder, K. J. (1974). A cognitive determinant of favorability of impression. *The Journal of Social Psychology*, *94*, 71-81.

Frederickson, B. L. & Carstensen, L. L. (1998). *Choosing social partners: How old age and anticipated endings make people more selective.* In M. Lawton, T. A. Salthouse (Eds.), Essential papers on the psychology of aging (511-538). New York, NY US: New York University Press.

Fredrickson, B. L. (2001). The role of positive emotions in positive psychology: The broaden-and-build theory of positive emotions. *American Psychologist*, *56*, 218-226. doi:10.1037/0003-066X.56.3.218.

Fredrickson, B. L. & Branigan, C. (2005). Positive emotions broaden the scope of attention and thought-action repertoires. *Cognition And Emotion*, *19*, 313-332. doi:10.1080/02699930441000238.

Frings, D., Hurst, J., Cleveland, C., Blascovich, J. & Abrams, D. (2012). Challenge, threat, and subjective group dynamics: Reactions to normative and deviant group members. *Group Dynamics: Theory, Research, And Practice*, *16*, 105-121. doi:10.1037/a0027504.

Froh, J. J., Kashdan, T. B., Ozimkowski, K. M. & Miller, N. (2009). Who benefits the most from a gratitude intervention in children and adolescents? Examining positive affect as a moderator. *The Journal Of Positive Psychology*, *4*, 408-422. doi:10.1080/17439760902992464.

Fuhrman, R. W., Flannagan, D. & Matamoros, M. (2009). Behavior expectations in cross-sex friendships, same-sex friendships, and romantic relationships. *Personal Relationships*, *16*, 575-595. doi:10.1111/j.1475-6811.2009.01240.x.

Ganikos, M. (2010). Organ donation: An overview of the field. In J. T. Siegel, E. M Alvaro (Eds.), *Understanding Organ Donation: Applied Behavioral Science Perspectives* (13-39). Hoboken, NJ US: Blackwell Publishing.

Gonzalez, A. V., Siegel, J. T, Alvaro, E. M. & O'Brien (in press). Depression and Physician Patient Communication Among Hispanic End-Stage Renal Disease Patients. *Journal of Health Communication.*

Gordon, E. J. (2001). "They don't have to suffer for me": Why dialysis patients refuse offers of living donor kidneys. *Medical Anthropology Quarterly, 15*, 245-267.

Grolnick, W. S., Friendly, R. W. & Bellas, V. M. (2009). Parenting and children's motivation at school. In K. R. Wenzel, A. Wigfield (Eds.), *Handbook of motivation at school* (279-300). New York, NY US: Routledge/Taylor & Francis Group.

Greenberg, J., Pyszcynski, T. & Solomon, S. (1986). The causes and consequences of a need for self-esteem: A terror management theory. In R. F. Baumeister (Ed.) *Public self and private self* (189-212). New York: Springer-Verlag.

Gurland, S. T., Grolnick, W. S. & Friendly, R. W. (2012). The role of expectations in children's experience of novel events. *Journal of Experimental Child Psychology, 113*, 305-321.

Hale, C. L. & Delia, J. G. (1976). Cognitive complexity and social perspective-taking. *Communication Monographs, 43*, 195-203. doi:10.1080/03637757609375932.

Harkness, K. L. & Lumley, M. N. (2007). Child abuse and neglect and the development of depression in children and adolescents. In J. R. Abela & B. L. Hankin (Eds.), Handbook of depression in children and adolescents (466–488). New York: Guilford.

Harvey, J. H., Harkins, S. G. & Kagehiro, D. K. (1976). Cognitive tuning and the attribution of causality. *Journal of Personality and Social Psychology, 34*, 708-715. doi:10.1037/0022-3514.34.4.708.

Heider, F. (1958). *The psychology of interpersonal relations.* Hoboken, NJ US: John Wiley & Sons Inc. doi:10.1037/10628-000.

Henderson, M. D., de Liver, Y. & Gollwitzer, P. M. (2008). *Journal of Personality and Social Psychology, 94*, 396-411.

Henning, P. B. (2011). Disequilibrium, development and resilience through adult life. *Systems Research and Behavioral Science, 28*, 443-454.

Higgins, E. T. (1989). Self-discrepancy: A theory relating self and affect, *Psychological Review, 94*, 319-340.

Hofmann, W., Friese, M. & Wiers, R. W. (2008). Impulsive versus reflective influences on health behavior: A theoretical framework and empirical review. *Health Psychology Review, 2*, 111-137.

Hogg, M. A. (2007). Uncertainty-identity theory. In M. P. Zanna (Ed.), *Advances in experimental social psychology*, (Vol. 39, 69–126). San Diego, CA: Academic Press.

Hogg, M. A. (2009). Managing self-uncertainty through group identification. *Psychological Inquiry, 20*, 221–224.

House, W. C. & Perney, V. (1974). Valence of expected and unexpected outcomes as a function of locus of goal and type of expectancy. *Journal of Personality and Social Psychology, 29*, 454-463. doi:10.1037/h0036123.

Inhelder, B. & Piaget, J. (1958). *The growth of logical thinking.* London, England: Routledge & Kegan Paul.

Ionescu, T. (2012). Exploring the nature of cognitive flexibility. *New Ideas in Psychology, 30*, 190-200.

Isen, A. M., Daubman, K. A. & Nowicki, G. P. (1987). Positive affect facilitates creative problem solving. *Journal of Personality and Social Psychology, 52*, 1122-1131. doi:10. 1037/0022-3514.52.6.1122.

Kelley, D. L. & Burgoon, J. K. (1991). Understanding marital satisfaction and couple type as functions of relational expectations. *Human Communication Research, 18*, 40-69. doi:10. 1111/j.1468-2958.1991.tb00528.x.

Kessen, W. (1971). Early cognitive development: Hot or cold? In T. Mischel (Ed.), *Cognitive development and epistemology.* New York: Academic Press.

Kimmel, P. L. (2001). Psychosocial factors in dialysis patients. *Kidney International, 59*, 1599-1613.

Koenig, F. W. & King, M. B. (1964). Cognitive simplicity and outgroup stereotype. *Social Forces, 42*, 324-327. doi:10.2307/2575536.

Kohli, S., Batra, P. & Aggarwal, H. K. (2011). Anxiety, locus of control, and coping strategies among end-stage renal disease patients undergoing maintenance hemodialysis. *Indian Journal of Nephrology, 21*, 177-181.

Kregarman, J. J. & Worchel, P. (1961). Arbitrariness of frustration and aggression. *The Journal of Abnormal and Social Psychology, 63*, 183-187. doi:10.1037/h0044667.

Kranenburg, L., Zuidema, W., Weimer, W., Hilhorst, M, Ijzermans, J., Passcier, J. & Busschbach, J. (2009). Strategies to advance living kidney donation: a single center's experience. *Progress in Transplantation, 19*, 71-75.

Krosnick, J. A. & Petty, R. E. (1995). Attitude strength: An overview. In R. E. Petty, J. A. Krosnick (Eds.), *Attitude strength: Antecedents and consequences* (1-24). Hillsdale, NJ England: Lawrence Erlbaum Associates, Inc.

Kruglanski, A. W. & Webster, D. M. (1996). Motivated closing of the mind: 'Seizing' and 'freezing.'. *Psychological Review, 103*, 263-283. doi:10.1037/0033-295X.103.2.263.

Kugler, M. B., Cooper, J. & Nosek, B. A. (2010). Group-based dominance and opposition to equality correspond to different psychological motives. *Social Justice Research, 23*, 117-155. doi:10.1007/s11211-010-0112-5.

Lazarus, R. S. (1991). Progress on a cognitive-motivational-relational theory of emotion. *American Psychologist, 46*, 819-834. doi:10.1037/0003-066X.46.8.819.

Levealahti, H., Tishelman, C. & Ohlén, J. (2007). Framing the onset of lung cancer biographically: Narratives of continuity and disruption. *Psycho-Oncology, 16*, 466-473.

Lewandowski, J. A., Rosenberg, B. D., Parks, M. J. & Siegel, J. T. (2011). The effect of informal social support: Face-to-Face versus computer-mediated communication. *Computers in Human Behavior, 27*, 1806-1814.

Lewin, K. (1936). Psychology of success and failure. *Occupations, 14*, 926-930.

Lewin. K. (1941). Self-hatred among Jews. In K. Lewin (Ed.), *Resolving social conflicts: Selected papers on group dynamics* (186—200). New York: Harper & Brothers.

Lewin, K. (1946). Behavior and development as a function of the total situation. In L. Carmichael (Ed.), *Manual of child psychology* (791-844). Hoboken, NJ US: John Wiley & Sons Inc. doi:10.1037/10756-016.

Lewin, K. (1951). In D. Cartwright (Ed.), *Field theory in social science: Selected theoretical papers by Kurt Lewin.* New York: Harper & Row.

Lewin, K. (1959). *Field Theory in Social Science.* New York: Harper & Bros, 1959.

Lewis, K. (1998). Emotional adjustment to a chronic illness. *Lippincott's Primary Care Practice, 2*, 38-51.

Lipman-Blumen, J. (1973). Role de-differentiation as a system response to crisis: Occupational and political roles of women. *Sociological Inquiry*, *2*, 105-129.

Lovinger, J. (1976). *Ego development.* San Francisco, CA: Jossey-Bass.

Lyubomirsky, S., Tucker, K., Caldwell, N. & Berg, K. (1999). Why ruminators are poor problem solvers: clues from the phenomenology of dysphoric rumination. *Journal of Personality and Social Psychology*, *77*, 1041-1060.

MacGeorge, E. L., Homan, S. R., Dunning Jr., J. B., Elmore, D., Bodie, G. D., Evans, E., . . . Geddes, B. (2008). Student evaluation of audience response technology in large lecture classes. *Education Technology Research Development*, *56*, 125-145.

Marien, H., Aarts, H. & Custers, R. (2012). Being flexible or rigid in goal-directed behavior: When positive affect implicitly motivates the pursuit of goals or means. *Journal of Experimental Social Psychology*, *48*, 277-283.

Martin, L. L. & Tesser, A. (1989). Toward a motivational and structural theory of ruminative thought. In J. S. Uleman, J. A. Bargh (Eds.), *Unintended thought* (306-326). New York, NY US: Guilford Press.

McLaughlin, K. A. & Hatzenbuehler, M. L. (2009). Stressful life events, anxiety sensitivity, and internalizing symptoms in adolescents. *Journal of Abnormal Psychology*, *118*, 659-669. doi:10.1037/a0016499.

Meier-Krische H. Y., Arndorfer, J. A. & Kaplan, B. (2002). The impact of body mass index on renal transplant outcomes: A significant independent risk factor for graft failure and patient death. *Transplantation*, *73*, 70-74.

Mendes, W., Blascovich, J., Hunter, S. B., Lickel, B. & Jost, J. T. (2007). Threatened by the unexpected: Physiological responses during social interactions with expectancy-violating partners. *Journal of Personality and Social Psychology*, *92*, 698-716. doi:10.1037/0022-3514.92.4.698.

Moriya, J. & Tanno, Y. (2009). Competition between endogenous and exogenous attention to nonemotional stimuli in social anxiety. *Emotion*, *9*, 739-743. doi:10.1037/a0016817.

Moskowitz, G. B. (2009). The compensatory nature of goal pursuit: From explicit action to implicit cognition. In G. B. Moskowitz, H. Grant (Eds.), *The psychology of goals* (304-336). New York, NY US: Guilford Press.

Nakhleh, R. E., Myers, J. L., Allen, T. C., DeYoung, B. R., Fitzgibbons, P. L., Funkhouse, W. K., … & Silverman, J. F. (2011). *Archives of Pathology and Laboratory Medicine*, *136*, 148-154.

Neipp, M., Karavul, B., Jackobs, S., zu Vilsendorf, A. M., Richter, N., Becker, T., ... & Klempnauer, J. (2006). Quality of life in adult transplant recipients more than 15 years after kidney transplantation. *Transplantation*, *81*, 1640-1644.

Nissim, R., Rennie, D., Fleming, S., Hales, S., Gagliese, L. & Rodin, G. (2012). Goals set in the land of the living/dying: A longitudinal study of patients living with advanced cancer. *Death Studies*, *36*, 360-390.

Nordgren, L. F. & Chou, E. Y. (2012). A Devil on each shoulder: When (and why) greater cognitive capacity impairs self-control? Social Psychological and Personality Science, 0, 1-5, doi: 10.1177/1948550612451622.

Pennell, G. (1996). Integrating complexity into the study of life events: Comment on Suedfeld and Bluck (1993). *Journal Of Personality And Social Psychology*, *71*, 777-780. doi:10.1037/0022-3514.71.4.777.

Perls, F. S., Hefferline, R. F. & Goodman, P. (1951). *Gestalt therapy: Excitement and growth in the human personality.* New York: Julian Press.

Petty, R. E. & Krosnick, J. A. (1995). *Attitude strength: Antecedents and consequences.* Hillsdale, NJ England: Lawrence Erlbaum Associates, Inc.

Pinquart, M., Nixdorf-Hänchen, J. C. & Silbereisen, R. K. (2005). Associations of age and cancer with individual goal commitment. *Applied Developmental Science, 9,* 54-66. doi:10.1207/s1532480xads0902_2.

Plessow, F., Schade, S., Kirschbaum, C. & Fischer, R. (2012). Better not to deal with two tasks at the same time when stressed? Acute psychosocial stress reduces task shielding in dual- task performance. *Cognitive, Affective & Behavioral Neuroscience, 12,* 557-570. doi: 10.3758/s13415-012-0098-6.

Polonsky, W. H., Fisher, L., Guzman, S., Sieber, W. J., Phillis-Tsimikas, A. & Edelman, S. V. (2010). Are patients' initial experiences at the diagnosis of type 2 diabetes associated with attitudes and self-management over time? *The Diabetes Educator, 36,* 828-834.

Power, J., Brown, L. & Ritvo, P. (2008). A qualitative study examining psychosocial distress, coping, and social support across the stages and phases of epithelial ovarian cancer. *Health Care for Women International, 29,* 366-383.

Pradel, F. G., Suwannaprom, P., Mullins, C. D., Sadler, J. & Bartlett, S. T. (2008). Short-term impact of an educational program promoting live donor kidney transplantation in dialysis centers. *Progress in Transplantation, 18,* 263-272.

Prislin, R. (1996). Attitude stability and attitude strength: One is enough to make it stable. *European Journal of Social Psychology, 26,* 447-477. doi:10.1002/(SICI)1099-0992(199605)26:3<447::AID-EJSP768>3.0.CO;2-I.

Pyszczynski, T. A. & Greenberg, J. (1981). Role of disconfirmed expectancies in the instigation of attributional processing. *Journal Of Personality And Social Psychology, 40,* 31-38. doi:10.1037/0022-3514.40.1.31. Raup, R. B. (1925). *Complacency: The foundation of human behavior.* Macmillan: New York.

Richter, C. P. (1943). Total self-regulatory functions in animals and human beings. *Harvey Lecture Series, 38,* 1942-1943.

Rodrigue, J. R., Cornell, D. L., Kaplan, B. & Howard, R. J. (2008). A randomized trial of a home-based educational approach to increase live donor kidney transplantation: effects in blacks and whites. *American journal of kidney diseases: the official journal of the National Kidney Foundation, 51,* 663-670.

Rodrigue, J. R., Bonk, V. & Jackson, S. (2001). Psychological considerations of living organ donation. In *Biopsychosocial perspectives on transplantation* (59-70). Springer: New York.

Rosenberg, M. (1989). *Society and the adolescent self-image.* (Rev.ed.). Middeltown, CT: Wesleyan University Press.

Rosenberg, B. D., Lewandowski, J. A. & Siegel, J. T. (in press). Goal disruption theory, military personnel, and the creation of merged profiles: A mixed method >investigation. *Journal of Mixed Methods Research.*

Rosenthal, T. L. & Zimmerman, B. J. (1976). Organization and stability of transfer in vicarious concept attainment. *Child Development, 47,* 110-117. doi:10.2307/1128289.

Rotter, J. B. (1954). *Social learning and clinical psychology.* Upper Saddle River, NJ: Prentice- Hall.

Routledge, C. & Juhl, J. (2012). The creative spark of death: The effects of mortality salience and personal need for structure on creativity. *Motivation And Emotion*, *36*, 478-482. doi:10.1007/s11031-011-9274-1.

Schneider, S. L. (2001). In search of realistic optimism: Meaning, knowledge, and warm fuzziness. *American Psychologist*, *56*, 250-263. doi:10.1037/0003-066X.56.3.250.

Seidel, A. J., Franks, M. M., Stephens, M. & Rook, K. S. (2012). Spouse control and type 2 diabetes management: Moderating effects of dyadic expectations for spouse involvement. *Family Relations: An Interdisciplinary Journal Of Applied Family Studies*, *61*, 698-709. doi:10.1111/j.1741-3729.2012.00719.x.

Selye, H. (1956). *The stress of life*. New York: McGraw-Hill.

Shows, W., Gentry, W. & Wyrick, L. (1974). Social constriction in psychiatric patients: a normative study. *The American Journal of Psychiatry*, *131*, 1287-1288.

Siegel, J. T. & Alvaro, E. A., (Eds.). (2010). *Understanding Organ Donation: Applied Behavioral Science Approaches (*313-330). Malden: MA, Blackwell-Wiley.

Siegel, J. T. & Burgoon, J. K. (2002). Expectancy theory approaches to prevention: Violating adolescent expectations to increase the effectiveness of public service announcements. In W. D. Crano, M. Burgoon (Eds.), *Mass media and drug prevention: Classic and contemporary theories and research* (163-186). Mahwah, NJ US: Lawrence Erlbaum Associates Publishers.

Siegel, J. T. (2004). The imaginary audience, the personal fable, and a rival hypothesis: An alternative explanation for behavior typical of adolescence. Ph.D. dissertation, University of Arizona, United States – Arizona. Retrieved 13 March, 2013, from Dissertations & Theses: Full Text. (Publication No. AAT 3158156).

Siegel, J. T. (2011). Dying for romance: Risk taking as purposive behavior. *Psychology, Health and Medicine*, *16*, 719-726.

Siegel, J. T., Alvaro, E. M., Crano, W. D., Skendarian, J., Lac, A. & Patel, N. (2008). Reducing inhalant use by changing socio-personal expectations. *Prevention Science*, *9*, 153-165.

Siegel, J. T., Alvaro, E. A., Hohman, Z. A. & Mauer, D. (2011). "Can you spare an organ?" Exploring Hispanic Americans' willingness to discuss living organ donation with loved ones. *Health Communication*, *26*, 754-764.

Siegel, J. T., Alvaro, E., Lac, A., Crano, W. D., Alexander, S. (2008). Intentions of becoming a living organ donor among Hispanics: A theoretical approach exploring differences between living and non-living organ donation, *Journal of Health Communication*, *13*, 80-99.

Siegel, J. T., Crano, W. D., Alvaro, E. A., Lac, A, Rast, D. & Kettering, V. (2012). Dying to be popular: Why do adolescents go to extremes? In M. A. Hogg & Blaylock, D. (Eds.), *Extremism and the psychology of uncertainty* (163-186). Malden, MA: Wiley-Blackwell.

Simmons, R. G., Hickey, K., Kjellstrand, C. M. & Simmons, R. L. (1971). A kidney from the family. *British Medical Journal*, *4*, 229.

Simmons, R. G. & Klein, S. D. (1972). The search for kidney donors. *The American Journal of Psychiatry*, *129*, 687-692.

Skenderian, J., Siegel, J. T., Crano, W. D., Alvaro, E. & Lac, A. (2008). Expectancy violations and adolescents' intentions to use marijuana. *Psychology of Addictive Behaviors*, *22*, 563-569.

Smock, C. D. (1955). The influence of psychological stress on the 'intolerance of ambiguity.'. *The Journal Of Abnormal And Social Psychology, 50,* 177-182. doi:10.1037/h0047951.

Spital, A. & Jacobs, C. L. (2007). The beauty of the gift: the wonder of living organ donation. *Clinical transplantation, 21,* 435-440.

Tarantino, A. (2000). Why should we implement living donation in renal transplantation? *Clinical Nephrology, 53,* 55-63.

Thompson, R., Wiley, T. A., Lewis, T., English, D. J., Dubowitz, H., Litrownik, A. J. & ... Block, S. (2012). Links between traumatic experiences and expectations about the future in high risk youth. *Psychological Trauma: Theory, Research, Practice, And Policy, 4*(3), 293-302. doi:10.1037/a0023867.

Tolman, E. C. (1925). The nature of fundamental drives. *The Journal of Abnormal and Social Psychology, 20,* 349-358.

Tolman, E. C. (1926). A behavioristic theory of ideas. *Psychological Review, 33,* 352-369.

Tolman, E. C. & Honzik, C. H. (1930). Introduction and removal of reward, and maze performance in rats. *University of California Publications in Psychology, 4,* 257-275.

Tolman, E. C. (1932). *Purposive behavior in animals and men.* New York, NY: Century.

Tolman, E. C. (1933). Sign-Gestalt or conditioned reflex. *Psychological Review, 40,* 246-255.

Tolman, E. C. (1955). Principles of performance. *Psychological Review, 62,* 315-326.

Tolman, E. C. (1959). Principles of purposive behavior. *Psychology: A study of a science, 2,* 92- 157.

Tomaka, J., Blascovich, J., Kelsey, R. M. & Leitten, C. L. (1993). Subjective, physiological, and behavioral effects of threat and challenge appraisal. *Journal of Personality and Social Psychology, 65,* 248-260. doi:10.1037/0022-3514.65.2.248.

Thomson, A. L. & Siegel, J. T. (2013). A Moral Act, Elevation, and Prosocial Behavior: Moderators of Morality. *Journal of Positive Psychology, 8,* 50-64.

Trope, Y. & Pomerantz, E. M. (1998). Resolving conflicts among self-evaluative motives: Positive experiences as a resource for overcoming defensiveness. *Motivation And Emotion, 22,* 53-72. doi:10.1023/A:1023044625309.

van Rompay, T. L., de Vries, P. W., Bontekoe, F. & Tanja-Dijkstra, K. (2012). Embodied product perception: Effects of verticality cues in advertising and packaging design on consumer impressions and price expectations. *Psychology & Marketing, 29,* 919-928. doi:10.1002/mar.20574.

`Waterman, A. D., Rodrigue, J. R., Purnell, T. S., Ladin, K. & Boulware, L. E. (2010). Addressing racial/ethnic disparities in live donor kidney transplantation: Priorities for research and intervention. *Seminars in Nephrology, 30,* 90-98.

Weiner, B. (1980). May I borrow your class notes? An attributional analysis of help giving in an achievement-related context. *Journal of Educational Psychology, 72,* 676 – 681.

Weiss, D. S. (2004). The impact of event scale-revised. In J. P. Wilson & T. M. Keane (Eds.), *Assessing psychological trauma and PTSD: A practitioner's handbook* (2nd ed., 168–189). New York: Guildford.

Wiggins, J. A. (1965). Interaction structure, frustration, and the extensiveness and intensity of aggression. *Sociometry, 28,* 89-99. doi:10.2307/2786088.

Wolff, H. & Moser, K. (2008). Choice, accountability, and processing in escalation situations. *Journal of Psychology, 216,* 235-243.

Yaniv, I. & Choshen-Hillel, S. (2012). Exploiting the wisdom of others to make better decisions: Suspending judgment reduces egocentrism and increases accuracy. *Journal Of Behavioral Decision Making*, *25*, 427-434. doi:10.1002/bdm.740.

Young, W. R. & Hollands, M. A. (2012). Newly acquired fear of falling leads to altered eye movement patterns and reduced stepping safety: A case study. *Plos ONE*, *7*, doi:10.1371/journal.pone.0049765.

Zander, A. F. (1944). A study of experimental frustration. *Psychological Monographs*, *56*, i-38.

Zotter, D. L. & Crowther, J. H. (1991). The role of cognitions in bulimia nervosa. *Cognitive Therapy and Research*, *15*, 413-426.

In: Organ Donation and Transplantation
Editor: Mary Anne Lauri
ISBN: 978-1-62948-257-6

Chapter 8

I DO BUT I DON'T ... THE YES, BUT FACTOR IN ORGAN DONATION AND TRANSPLANTATION

***Gail Moloney*[*1], *Iain Walker*[†2] *and Tegan Charlton*[‡1]**
[1]Psychology, Southern Cross University, Coffs Harbour, NSW, Australia
[2]CSIRO, Social and Economic Sciences Program, Perth, WA, Australia

ABSTRACT

In Australia, the number of people requiring life-saving organ transplants greatly exceeds organ donation rates. In an attempt to address this disparity, health campaigns promote the idea that a donated organ is a gift – a gift of life. This sentiment is consistently endorsed by the majority of Australians, and is expected by many to translate into high donation rates. In this chapter we present research that has explored the disjuncture between donation rates and needs by conceptualising lay understandings about donation and transplantation as socially derived knowledge within the theory of social representations (Moscovici, 1984). We argue that what is perceived to be an alarming disjuncture is an artefact of linear thought, and not necessarily how the issue is socially understood. We argue that contradiction defines social thinking and, thus, how donation and transplantation is understood. Rather than conceptualising the difference between donation rates and needs as a linear distance that can be reduced by associating donation with a gift of life, we contend that low donation rates and high donation needs represent different aspects of a single representation containing contradictory elements. From this position, we translate our findings into strategies and practices for talking about donation.

* gail.moloney@scu.edu.au.
† Iain.A.Walker@csiro.au.
‡ t.charlton.11@student.scu.edu.au.

INTRODUCTION

An 18 year old boy dies instantly as a result of severe trauma to his head after the car he was driving collided with a truck. Within a medical framework, it appears not only logical but imperative that the organs from this young man are donated to alleviate the suffering of a few of the 1600 people in Australia who desperately need an organ transplant (Donate Life, 2011). In this paper we question the logicality of this argument by challenging the assumption of linear causality that seductively suggests that an expressed positive attitude towards organ donation will translate to actual donation behaviour.

In questioning that a favourable attitude will, by course, translate to actual donation we sought firstly to understand the reality of organ donation and transplantation in the non-medical world (Moloney & Walker, 2000; 2002; Moloney, Hall, & Walker, 2005). Articulated through the theory of social representations, we talk here of the socially derived and collectively concerted values, beliefs and behaviours associated with this issue (Moscovici, 1984).

Social representations serve a multiplicity of functions. They explain why things are the way they are, allow the justification of evaluative and moral judgments, position and prescribe social identities, and allow the naming and classifying of novel, or challenging ideas, people and things (Bauer & Gaskell, 1999). Emerging through interaction between individuals, groups and institutions, the constitutive nature of representations facilitates communication and emerges through communicative processes (Moscovici, 1988).

Conceptualised as such, organ donation becomes more than an individual attitude or behaviour; it is a shared understanding constructed through verbal and non-verbal interactions within a group, society or collective. This does not negate individual thought or experience; rather it makes apparent that the frameworks of what we understand emanate through communication (Moscovici, 1973; 1988). What is important here is that the meanings associated with an issue such as organ donation are created through social exchange, and are therefore fluid and negotiable as opposed to static and defined (see Moscovici, 1988).

Central to this approach is the tenet that social representations are not a vulgarisation, a distortion, or a diffusion of scientific knowledge; rather they are the ways in which 'objects are understood in the public domain' (Bauer & Gaskell, 2008, p. 338). This highlights that social representations may well be qualitatively different from their scientific counterpart in a sense that is not necessarily linear or predictable. In short, representations are simply how the issue is understood in the public domain (Bauer & Gaskell, 2008). This tenet is crucial to the argument we present here.

In our early work (Moloney, Hall & Walker, 2005), we pursued the question of how organ donation and transplantation was socially understood, by asking people what their first thoughts were when they thought of organ donation. Interestingly, irrespective of whether the response was to organ donation, organ transplantation, or both organ donation and transplantation, the elicited associations were always contradictory in affect. That is, when respondents were asked to write the first 5 words that sprung to mind[4], the elicitations coalesced around positive evaluative ideological responses such as *life, worthwhile, benefit to humanity, a gift*, and negatively-connoted social practices such as *death, operation, accident,*

[4] Participants were randomly assigned to respond to either organ donation, organ transplantation or organ donation and transplantation (see Moloney et al., 2005).

and *spare parts*. Together, the elicitations suggested a consensual, but contradictory, semantic network of meanings associated with this issue.

These dilemmatic elicitations were also a central feature of respondents' discourse in our 2002 study that examined how people talk about organ donation and transplantation (Moloney & Walker, 2002). Qualifiers allowed the "illogicality" of the seeming contradiction of simultaneously holding a position endorsing the practice, meritoriously interpreted as a benefit to society, with a position expressing concerns over issues such as mutilation of the body and the validity of brain death. The two 'contradictory' positions were reconciled within the one representation. For example, a pro-donation stance such as *Organ donation is a service to humanity* was coupled with or followed by a qualifying statement such as *thinking of them as hunk of meat, like a piece of sheep – that is what doctors think* (Moloney & Walker, 2002. p.309).

Our early work also traced the genesis and change of the social representation (Moloney & Walker, 2000), showing how initially the possibility of transplanting organs from one human to another was anchored in existing representations at the time, and how donation and transplantation came to be iconised. Major, well-publicised events such as the advent of immune-suppressant drugs and the subsequent long term success of heart transplants led to identifiable changes in how this issue was socially represented. Social representations are constantly changing, partly in response to events in the social environment, and partly in response to internal tensions.

For these reasons, we recently conducted another word association task, curious to know how the issue of organ donation was now socially understood. This new study was conducted seven years after our original study, and was completed by respondents who resided in a regional area on the East Coast of Australia as opposed to an urban city on the West Coast, where our 2005 study was conducted (Charlton, 2012). In total, 1189 associations were elicited from 533 participants. After cleaning and homogenisation, the most frequency occurring word categories were retained for further analysis[5] (see Charlton, 2012 for further details). The semantic relationship of these elicitations is shown in the solution from a Multi-Dimensional Scaling (MDS) analysis of the extent that each of the most frequently occurring word categories co-occurred in any one respondent's elicitations (Figure 1).

We were surprised to note the similarity between our earlier data of 2005 and the more recent data of 2012. In the latter data set shown in Figure 1, elicitations in response to the stimulus phrase *Organ Donation* were again contradictory in affect, and dominated by the words *life* and *death*. The semantic network appears as much about *life*, *saving lives*, *help,* and *selfless* as it is about *death*, *accident*, *grief* and *pain*. The robustness of the similarity between the early and latter data sets, particularly in relation to centrality of *life* and *death,* suggested to us that little had changed in how this issue was socially represented.

There was, however, one noticeable absence in the word association data of 2012 compared to 2005, and that was the elicitation of the phrase *spare part*. In our 2005 data *spare part was* frequently associated with all stimulus words. It was also a central feature of the discourse in our 2002 focus group discussions. We suggest that whilst the core ideas and values central to the representation have not changed since 2005, the manifestation of these

---

[5] These word categories had a frequency magnitude above 1. Frequency Magnitude = 100/ sum of all frequencies in data set * raw frequency of term. A percentage figure that takes the axiomatic frequency count and relates it to the size of the data set from which the frequency value was derived (see Callaghan, Moloney & Blair, 2012).

core ideas in language in 2012 has. Thus, the absence of the term *spare part* may reflect the lack of discursive use of this term today given that other mechanistic terms such as cutting, disfigurement[6] were elicited in our 2012 data set (see Core theory: Abric, 1993). This latter point may also be tied to the sample characteristics (2012 sample comprised university staff and students whilst the 2005 comprised of community members) or the currency of the phrase in 2012.

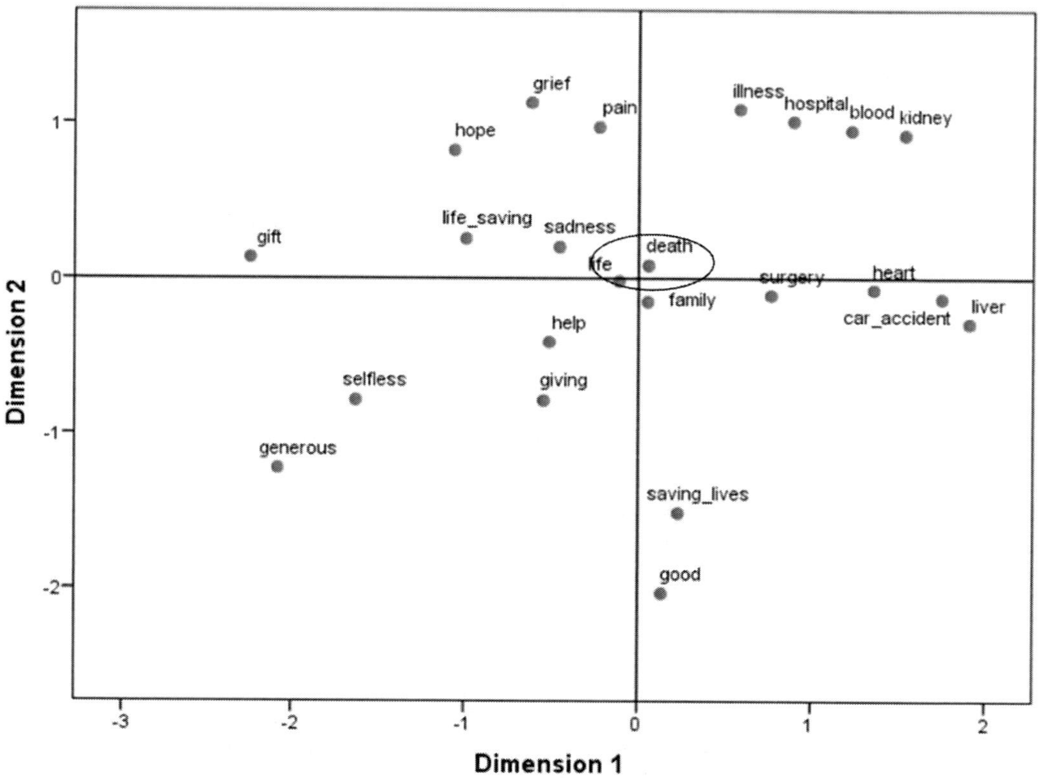

Figure 1. Two-Dimensional MDS solution of co-occurrence matrix for words elicited to stimulus phrase Organ Donation: S-Stress =.19, RSQ = 79[7]. The ellipse shows elicitations with highest frequency of co-occurrence.

Organ Donation and Contradictory Thinking

Theoretically, contradictory or dilemmatic thinking is both a part and a product of the co-construction of social knowledge through the Self-Other-Object as depicted in the representation triad in Figure 2 (Markova, 2006; also Billig, 1987; Billig, Condor, Edwards, Gane, Middleton & Radley, 1988).

The representational triad of the Self-Other-Object typifies how an individual's knowledge of a social object, such as organ donation, is mediated by relevant others. Put

[6] See Charlton (2012) for further detail.

[7] Diagonal of co-occurrence matrix was the absolute frequency of occurrence. Euclidean were distances used.

simply, the frameworks within which an issue is understood are first and foremost socially-derived. This implies consensus otherwise the collectively concerted understandings that constitute a social representation could not exist. Consensus here refers to consensual reality as opposed to majority agreement (Rose, Efraim, Gervais, Joffe, Jovchelovitch & Morant. 1995; Moloney et al., 2005).

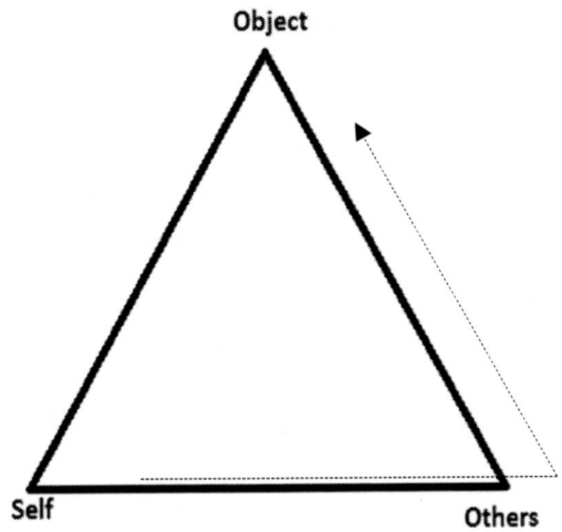

Figure 2. Self-Others-Object representational triad: See Bauer & Gaskell, (1999); Markova (2006); Wagner & Hayes (2005)

Consensual reality pertains to the shared, historically-derived meanings about a social object that provide a mutual framework for people to discuss, argue and negotiate within (Rose et al., 1995). Consensual reality does not imply that individuals hold the same views about an issue, but rather that individuals have a tacit awareness and understanding as to how that issue is understood by the group, society or collective. Disagreement with, and negotiation about and around, these socially derived understandings can occur because this mutual understanding provides the parameters for communication (Rose, et al., 2005; Moloney 2007)

Representations emerge at times of challenge, at points where the goals of different groups cross or "societal fault-lines" occur, as collective ways of coping with something new or unfamiliar (Bauer & Gaskell, 1999, p.178). In 1967, Christian Barnard's ground breaking heart transplant propelled medical views about organ donation and transplantation into the lay world, challenging the non-medical world as the implications of what had been performed were reconciled with the inconceivable nature of the procedure (Moloney & Walker, 2000). Nearly 40 years later, the tension between the benefit and the practise still exists. We use the concept of themata to explain why.

Themata

From a dialogical argument, antinomies are central to human thought and communication (Markova, 2003). Conceptualised interdependently, these oppositional taxonomies have been posited to serve as the focal point for emergent social representations. By this we mean they give both structure and form to how social understandings about an issue form within a group, society or collective. As source ideas they are generative; they emerge and re-emerge with the social context of the time allowing old ideas to be blended with the new, the past with the present, and the traditional with the modern. Themata such as edible/inedible, self/other, left/right; clean/dirty have continually underpinned the ways in which social issues have been and are understood (Moscovici & Vignaux, 1994).

Politics, for example, is frequently delineated by the left/right dichotomy irrespective of time and place. What we should and should not touch coalesces around themata of clean/dirty and pure/impure (Callaghan, Moloney & Blair, 2012); these themata have also been shown to underpin social delineations of majority/minority groups (Moscovici, 2009). Themata of morality/immortality underpinned first the Gay Related Immune Syndrome (GRIDS) and then the Auto Immune Deficiency Syndrome (AIDS) (Markova, 2003); similarly, Self/Other themata underpin how we negotiate around mental illness (Foster, 2006).

Recently, it has been argued that the interdependence between each of these oppositional taxonomies gives rise to many of the contradictory social understandings held about an issue (Moloney, Williams & Blair, 2012). Whilst each oppositional taxonomy has been interpreted as being generative of separate representations (Moscovici, 2009), Moloney et al., argue that the tension between oppositional taxonomies also gives the representational field its dynamic, dilemmatic nature - at times it is congruent, at other times incongruent; sometimes it is fragmented and ambivalent; but through all there presides a consensual reality that socially defines the issue (Rose, et al., 1995, p.153; Moloney et al, 2012). Following this line of argument, we propose that the salience of the social context at any one time, elicits different aspects of the representational field of organ donation and transplantation and, in so doing, accommodates the co- existence of these contradictory understandings (Moloney et al., 2005)

Themata, Representations and Organ Donation

The similarity between our earlier research (Moloney & Walker, 2002; Moloney, Hall, & Walker, 2005) and our more recent work in 2012, suggests little has changed in how organ donation is socially understood - in relation to our samples at least. In both word association tasks, *life* and *death* dominated the elicitations, and in our 2002 study these were central to how people talked about the issue. It seems to us that underpinning this contradictory field are the thema of self/other and life/death.

When organ donation and transplantation is considered in relation to *others*, a strong positive normative view is elicited. Respondents were, we believe, genuinely in favour of organ donation and fully aware of the benefits it offered others. Coupled with this, however, is another perspective that doesn't negate the positive normative stance but coexists and qualifies it, driven by how organ donation is understood in relation to the self. Respondents struggle with the image of organs being removed from a loved one's body, the validity of a medically-determined brain death, and the circumstances in which the donation of organs is now a possibility.

We believe that social understandings of this issue will always be marked by a tension between life/death and self/other. In some contexts, life and others will prevail, but equally in other contexts, the potency of death and its relationship to self (be that one's self or one's family) will overshadow what a pro-donation decision could offer others.

Implications for Practice

When the barometer for understanding the public's reaction to organ donation and transplantation is medically derived, the expectation is that donation rates should match the number of organs required because scientifically there is no reason for them not to (see Bauer & Gaskell, 2008). Within this paradigm, positive attitudes to organ donation should, by course, translate into actual donation behaviour.

However, when the issue of organ donation and transplantation is conceptualised within a social representation framework, the positive attitudes expressed are considered to be only one constituent of the system of beliefs, values and practices that are the representation (Moscovici, 1973, p. xiii). As such, the *paradox* of the disparity between favourable attitudes towards organ donation and transplantation and the *dismal* rate of actual organs donated, simply does not exist. The representational field that is organ donation and transplantation is, we argue, clearly heterogeneous, characterised by tension, ambiguity and contradiction.

To say that the majority of people within a society support organ donation and transplantation is to make salient only one aspect of the system of beliefs, values and practices. It is true that when asked, most people will say they do support organ donation. However, when asked to elaborate on that statement, or asked in a relation to a different context a *but* emerges qualifying this pro-donation stance.

This linear view of the relationship between knowledge in the medical domain and knowledge in the community leads to a view that organ donation rates can be increased by translation of knowledge from the reified world of science into the universal discourse of the community. Models are constructed that delineate the 'barriers' to increased 'knowledge' on the assumption that this will then increase donation rates. Recent 'meta' analyses of qualitative research on organ donation has attempted to trawl the qualitative literature for clues about how and why the community thinks as it does about organ donation (e.g., Irving, Tong, Jan, Cass, Rose, Chadban, Allen, Craig,Wong, & Howard, 2012; Morgan et al., 2005; Newton, 2011). These reviews identify factors such as 'religion' and 'culture' as background explanatory variables that help to explain participants' views. In doing so, though, they assume a linear and unidirectional view about how to influence people's views (and ultimately their behaviours) about donation. They continue to assume a separation between attitudes and behaviours. They continue to assume that identifying and overcoming 'barriers' will lead to an increase in donation rates. This is too simple, still.

Conclusion

Our earlier studies showed that people's views about donation are complex and contradictory. This conclusion is supported by the data freshly presented in this chapter. Social representations theory provides an alternative model for comprehending the ideological space around organ donation. In this, attitudes and behaviours (decisions to donate or not) are part of the same representation; they are not separate constructs. We note that this view is not dissimilar to some early accounts of attitudes (e.g., Campbell, 1963) or to contemporary alternative measurement models such as Rasch modelling (Andrich, 1988).

Organ donation, as a representation, contains within it a range of attitudinal and behavioural positions, not all of which are consistent. Indeed, our studies show clearly that the representation field is characterised by fundamentally contradictory elements. The central components *life* and *death* are as contradictory as can be imagined! Although contradictory, they are still fundamentally and inextricably co-constituted. This primal point is what creates the dilemmatic tension that allows people, individually and in groups, to create expressed positions anew, to apparently shift positions easily and quickly, to show deep ambivalence about organ donation, and to express disconnection between what they might say about donation and what they decide to do about donation (Billig, 1987; Billig et al., 1988).

Endeavours aimed at increasing the number of people willing to have their organs, and their loved ones' organs, donated to someone else, will, we argue, always flounder until this fundamental point of contradiction and dilemma is grasped. Understanding this point we believe will give rise to a new understanding of the dynamism of people's views and behaviours about organ donation and transplantation.

References

Abric, J. C. (1993). Central System, Peripheral System: Their Functions and Roles in the Dynamics of Social Representations. *Papers on Social Representations, 2*, 75-128.

Andrich, D. (1988). *Rasch models for measurement*. London: Sage.

Bauer, M., & Gaskell, G. (2008). Social representations Theory: A progressive research programme for social psychology. *Journal for the Theory of Social Behaviour, 38*, 335-353.

Bauer, M. W., & Gaskell, G. (1999). Towards a Paradigm for Research on Social Representations. *Journal for the Theory of Social Behaviour, 29*(2), 163-186.

Billig, M. (1987). *Arguing and thinking: A rhetorical approach to social psychology.* Cambridge, UK: Cambridge University Press.

Billig, M., Condor, S., Edwards, D., Gane, M., Middleton., D. & Radley, A. (1988) *Ideological dilemmas; a social psychology of everyday life*. London: Sage.

Callaghan, P., Moloney, G., & Blair, D. (2012). Contagion in the representational field of water-recycling: Informing new environment practice through social representation theory. *Journal of Community and Applied Social Psychology, 22*, 20-37.

Campbell, D (1963) *Social Attitudes and Other Acquired Behavioral Dispositions.* New York: McGraw-Hill.

Castro, P. (2008). Social representation, change and resistance: On the difficulties of generalising new norms. *Culture and Psychology*, *14*, 475-497.

Charlton, T. (2012). *Organ Donation: Consent Systems, Knowledge of Wishes and Next-of-kin. Unpublished manuscript*. Coffs Harbour: Southern Cross University.

Donate Life (2011). *Facts and statistics: Organ, eye and tissue donation facts.* Retrieved from *http://www.donatelife.gov.au/discover/facts-a-statistics*

Foster, J. (2006). Media Presentation of the Mental Health Bill and Representations of Mental Health Problems. *Journal of Community & Applied Social Psychology, 16*, 285-300

Guimelli, C. (1998). "Differentiation Between the Central Core Elements of Social Representations: Normative vs. Functional Elements." *Swiss Journal of Psychology, 57*: 209-224.

Irving, M. J., Tong, A., Jan, S., Cass, A., Rose, J., Chadban, S., Allen, R, Craig, J., Wong, G., & Howard, K. (2012). Factors that influence the decision to be an organ donor: A systematic review of the qualitative literature. *Nephrol. Dial. Transplant. 27*, 2526-2533.

Markova, I. (2003). *Dialogicality and social representations. The dynamics of mind.* Cambridge: Cambridge University Press.

Markova, I. (2006). "On the Inner Outer in Dialogue." *International Journal for Dialogical Science, 1,* 125-147.

Markova, I. (2008). The epistemological significance of the theory of social representations. *Journal for the theory of social behaviour, 38*(4), 461-487.

Moloney, G. Hall, R. & Walker, I. (2005). Social representations and themata: The construction and functioning of social knowledge about donation and transplantation. *British Journal of Social Psychology, 44(3) 415-441.*

Moloney, G., & Walker, I. (2002). Talking about transplants: Social representations and the dialectical, dilemmatic nature of organ donation and transplantation. *British Journal of Social Psychology*, *41*, 299 – 320.

Moloney, G., & Walker, I. (2000). Messiahs, pariahs, and donors: The development of social representations of organ transplants. *Journal for the Theory of Social Behaviour*, *30*, 203-227.

Morgan, S. E., Harrison, T. R., Long, S. D., Affifi, W. A., Stephenson, M. S., & Reichert, T. (2005). Family discussions about organ donation: How the media influences opinions about donation decisions. *Clinical Transplant.*, *19*, 674-682

Moscovici (2009) *Perspectives on minority influence. European studies in social psychology.* Cambridge: Cambridge University Press.

Moscovici, S. (1988). Notes Towards a Description of Social Representations. *European Journal of Social Psychology, 18*, 211-250.

Moscovici, S. (1984). The Phenomenon of Social Representations. *Social Representations.* R. M. Farr and S. Moscovici. Cambridge/Paris, Cambridge University Press/Maison des Sciences de l'Homme: 3-69.

Moscovici, S. (1973). Foreword. In C. Herzlich (Ed.), *Health and Illness*. London: Academic Press.

Moscovici, S., & Vignaux, G. (1994). Le Concept de Themata. In C. Guimelli (Ed.), *Structures et Transformations des Representations Sociales* (pp. 25-72). Neuchatel: Delachaux et Niestle.

Rose, D., Efraim D., Gervais, M., Joffe H., Jovchelovitch, S., & Morant, N. (1995). Questioning Consensus in Social Representations Theory. *Papers on Social Representations, 4*, 150-155.

Wagner, W., J. Valencia, et al. (1996). "Relevance, Discourse and the 'Hot' Stable Core of Social Representations - A Structural Analysis of Word Associations." *British Journal of Social Psycholog,y 35*,331-351.

Wagner, W. and N. Hayes (2005). *Everyday Discourse and Common Sense: The Theory of Social Representations.* New York, Palgrave Macmillan.

In: Organ Donation and Transplantation
Editor: Mary Anne Lauri
ISBN: 978-1-62948-257-6

Chapter 9

BUILDING TRUST TO ENCOURAGE DONORS: EXAMINING WAYS TO INCREASE DONATION AMONG AFRICAN AMERICANS

Amber Marie Reinhart*
University of Missouri, St Louis, US

ABSTRACT

Reports show the waiting list for organ transplants is growing three times faster than the rate of available donors (Morgan & Miller, 2001) and recent data shows that donation rates have peaked and are now slightly decreasing each year (DuBay et al., 2012). These reports are especially alarming for African Americans, who represent 30% of those candidates on the transplant waiting list, and who often wait for a donor match twice as long as any other racial group (UNOS, 2013). This chapter explores the complex reasons why there are a disproportionate number of African American donors. The chapter investigates four overall barriers to increasing African American donors; lack of awareness and knowledge about organ donation, medical distrust, religious and bodily concerns, and medical missteps. Next, I examine what thirteen past health campaign interventions have done successfully to increase the number of donors and outline some of the optimal approaches and recommendations for future interventions.

INTRODUCTION

African Americans represent roughly 14% of the US population (US Census Bureau, 2011) and are the largest group of minorities in need of an organ transplant within the United States (UNOS, 2013). As of April 01, 2013 there are currently a total of 117,776 individuals on the waiting list for available organ donors and sadly about 7,000 of those individuals will

* Corresponding author: Email: reinhartam@umsl.edu.

die while waiting for a donor match (UNOS, 2013). A staggering 30% of those candidates waiting on the transplant list are African Americans (UNOS, 2013) and they often wait twice as long as any other racial/ethnic group with African American patients waiting, on average, for 1,185 days to receive a kidney transplant compared to 605 days for Caucasian patients (Robinson, Perryman, Thompson, Amaral, & Arriola, 2012; Siminoff & Sturm, 2000). Even more alarming is that fact that the waiting list for organ transplants is growing three times faster than the rate of available donors (Morgan & Miller, 2001) and recent data shows that donation rates have peaked and are now slightly decreasing each year (DuBay et al., 2012). Taken together, it is easy to see why increasing not only the number of donors overall, but more specifically the number of African American donors, is a public health imperative. This chapter explores the multifaceted reasons why African American donors are in short supply. Optimal approaches for future campaigns are also discussed, as well as a brief review of the successful past efforts and campaigns to increase African American donors.

African Americans continue to be under-represented among those receiving a transplant and over-represented on the transplant list for several reasons. One major reason is that African Americans have a significantly higher prevalence than Caucasians for developing certain medical conditions, such as diabetes (1.5 times more likely) and hypertension (17 times more likely), which often progress into end-stage renal disease (Higgins & Fishman, 2006). The prevalence for developing those conditions leaves African Americans four times more likely than Caucasians to get end-stage renal disease, which eventually leads to the need for kidney dialysis, and finally a kidney transplant in order to stay alive (USRDS, 2009). So, even though African Americans may donate in proportion to their representation within the population (OPTN, 2010), their current rates of donation fail to keep up with their disproportionately higher need for transplantation due to predisposed health conditions (Robinson et al., 2012).

Another cause for the discrepancy between the growing demand and available supply of donors is the problem with donor matching. After kidney transplantation, African Americans have 10-20% graft survival rates, which is lower than any other racial/ethnic group, and makes finding the best-suited donor match very important (Callender, Miles, Hall, & Gordon, 2002). The kidney matching process is "heavily dependent" on the correspondence of human lymphocyte antigens (HLA), a protein complex, and research has shown that members of the same racial/ethnic group are the best HLA matches for other members of the same group (Robinson et al., 2012, p. 365). Since successful transplantation is often improved by matching organs between members of the same racial group due to tissue matching and issues of histocompatibility, African Americans receive the best possible chance of a successful donor match when receiving organs from other African Americans, but if not enough donors are on the list, many African Americans will die waiting for a suitable match (Higgins et al., 2006).

All of these issues answer the question of why there are so many African Americans on the waiting list, but they fail to address the other side of the equation – why are there so few African American donors when such a high need exists? African Americans agree to become donors at about half the rate Caucasians agree to donate (Siminoff & Sturm, 2000) and researchers have found the answer to the question of "why are there fewer African American donors?" to be complex and difficult to address in a single intervention.

REASONS FOR THE DISPROPORTIONATE NUMBER OF DONORS

In early pilot studies on reasons for low donation rates among African Americans, Callender and his colleagues (1991) identified several primary reasons for the lower donation rate, ranging from lack of awareness to a preference that organs be given to other African Americans. Taking into account the sound research from Callender et al. (1991), and addressing one relevant barrier Callender did not address (missteps within the medical community), I see 4 overall barriers to increasing the number of African American donors: lack of awareness/knowledge, medical distrust, religious and bodily concerns, and medical missteps.

Lack of Knowledge/Awareness

Evidence of knowledge gaps about organ donation in the African American community dates all the way back to Callender and colleagues (1982) pilot study and has been cited repeatedly as one of the primary rationales for the lack of positive attitudes toward donation (Callender, 1991, 2002; Morgan, 2006; Morgan & Cannon, 2003; Morgan & Miller, 2002; Siminoff, Lawrence, & Arnold, 2003). One's explicit knowledge about organ donation, as well as one's knowledge on the need for donors on the transplant lists, has been shown to be associated with their willingness donate organs (DeJong et al., 1998; Morgan, Miller, & Arasaratnam, 2003; Reitz & Callender, 1993). However, erroneous beliefs about organ donation seem to be more pervasive among African Americans than any other racial group. A majority of African Americans are unaware of the real need for donors and instead filled with mistaken opinions on the donation process (Hall et al., 1991; Morgan et al., 2003). With the well-established link between knowledge and wiliness to donate, working to improve knowledge and dispel misconceptions is an important area to consider when looking for ways to increase African American donors (Feeley, 2007; Horton & Horton, 1990; Kopfman & Smith, 1996; McNamara et al., 1999; Morgan, 2004; Morgan & Miller, 2002; Morgan et al., 2003).

Related to a lack of knowledge about donation in general is also a lack of understanding the concept of brain death. Most deceased organ donors are brain dead, meaning that they have endured a total and irreversible loss of all brain function and are now to be considered both clinically and legally dead (HRSA, 2012a). In spite of the fact that brain death is absolute and their loved one is deceased, medical advances allow ventilation machines and medications to keep the patient's heart beating and blood flowing to their organs leaving some family members confused. They begin to think their loved one is still alive and able to recover since they can see their loved one's chest move and the patient feels warm to the touch. Regrettably this is not the case since brain death is not the same as a coma or vegetative state from which someone may recover (DeJong et al., 1998). Understandably this can be a difficult concept for people to wrap their heads around and comprehend completely, especially when the loss of a loved one is sudden and they are being asked to make a decision on donation (Horton & Horton, 1990; Radecki & Jaccard, 1997; McNamara et al., 1999; Siminoff, Burant, Younger, 2004; Siminoff & Chillag, 1999).

A study by Siminoff and colleagues (2003) found that out of 403 families of organ donor-eligible patients who reported that someone at the hospital told them the patient was brain dead only 114 (28.3%) of those families were able to provide a completely correct definition of brain death. Another study by Franz, DeJong, Wolfe, Reitsma, & Beasley, (1997) uncovered that among 164 families of medically suitable donor candidates only 61% of the donor and 53% of the non-donor respondents said they had received an explanation of brain death. Franz et al. (1997) reported the next of kin who decided against donation had far less understanding of brain death than those who decided in favor of donation. This highlights the vast importance of medical professionals properly explaining the donation process and brain death. However, further complicating the matter, studies have found that medical staff can have a difficult time understanding and explaining the concept of brain death making it a substantial barrier to gaining family consent for donation (DuBois & Anderson, 2006; Evanisko et al., 1998).

Medical Distrust

One can easily see how important accurate explanations from medical professionals are when trying to obtain family consent, but those discussions are of no use if the eligible donor's next of kin don't believe what the professionals are telling them. Medical distrust is another prevalent barrier to donation among African Americans and has been discovered in several studies as a major deterrent to donation (Davidson & Deveney, 1991; Callender et al., 1982; Minniefield, Yang, & Muti, 2001; Sanner, 1994; Siminoff, Burant, & Ibrahim, 2006; Yuen et al., 1998). Medical distrust can encompass misgivings of the medical community in general (Kurz et al., 2007; Morgan & Cannon, 2003), deep suspicions in what African Americans perceive to be an untrustworthy organ allocation system (Schutte & Kappel 1997; Siminoff & Arnold, 1999), and fear of continued racism in the medical community (Yuen et al., 1998).

Many non-donors, regardless of their racial backgrounds, are under the false impression that if one declares themselves an organ donor medical professionals will not work as hard to save them in an emergency situation and instead take their organs for donation (Callender, Miles & Hall, 2002; Morgan & Miller, 2002). A study by Minniefield and Muti (2002) found that 100% of 25- to 35-year olds, both African Americans and other ethnicities, had a fear of not getting adequate medical attention if they were found to be organ donors. Another study by Yuen et al. (1998) found more African American respondents than Caucasian respondents believe this fallacy and agreed with the statement, "Doctors would not try as hard to save me if they knew I was an organ donor"(p. 16). This finding has been replicated in several other studies and provides a powerful barrier to signing the back of a driver's license for many would-be donors (Callender et al., 1991; Siminoff & Sturm, 2000). This misconception may seem silly to those well versed in medicine or donation, but within the context of how the medical community has historically treated African Americans, the fallacy stops seeming farfetched and becomes much more comprehensible.

Many researchers point to the atrocities of the Tuskegee Syphilis Study as the start of medical distrust among African Americans, and while that atrocity is certainly a contributing factor, the problem of institutionalized racism within the medical field started much earlier with non-voluntary medical experimentation on slaves during the antebellum period (Gamble, 1997). Slaves endured excruciating pain during these medical experiments and many died as a result. During that time period doctors would also dig up the graves of the slaves for dissection, leaving not even dead African Americans safe from medical experimentation Gamble, 1997). These horrific practices continued even after the Civil War with grave robbers regularly stealing bodies of African Americans in the South to use as anatomy cadavers in Northern medical schools and a myriad of African American folktales about "night doctors" or "Klu Klux Klan doctors" who would kidnap African Americans, at night and usually in urban areas, to kill them and use their cadavers in medical experiments (Gamble, 1997, p. 1774).

By far the single worst case of unethical medical practice is the Tuskegee Syphilis Study. In 1932, the Public Health Service, working with the Tuskegee Institute, knowingly withheld treatment from 399 African American men with syphilis to study the long-term effects of the disease (CDC, 2012). The men were misled about the reasons for the study, not informed of the appalling risks to themselves or their families, and not given penicillin after the drug was identified in the 1940s as a cure for the disease. The study lasted over 40 years and over that time period many of the participants needlessly died of syphilis, their wives contracted the disease, and their children were born with congenital syphilis (CDC, 2012). As though the study itself is not appalling enough a more sickening myth has been perpetuated over the years by news anchors, television dramas, and books written on the topic that the men in the Tuskegee study were injected with syphilis, leading many African Americans to use the study as an example of premeditated genocide (Gamble, 1997). Whether pointing to the real atrocities of Tuskegee or the persistent myths surrounding the historical event it is clear to see why African Americans are justified in their past distrust of the medical community.

Given all of the negative history it is not surprising to find that some African Americans feel their lives are devalued by medical professionals and want assurances that if they do become donors their organs will go to other African Americans (Callender et al., 1991; Hall, Callender, Yeager, Barber Jr., Dunston, & Pinn-Wiggins, 1991; Minniefield et al., 2001; Reitz & Callender, 1993). However, that is an assurance the current organ procurement policies cannot make and the lack of assurances represent another roadblock that keep African Americans from donating because they fear the donation system is unjust and their organs will go to more wealthy or Caucasian donors (Callender et al., 1991; Hall et al., 1991; Morgan, 2006). All of these reasons represent an overarching theme of distrust that leads to fewer donors.

Religious and Bodily Concerns

There are several studies outlining the myriad of religious and spiritual beliefs that have been shown to present obstacles to donation (Arriola, Robinson, Thompson, & Perryman, 2010; Minniefield & Muti, 2002; Morgan et al., 2003; Morgan & Miller, 2002; Morse et al., 2009; Rubens, 1996). A desire to maintain bodily integrity (Davidson & Devney, 1991) and fear of mutilation (Morgan & Miller, 2002) are concerns expressed by both potential donors and next of kin. Combined those two concerns provide both barriers to getting people to become donors themselves and to getting families to consent to donation as well (Horton &

Horton, 1990; McNamara, et al., 1999; Morgan et al., 2003; Rubens, 1996; Sanner, 1994). Also related to bodily concerns are anxieties about feeling pain after death when donating, the "ick" factor of donation, and concerns about entering a hospital and having your organs taken while you are still alive (Minniefield & Muti, 2002; Morgan, Stephenson, Harrison, Afifi, & Long, 2008; Quick, LaVoie, Scott, Bosch, & Morgan, 2012). To some extent these bodily concerns can be properly addressed through educational campaigns, but there are some fears, such as the "ick" factor, that need more nuanced approaches to quell those concerns.

Religious beliefs are a guiding force for some African American families, and given that previous studies (Morgan & Miller, 2002; Robinson et al., 2012) have shown that one's religious beliefs are fundamental when determining one's attitudes toward organ donation, it is essential for donation campaigns to correct any religious fallacies that may exist within African American families. For example, a number of African Americans believe there are religious prohibitions or objections toward donation (Palmer, 2007; Schutte & Kapel, 1997; Rubens, 1996), even though almost all major religions support donation or believe it is a matter of personal conscience (HRSA, 2012b). However, when a church is silent on the matter of donation many parishioners may take that silence as disapproval and not feel any spiritual impetus for becoming a donor (Morgan, 2006). Not wanting to disturb the body of a donor after death or the belief that one's body should remain in tact and whole for burial are negatively correlated with African Americans' willingness to donate and such beliefs are far more common within the African American community presenting another barrier to donation (McNamara et al., 1999; Morgan, 2006; Rubens, 1996). Given how deeply religious some African Americans are, calming these religious fears and correcting the inaccurate beliefs about body mutilation could go a long way toward increasing donors.

Medical Missteps

Not all of the barriers to increasing donation are related to the lack of knowledge or inaccurate beliefs of African Americans about donation; a portion of the donation problem can be attributed directly to the medical community itself. Arnold, Puswella, and Devita's (2005) data suggest that health care providers were less likely to talk to African Americans versus Caucasians about organ donation and spoke differently about donation to the different racial groups. Other studies have found a self-fulfilling defeatist attitude from medical professionals when approaching African American families about donation (Reitz & Callender, 1993; Siminoff, Arnold, & Caplan, 1995; Siminoff & Sturm, 2000). Plawecki and Plawecki, (1989) stressed the need for nurses approaching African American families about organ donation to better understand and appreciate the African American belief system and culture, after many documented and failed attempts. With African Americans less likely than Caucasians to be referred or evaluated for transplantation, to receive education on the topic, or to get a deceased donor or living kidney transplant it is easy to see how the problem is compounded by issues on both sides of the donor requests (Alexander & Sehgal, 1998; Guadagnoli et al., 1999; Hartwig, Hall, Hathaway, & Gaber, 1993; Kurz, Scharff, Terry, Alexander, & Waterman, 2007).

Past Donation Campaign Focusing on African Americans: What Works?

Before making recommendations on what should be done in the future to improve the donation rates among African Americans it is important to look at what has succeeded and failed in past interventions. Recognizing the urgent need to increase donors, starting in 2002, the Health Resources and Services Administration (HRSA), as well as the National Institute of Diabetes and Digestive and Kidney Diseases, both requested proposals outlining programs that would increase donation among minorities, African Americans in particular (Hall, Robbins, Paiva, Knott, Harris, & Mattice, 2007). Since then there have been a handful of studies published that use some type of intervention or campaign to increase donor rates among African Americans. A review of those studies was done to look at the type of segmented audience used, basic description of study design, and key findings. Table 1 details the 13 studies reviewed. Studies concerned with learning about the attitudes, beliefs, and intentions of African Americans were not included for this brief review.

As previously noted, there have been few campaigns that specifically target African Americans and those studies often lack sound evaluation procedures, report small effects, and lack a theoretical focus (Hall et al., 2007; Harrison et al., 2001; Morgan, 2006; Thomas, 2000). Sound evaluation procedures and a theoretical focus to guide the campaign are certainly aspects future campaigns should seek to include, but there are also some facets of those past interventions that should be reviewed and integrated into future campaigns.

First, past campaigns have shown an effective interpersonal channel can be to use lay or peer educators to deliver donation messages aimed at increasing African American donors (Callender & Miles, 2010; Feeley et al., 2009; Harrison et al., 2011; Resnicow et al., 2012). Harrison et al. (2011) had peer educators who engaged people at driver's licensing bureaus in conversations about organ donation and were trained on appropriate communication strategies to dispel myths on organ donation. African Americans in particular were most affected by the interpersonal component of this campaign and responded well to speaking face-to-face with another African American on the subject of donation (Harrison et al., 2009). Another approach from Feeley et al. (2009) had college students educating one another about donation through campus-wide campaigns. In addition to interpersonal communication, small discussion groups can also provide a productive way to talk through misgivings African Americans have about donation (Andrews et al, 2012; Thompson, 1993; Townsend et al., 1990). Andrews et al. (2012) increased minority registration through the use of peer leaders within African American churches who showed a pro-donation DVD tailored to African American churches and led small group discussions within the church about organ donation. Both small group discussions and interpersonal conversations offer a unique opportunity to teach African Americans about the real facts on donation, dispel any myths about donation, communicate a need for organ donors within a community, and deliver those messages from another African American, thereby getting through several barriers with one campaign component.

Next, another proven strategy from previous campaigns involves using organ procurement organizers of the same racial background, which as previously described can be a straightforward way to increase family consent (Gentry et al., 1997; Gravel et al., 1996; Shafer et al., 1997). Finally, multi-channel campaigns are more successful than single channel ones and tend to elicit larger effect sizes (Callender & Miles, 2010; Feeley et al., 2009; Harrison et al., 2011). Harrison et al. (2011) saw the largest gains from the interpersonal component of their driver's licensing bureau campaign, but donor registration also increased through the use of their mass mediated and point-of-decision materials demonstrating the utility of including all three components within one campaign.

Table 1. Key Findings of Organ and Tissue Donation Campaigns Targeting African Americans

Author(s) – Year Published	Population/Sample	Study Design	Key Findings
Andrews, Zhang, Magee, Chapman, Langford, & Resnicow - 2012	Twenty-two predominantly African American churches in Southeast Michigan	Randomized, controlled intervention. Intervention groups were presented with information on organ donation from peer leaders and a tailored DVD versus control group who received information on increasing consumption of fruits and vegetables	After adjusting for demographics, the intervention and comparison groups did not differ on any of the 3 attitude scales. At one-year posttest members of the intervention church were 1.23 times more likely to have signed a donor card (n=163) versus the control group (n=48).
Harrison, Morgan, King, & Williams - 2011	People going into a DMV in two diverse counties of Michigan (Wayne County & Oakland County) over a 2-month period in 2009	Three-prong campaign using mass media, point-of-decision, and interpersonal components to increase organ registry sign-ups at DMVs	The campaign increased African American registration by 700% from baseline.
Arriola, Robinson, Thompson, & Perryman - 2010	Nine predominantly African American churches	Randomized, controlled intervention. Intervention group was presented with Project ACTs educational materials (video and written materials)	Significant interaction between condition and time on readiness to talk with family – those in the intervention group were 1.64 times more likely to be in action or maintenance at follow-up than those in the control group
Resnicow et al. - 2010	Hair salons in urban Michigan areas	Randomized, controlled intervention. Intervention group was presented with a four-session brief motivational intervention that encouraged donation versus the comparison group who received four-sessions of health chats focusing on chronic illnesses	After the intervention rates of self-reported positive donation status were 19.8% for the intervention group and 16% for the comparison group. Intervention participants were 1.7 times more likely to report positive donation status and enrollment rates were 4.8% for intervention participants versus 2% for control participants.
Callender & Miles - 2010 (There are several articles	African Americans in 36 U.S. cities and four historically Black colleges from	The National Minority Organ Tissue Transplant Education Program (MOTTEP) is a	Between 1990 and 2008, minority donations percentages have doubled (15% to 30%). African-American organ donors

Author(s) – Year Published	Population/Sample	Study Design	Key Findings
by Callender and colleagues that present findings from previous years of the program, this is the most recent)	1982-2008	grassroots effort emphasizing community education and empowerment combined with the use of mass media. Interventions using racially similar messengers who were affected by donation, a mass mediated campaign, and a racially sensitive marketing campaign	per million (ODM) have quadrupled from 8 ODM to 53 ODM between 1982 and 2008. Overall there was an improvement in knowledge, attitudes toward donation, willingness to sign a donor card, and increase in family discussions on donation. Increase in registered donors.
Feeley, Anker, Watkins, Rivera, Tag, & Volpe - 2009	Six college campuses across New York City	Peer-to-peer campaign. Peer educators learned about donation through active learning methods and implemented campus-wide campaigns to recruit fellow students	Donor registration and family communication improved over time. Across 6 campuses, campaigners were able to recruit 1019 students as registered donors
Kopfman, Smith, Morrison, Massi, & Yoo -2002	College students at 2 Midwestern Universities	Quasi-experimental design. Subjects were presented with fact-based messages and then asked questions about donation beliefs and preferences	African Americans wand Caucasians did not differ on 4 variables (experienced more anxiety, experienced more unfavorable thoughts, reported a great number of unfavorable emotions, and evaluated pro-donation messages more negatively) that were believed to explain observed differences in prior action, thought, or intent to donate
Shafer et al. - 1997	All eligible minority donors at the Ben Taub General Hospital in Houston, Texas from 1993-1996	Longitudinal study of two full-time in-house coordinators (IHC), hired by Life-Gift, whose job was to closely manage and coordinate the consent process, and to assist the organ procurement coordinators in donor management. Race-specific requestors were used a majority of the time	The African-American consent rate increased from the 3-year average (1993 to 1995) of 35% to the 1996 consent rate of 73%, representing a 114% increase in consent rate. There was a 153% increase in African-American organ donors from the prior 3-year average of 6.3 African-American donors per year to 16 African-American donors recovered in 1996.
Gentry, Brown-Holbert & Andrews - 1997	All African American donor requests from 1988-1996 at the Organ Procurement Organization (OPO) in North Texas	Longitudinal study of an OPO after adding in an African American requestor who later became a full-time organ procurement coordinator and handled all requests from other African Americans and a public	Demonstrated the benefit of targeting a specific community with a full-time OPO of the same ethnicity. There was a significant increase in African American consent rates and organ donations after the intervention, with consent rates rising from 0% to 60% in

Table 1. (Continued)

Author(s) – Year Published	Population/Sample	Study Design	Key Findings
		education coordinator who designed and implemented public education programs	1994 and up to 80% in 1995. Total African American donors rose from 0 to 12 by 1994
Gravel & Szeman-1996	All donor requests from at the University of Michigan Medical Center from 1988-1993	Longitudinal assessment of donor requests from 1988-1990, before the model was introduced, and those from 1991-1993, after the model. Used the Transplant Center Development Model, which facilitates the donation process, specializes staff education, and promotes administrative involvement specializes staff education, and promotes administrative involvement	After the Transplant Center Development Model was implemented in 1991, the organ referral mean increased 47%, the organ donation mean 50%, and the tissue donation mean 117%
Kappel, Whitlock, Parks-Thomas, Hong, & Freedman - 1993	African Americans in the Midwest between 1988-1991	Longitudinal assessment of educational intervention in churches	Referral and donation rates of African American donors increased from 31% in 1988 to 48% in 1992.
Thompson - 1993	African American teens and adults in St. Louis, MO	Pilot study with pre-discussion survey and group discussions. The group discussion format was adapted from focus group techniques used in social marketing research and focused on the concerns of the undecided and those opposed to donation	Teens (73%) were more willing than adults (35%) to sign organ donor cards. Adults indicated more indecision than did teens, with 27% undecided regarding signing a donor card.
Townsend, Rovelli, & Schweizer - 1990	Convenience sample primarily of African American adults	Small, informal discussion groups	A significant increase in the acceptance of organ donation from 20% before the discussions to 60% after the discussions. Also saw an increase in family discussions about donation following the intervention.

There are also other studies on organ donation in general that were effective in increasing donors and those hypotheses should be tested solely on African American audiences to see if the study results are replicable within this single racial group. For example, isolating specific psychological traits, such as decision efficacy, which pertains to a type of self-efficacy where participants feel cognitively and emotionally capable of making the decision to become a donor should be explored to see if this efficacy is lacking more in the African American culture (Anker, Feeley, & Kim, 2010). Campaign designers should also look at certain message features, such as narrative versus statistical and gain-framed versus loss-framed (Feeley, Marshall, Reinhart, 2006; Reinhart, Marshall, Feeley, & Tutzauer, 2007) to see which messages receive more positive reactions and increase knowledge to become a donor in order to craft the most persuasive messages for each campaign component.

OPTIMAL APPROACHES FOR THE FUTURE

After reviewing the varied pieces to past interventions, it would then make sense to advocate for multi-faceted campaigns that help to lessen the gap in available donors and those on the waiting lists. These campaigns need to include components that work on improving knowledge about donation and at the same time eliminating donation misconceptions and myths within the African American community. Effective outreach strategies and persuasive campaigns will also need to specifically address salient issues for African Americans (such as mistrust of the allocation system and assurances that various religions support donation), while also increasing family discussions about donation and advancing the medical community's approach to recruitment of African American donors.

Increasing Knowledge & Trust, While Dispelling Myths & Misconceptions

Communicating about donation remains a vital area of focus and increasing the knowledge African Americans have about donation and the growing need for donors is essential to any successful campaign (Afifi et al., 2006; Quick et al., 2012). A proven strategy for improving knowledge among African Americans involves using interpersonal components within a campaign. Harrison et al.'s (2011) campaign within the driver licensing bureaus saw a 700% increase above baseline in organ donation and the interpersonal component was credited for generating the highest number of new registrations and being particularly important to the African Americans who decided to register. Several other studies stress the importance of an interpersonal component to campaigns and report interpersonal communication to moderate the effects of campaign messages on desired outcomes (Feeley & Moon, 2002; Morgan, 2009; Morgan & Miller, 2002).

Another element that could be added into an interpersonal component of a campaign would be including African Americans whose lives have been touched by donation, either through receiving an organ or having a family member who donated organs. Minniefield, Yang, and Muti (2001) found that African Americans were three times less likely than Caucasians to know a person who had been an organ donor. Increasing the connections between those who have been touched by donation with those who have yet to become a donor could go a long way toward making donation seem more normative in the African American community, while at the same time dispelling the myth that African Americans are not organ recipients.

Religious beliefs are central to shaping attitudes, intentions, and behaviors regarding donation and since religious institutions play a prominent role in the lives of most African Americans overcoming any religious misconceptions people may have is imperative to increasing donors (Morgan & Miller, 2002; Robinson et al., 2012). One approach is to include religious leaders within the intervention. Campaigns can encourage religious leaders to act as lay educators in their sermons, add donation as a topic for their pastoral counseling, and actively work to clarify mistaken beliefs within their congregations. All of these efforts can improve overall knowledge on donation, relieve issues of medical distrust on the topic of donation, and positively impact African Americans' donation rates (Atkins et al., 2003; Davis et al., 2005; Morse et al., 2009; Robinson et al., 2012). Given that Purnell, Powe, Troll, Wang, LaVeist, & Boulware (2011) found a majority of those who had not yet become donors preferred disclosing their donation intentions via personal discussions with religious representatives, those representatives can also engage in conversations about intentions and encourage family discussion on the topic. Allowing people to disclose their donation intentions through personal discussions, rather than signing the back of their license or an online registry, may help to eliminate concerns about receiving poor medical treatment after being flagged as a registered donor.

Morgan (2006) found in addition to knowledge and attitudes, social norms were influential in African Americans' decision to donate. Past studies have found success involving workers in beauty salons (Linnan & Ferguson, 2007) and leaders in churches (Baskin, Resnicow, & Campbell, 2001) to help increase donor registration. Involving those people who are influential within the community and who could educate about and publicly embrace the topic of donation would allow a more community-wide approach to donation and certainly improve donation rates. Coupled with an interpersonal component that includes an African American who was involved with donation, becoming a donor would become a more normative behavior and involving community leaders in educating people about donation would help encompass donation as a community initiative, rather than something people do privately and don't discuss with others.

Increase Family Discussion

Increasing family discussions on donation has been singled out in several studies as an important component to successful campaigns and is especially important in the African American community (DeJong et al., 1995; Dodd-McCue & Tartagli, 2007; Morgan, 2006; Morgan et al., 2002; Schutte & Kappel, 1997; Siminoff & Sturm, 2000). Morgan et al. (2002) found more positive attitudes toward donation led to a greater willingness to talk about donation and increased knowledge about donation to positively impact one's wiliness to discuss donation, so educational campaigns should also seek to incorporate family discussion. These findings suggest those committed to the decision about becoming a donor feel more confident discussing their decision with others and, if knowledgeable about donation and donation myths, would be able to debunk any misconceptions or misgivings other family members may bring into family discussions on donation (Morgan et al., 2002). If this is the case, encouraging family talks about donation that are initiated by those who have already made the decision to become a donor could provide another normative, interpersonal influence to those who members of their family who have not yet become a donor and provide a trusted source of information who can provide factual information on donation, dismiss misconceptions, and aid in overcoming feelings of fear and medical mistrust.

Steps to Improve Communication from the Medical Community

Communication on donation from the medical community needs to focus not only on widening the knowledge on the topic, such as understanding brain death, but also lessening the distrust African Americans have toward the medical community. McNamara et al. (1999) found that African Americans were three to four times more likely to donate if they believed doctors do all they can to save a life before pursuing donation. Within the medical community, primary-care physicians are one option of someone within the medical field African Americans already trust and would be able to educate about donation, alleviate medial distrust, and correct misconceptions held about donation. These physicians are also in the unique position where, if they have a good relationship with the patient, can address feelings of medical mistrust and encourage donation far before an emotion-filled request from an organ procurement organization (OPO) after a loved one has passed away (Russell et al., 2012). Primary-care physicians would also be able to reach and educate an entire family and encourage family discussions about donation in an interpersonal way that could support a public education campaign (Yuen et al., 1998).

Using minority requestors that match the racial or ethnic background of the eligible donor has been shown to increase donation rates (Gravel et al., 1996; Gentry et al., 1997; Shafer et al., 1997) and is something many researchers believe all organ procurement organizations should seek to enact (McNamara et al., 1999; Minniefield, Yang, & Muti, 2001). Callender, Bey, Miles, & Yeager (1995) and even go so far as to recommend minority participation on all levels of the process to complement their plans for a national minority transplant strategy. If requestors of the same ethnicities were the norm, health care providers in critical care settings would have a better opportunity to quell concerns about bodily disfigurement, premature death, and the equity of the allocation system.

Siminoff & Sturm (2000) outline likely barriers health care professionals should prepare for when asking for consent to donation: not knowing the patient's wishes about donation, a need for more education about the organ shortage, and the need for reassurance that everything medically possible was done to save the patient's life. If family discussion rates rise the first barrier could be erased. Better public education campaigns using interpersonal components and authoritative and accurate information from one's primary care doctor can wipe out the second barrier, leaving organ procurement organization representatives to ensure the third barrier is properly addressed before the request is made to a patient's family. Research from both Gortmaker and colleagues (1998) and Arnold and colleagues (2005) point to four communication processes that positively correlate with donation rates, and should be used by medical professionals when making the donation requests. First, be sure to clearly explain any medical issues (such as brain death) and have the family accept the issues before discussing donation. Next, discuss specific topics of concern about donation and clear up any misconceptions about donation's effect on funerals or the cost. Third, allow the family ample time with the organ procurement organization staff (preferably of the same racial background) in a quiet and private place and involve the staff early on in the process. Finally, provide psychosocial support for the grieving family during and after the donation request. By enacting more sensitive approaches that first address any concerns or misconceptions families may have prior to making the donation request and giving the family ample support, families will feel more at ease when determining whether or not to donate a loved one's organ and donation rates would certainly rise.

Conclusion

The daunting task before health researchers and campaign developers then is to create public health campaigns and interventions that not only inspire more African Americans to sign statewide organ and tissue donation registries and discuss their donation wishes with loved ones, but at the same time fight against the barriers to donation and increase overall knowledge about the process. That is a hefty undertaking, but with the proper planning, researchers can create a multi-faceted approach that is grounded in a theoretical foundation and based on formative research and will be well on their way to increasing the number of African American donors and giving those African Americans on the waiting list the best chance for survival.

References

Afifi, W. A., Morgan, S. E., Stephenson, M. T., Morse, C., Harrison, T., Reichert, T. & Long, S. D. (2006). Examining the decision to talk with family about organ donation: Applying theory of motivated information management. *Communication Monographs*, *73*(2), 188-215.

Alexander, G. C. & Sehgal, A. R. (1998). Barriers to cadaveric renal transplantation among Blacks, women, and the poor. *Journal of the American Medical Association*, *280*(13), 1148-1152.

Andrews, A. M., Zhang, N., Magee, J. C., Chapman, R., Langford, A. T. & Resnicow, K. (2012). Increasing donor designation through black churches: results of a randomized trial. *Progress in Transplantation*, *22*(2), 161-167.

Anker, A. E., Feeley, T. H. & Kim, H. (2010). Examining the attitude–behavior relationship in prosocial donation domains. *Journal of Applied Social Psychology*, *40*(6), 1293-1324.

Arnold, R. M., Puswella, A. & Devita, M. (2005). Discussing organ donation with families; declaring brain death: The neurological criteria. *Journal of Palliative Medicine*, *8*(3), 639-641.

Arriola, K., Robinson, D. H., Thompson, N. J. & Perryman, J. P. (2010). Project ACTS: An intervention to increase organ and tissue donation intentions among African Americans. *Health Education & Behavior*, *37*, 264-274.

Atkins, L., Davis, K., Holtzman, S. M., Durand, R. & Decker, P. J. (2003). Family discussion about organ donation among African Americans. *Progress in Transplantation*, *13*(1), 28-32.

Baskin, M. L., Resnicow, K. & Campbell, M. K. (2001). Conducting health interventions in Black churches: a model for building effective partnerships. *Ethnicity & Disease*, *11*(4), 823.

Callender, C. O., Bayton, J. A., Yeager, C. & Clark, J. E. (1982). Attitudes among blacks toward donating kidneys for transplantation: a pilot project. *Journal of the National Medical Association*, *74*(8), 807-809.

Callender, C. O., Bey, A. S., Miles, P. V. & Yeager, C. L. (1995). A national minority organ/tissue transplant education program: the first step in the evolution of a minority strategy and minority transplant equity in the USA. *Trotter Review*, *9*(1), 8.

Callender, C. O., Hall, L. E., Yeager, C. L., Barber Jr, J. B., Dunston, G. M. & Pinn-Wiggins, V. W. (1991). Organ donation and blacks: a critical frontier. *New England Journal of Medicine*, *325*(6), 442-444.

Callender, C. O. & Miles, P. V. (2010). Minority organ donation: The power of an educated community. *Journal of the American College of Surgeons*, 210(5), 708-717.

Callender, C. O., Miles, P. V. & Hall, M. B. (2002). National MOTTEP: educating to prevent the need for transplantation. Minority Organ Tissue Transplant Education Program. *Ethnicity & Disease*, *12*(1), S1.

Callender, C. O., Miles, P. V., Hall, M. B. & Gordon, S. (2002). Blacks and whites and kidney transplantation: A disparity! but why and why won't it go away? *Transplantation Reviews*, *16*(3), 163-176.

Centers for Disease Control (CDC). (2012). *U.S. Public Health Service Syphilis Study at Tuskegee*. Retrieved on November 14, 2012 from http://www.cdc.gov/tuskegee/index.html

Davis, K., Holtzman, S., Durand, R., Decker, P. J., Zucha, B. & Atkins, L. (2005). Leading the flock: organ donation feelings, beliefs, and intentions among African American clergy and community residents. *Progress in Transplantation*, *15*(3), 211-216.

Davidson, M. N. & Devney, P. (1991). Attitudinal barriers to organ donation among Black Americans. *Transplantation Proceedings*, *23*(5), 2531-2532.

DeJong, W., Franz, H. G., Wolfe, S. M., Nathan, H., Payne, D., Reitsma, W. & Beasley, C. (1998). Requesting organ donation: an interview study of donor and nondonor families. *American Journal of Critical Care*, *7*(1), 13-23.

Dodd-McCue, D. & Tartaglia, A. (2007). African American consent and nonconsent cases: are there significant differences? *Progress in Transplantation*, *17*(3), 215-219.

DuBay, D., Redden, D., Haque, A., Gray, S., Fouad, M., Siminoff, L., Holt, C., Kohler, C. & Eckhoff, D. (2012). Is Decedent Race an Independent Predictor of Organ Donor Consent or Merely a Surrogate Marker of Socioeconomic Status? *Transplantation*, *94*(8), 873-878.

DuBois, J. M. & Anderson, E. E. (2006). Attitudes toward death criteria and organ donation among healthcare personnel and the general public. *Progress in Transplantation*, *16*(1), 65-73.

Evanisko, M. J., Beasley, C. L., Brigham, L. E., Capossela, C., Cosgrove, G. R., Light, J., Mellow, S., Poretsky, A. & McNamara, P. (1998). Readiness of critical care physicians and nurses to handle requests for organ donation. *American Journal of Critical Care*, *7*(1), 4-12.

Feeley, T. H. (2007). College students' knowledge, attitudes, and behaviors regarding organ donation: An integrated review of the literature. *Journal of Applied Social Psychology*, *37*(2), 243-271.

Feeley, T. H., Anker, A. E., Watkins, B., Rivera, J., Tag, N. & Volpe, L. (2009). A peer-to-peer campaign to promote organ donation among racially diverse college students in New York City. *Journal of the National Medical Association*, *101*(11), 1154-1162.

Feeley, T. H., Marshall, H. M. & Reinhart, A. M. (2006). Reactions to narrative and statistical written messages promoting organ donation. *Communication Reports*, *19*(2), 89-100.

Feeley, T. H. & Moon, S. I. (2009). A meta-analytic review of communication campaigns to promote organ donation. *Communication Reports*, *22*(2), 63-73.

Franz, H. G., DeJong, W., Wolfe, S. M., Reitsma, W. & Beasley, C. (1997). Explaining brain death: a critical feature of the donation process. *Journal of Transplant Coordination*, *7*(1), 14-21.

Gamble, V. N. (1997). Under the shadow of Tuskegee: African Americans and health care. *American Journal of Public Health*, *87*(11), 1773-1778.

Gentry, D., Brown-Holbert, J. & Andrews, C. (1997). Racial impact: Increasing minority consent rate by altering the racial mix of an organ procurement organization. *Transplantation Proceedings*, *29*(8), 3758-3759.

Gortmaker, S. L., Beasley, C. L., Sheehy, E., Lucas, B. A., Brigham, L. E., Grenvik, A., Patterson, R.H. & Garrison, N., McNamara, P. & Evanisko, M. J. (1998). Improving the request process to increase family consent for organ donation. *Journal of Transplant Coordination*, *8*(4), 210-217.

Gravel, M. T. & Szeman, P. (1996). Increasing referrals and donations using the Transplant Center Development Model. *Journal of Transplant Coordination*, *6*(1), 32-36.

Guadagnoli, E., McNamara, P., Evanisko, M. J., Beasley, C., Callender, C. O. & Poretsky, A. (1999). The influence of race on approaching families for organ donation and their decision to donate. *American Journal of Public Health*, *89*(2), 244-247.

Hall, L. E., Callender, C. O., Yeager, C. L., Barber Jr., J. B., Dunston, G. M. & Pinn-Wiggins, V. W. (1991). Organ donation in blacks: The next frontier. *Transplantation Proceedings* *23*(5), 2500-2504.

Hall, K. L., Robbins, M. L., Paiva, A., Knott, J. E., Harris, L. & Mattice, B. (2007). Donation intentions among African American college students: Decisional balance and self-efficacy measures. *Journal of Behavioral Medicine*, *30*(6), 483-495.

Hartwig, M. S., Hall, G., Hathaway, D. & Gaber, A. O. (1993). Effect of organ donor race on health team procurement efforts. *Archives of Surgery*, *128*(12), 1331-1135.

Harrison, T. R., Morgan, S. E., King, A. J. & Williams, E. A. (2011). Saving lives branch by branch: The effectiveness of driver licensing bureau campaigns to promote organ registry sign-ups to African Americans in Michigan. *Journal of Health Communication*, *16*(8), 805-819.

Higgins, R. S. D. & Fishman, J. A. (2006). Disparities in solid organ transplantation for ethnic minorities: Facts and solutions. *American Journal of Transplantation*, *6*(11), 2556-2562.

Horton, R. L. & Horton, P. J. (1990). Knowledge regarding organ donation: Identifying and overcoming barriers to organ donation. *Social Science & Medicine*, *31*(7), 791-800.

Kappel, D. F., Whitlock, M. E., Parks-Thomas, T. D., Hong, B. A. & Freedman, B. K. (1993). Increasing African American organ donation: The St Louis experience. *Transplantation Proceedings*, *25*(4), 2489-2490.

Kopfman, J. E. & Smith, S. W. (1996). Understanding the audiences of a health communication campaign: A discriminant analysis of potential organ donors based on intent to donate. *Journal of Applied Communication Research*, *24*(1), 33-49.

Kopfman, J. E., Smith, S. W., Morrison, K., Massi, L. & Yoo, H. J. (2002). Influence of race on cognitive and affective reactions to organ donation messages. *Transplantation Proceedings*, *34*(8), 3035-3041.

Kurz, R. S., Scharff, D. P., Terry, T., Alexander, S. & Waterman, A. (2007). Factors influencing organ donation decisions by African Americans: A review of the literature. *Medical Care Research and Review*, *64*(5), 475-517.

Linnan, L. A. & Ferguson, Y. O. (2007). Beauty salons: A promising health promotion setting for reaching and promoting health among African American women. *Health Education & Behavior*, *34*(3), 517-530.

McNamara, P., Guadagnoli, E., Evanisko, M. J., Beasley, C., Santiago-Delpin, E. A., Callender, C. O. & Christiansen, E. (1999). Correlates of support for organ donation among three ethnic groups. *Clinical Transplantation*, *13*(1), 45-50.

Minniefield, W. J. & Muti, P. (2002). Organ donation survey results of a Buffalo, New York, African-American community. *Journal of the National Medical Association*, *94*(11), 979.

Minniefield, W. J., Yang, J. & Muti, P. (2001). Differences in attitudes toward organ donation among African Americans and Whites in the United States. *Journal of the National Medical Association*, *93*(10), 372.

Morgan, S. E. (2004). The power of talk: African Americans' communication with family members about organ donation and its impact on the willingness to donate organs. *Journal of Social and Personal Relationships*, *21*(1), 112-124.

Morgan, S. E. (2006). Many facets of reluctance: African Americans and the decision (not) to donate organs. *Journal of the National Medical Association*, *98*(5), 695.

Morgan, S. E. (2009). The intersection of conversation, cognitions, and campaigns: The social representation of organ donation. *Communication Theory*, *19*(1), 29-48.

Morgan, S. E. & Cannon, T. (2003). African Americans' knowledge about organ donation: closing the gap with more effective persuasive message strategies. *Journal of the National Medical Association*, *95*(11), 1066.

Morgan, S. & Miller, J. (2002). Communicating about gifts of life: The effect of knowledge, attitudes, and altruism on behavior and behavioral intentions regarding organ donation. *Journal of Applied Communication Research*, *30*(2), 163-178.

Morgan, S. E., Miller, J. K. & Arasaratnam, L. A. (2003). Similarities and differences between African Americans' and Europeans Americans' attitudes, knowledge, and willingness to communicate about organ donation. *Journal of Applied Social Psychology*, *33*(4), 693-715.

Morgan, S. E., Stephenson, M. T., Harrison, T. R., Afifi, W. A. & Long, S. D. (2008). Facts versus feelings: How rational is the decision to become an organ donor? *Journal of Health Psychology*, *13*(5), 644-658.

Morse, C. R., Afifi, W. A., Morgan, S. E., Stephenson, M. T., Reichert, T., Harrison, T. R. & Long, S. D. (2009). Religiosity, Anxiety, and Discussions About Organ Donation: Understanding a Complex Systemof Associations. *Health Communication*, *24*(2), 156-164.

Organ Procurement and Transplantation Network (OPTN). (2010). Donors recovered in the U.S. by donor type: January 1, 1988-August 31, 2012. U.S. Department of Health and Human Services, Health Resources and Services Administration. Retrieved October 12, 2012 from http://optn.transplant.hrsa.gov/latestData/step2.asp

Palmer, T. E. (2007). Roles of religion and geography in organ donation in the African-American community. *Journal of the National Medical Association*, *99*(1), 94.

Plawecki, H. M., Freiberg, G. & Plawecki, J. A. (1989). Increasing organ donation in the black community. *American Nephrology Nurses' Association*, *16*(5), 321-324.

Purnell, T. S., Powe, N. R., Troll, M. U., Wang, N. Y., LaVeist, T. A. & Boulware, L. E. (2011). Donor designation: Racial and ethnic differences in US nondesignators' preferred methods for disclosing intent to donate organs. *Transplant International, 24*(10), 999-1007.

Quick, B. L., LaVoie, N. R., Scott, A. M., Bosch, D. & Morgan, S. E. (2012). Perceptions about organ donation among African American, Hispanic, and White high school students. *Qualitative Health Research*, *22*(7), 921-933.

Radecki, C. M. & Jaccard, J. (1997). Psychological aspects of organ donation: A critical review and synthesis of individual and next-of-kin donation decisions. *Health Psychology*, *16*(2), 183.

Reinhart, A. M., Marshall, H. M., Feeley, T. H. & Tutzauer, F. (2007). The persuasive effects of message framing in organ donation: The mediating role of psychological reactance. *Communication Monographs*, *74*(2), 229-255.

Reitz, N. N. & Callender, C. O. (1993). Organ donation in the African-American population: a fresh perspective with a simple solution. *Journal of the National Medical Association*, *85*(5), 353.

Resnicow, K., Andrews, A. M., Beach, D. K., et al. (2010). Randomized trial using hair stylists as lay health advisors to increase organ donation in African Americans. *Ethnicity & Disease*, *20*(3), 276-281.

Resnicow, K., Andrews, A. M., Zhang, N., Chapman, R., Beach, D. K., Langford, A. T. et al. (2011). Development of a scale to measure African American attitudes toward organ donation. *Journal of Health Psychology*, *17*, 389-398.

Robinson, D. H., Perryman, J. P., Thompson, N. J., Amaral, S. & Arriola, K. R. J. (2012). Testing the utility of a modified organ donation model among African American adults. *Journal of Behavioral Medicine*, *35*(3), 364-374.

Rubens, A. J. (1996). Racial and ethnic differences in students' attitudes and behavior toward organ donation. *Journal of the National Medical Association*, *88*(7), 417.

Russell, E., Robinson, D. H., Thompson, N. J., Perryman, J. P. & Arriola, K. R. J. (2012). Distrust in the Healthcare System and Organ Donation Intentions Among African Americans. *Journal of Community Health*, *37*(1), 40-47.

Sanner, M. (1994). A comparison of public attitudes toward autopsy, organ donation, and anatomic dissection. *Journal of the American Medical Association*, *271*(4), 284-288.

Schutte, L. & Kappel, D. (1997). Barriers to donation in minority, low-income, and rural populations. *Transplantation Proceedings*, *29*(8), 37463747.

Shafer, T., Wood, R. P., Van Buren, C. T., Guerriero, G., Davis, K., Reyes, D. A., ... & Levert-Cole, T. (1997). A success story in minority donation: the LifeGift/Ben Taub General Hospital In-House Coordinator Program. *Transplantation Proceedings*, *29*(8), 3753-3755.

Siminoff, L. A. & Arnold, R. (1999). Increasing organ donation in the African-American community: altruism in the face of an untrustworthy system. *Annals of Internal Medicine*, *130*(7), 607.

Siminoff, L. A., Arnold, R. M. & Caplan, A. L. (1995). Health care professional attitudes toward donation: effect on practice and procurement. *The Journal of Trauma and Acute Care Surgery*, *39*(3), 553-559.

Siminoff, L. A., Burant, C. J. & Ibrahim, S. A. (2006). Racial disparities in preferences and perceptions regarding organ donation. *Journal of General Internal Medicine*, *21*(9), 995-1000.

Siminoff, L. A. & Chillag, K. (1999). The fallacy of the “gift of life”. *Hastings Center Report*, *29*(6), 34-41.

Siminoff, L. A., Lawrence, R. H. & Arnold, R. M. (2003). Comparison of black and white families' experiences and perceptions regarding organ donation requests. *Critical Care Medicine*, *31*(1), 146-151.

Siminoff, L. A., Mercer, M. B. & Arnold, R. (2003). Families' understanding of brain death. *Progress in Transplantation*, *13*(3), 218-224.

Siminoff, L. A. & Sturm, C. M. S. (2000). African-American reluctance to donate: beliefs and attitudes about organ donation and implications for policy. *Kennedy Institute of Ethics Journal*, *10*(1), 59-74.

Thomas, S. B. (2000). The black organ and tissue donor shortage: A review of the literature. *Perspectives*, 11-23.

Thompson, V. L. (1993). Educating the African-American community on organ donation. *Journal of the National Medical Association*, *85*(1), 17.

Townsend, M. E., Rovelli, M. A. & Schweizer, R. T. (1990). Value of discussion groups in educating blacks about organ donation and transplantation. *Transplantation Proceedings*, *22*(2), 324-325.

US Census Bureau. (2011). *Quick Facts*. Retrieved on November 13, 2012 from: http://quickfacts.census.gov/qfd/states/00000.html

U.S. Department of Health and Human Services – Health Resources and Services Administration (HRSA). (2012a). *Organ donation and brain death*. Retrieved October 18, 2012 from http://www.organdonor.gov/about/braindeath.html

U.S. Department of Health and Human Services – Health Resources and Services Administration (HRSA). (2012b). *Religious views on donation*. Retrieved October 18, 2012 from http://www.organdonor.gov/about/religiousviews.html

United Network for Organ Sharing [UNOS]. (2013). Database on the Internet. Richmond, VA: United Network for Organ Sharing. Retrieved April 13, 2013, from: http://www.unos.org/

U.S. Renal Data System (USRDS). (2009). Retrieved October 2, 2012 from www.usrds.org

Yuen, C. C., Burton, W., Chiraseveenuprapund, P., Elmore, E., Wong, S., Ozuah, P. & Mulvihill, M. (1998). Attitudes and beliefs about organ donation among different racial groups. *Journal of the National Medical Association*, *90*(1), 13-18.

In: Organ Donation and Transplantation
Editor: Mary Anne Lauri

ISBN: 978-1-62948-257-6

Chapter 10

LASTING BONDS AND NEW CONNECTIONS: PUBLIC VIEWS ON THE DONOR-RECIPIENT-RELATIONSHIP AND THEIR IMPLICATIONS FOR THE ETHICS OF ORGAN TRANSPLANTATION

Mark Schweda*[*] *and Sabine Wöhlke
Department of Medical Ethics and History of Medicine,
University Medical Center Göttingen, Germany

ABSTRACT

Public campaigns, political debates and the academic expert discourse on organ donation tend to focus either on the motives of donors or on the needs of recipients. However, the relations between both sides are of high ethical relevance and need further empirical attention and theoretical reflection. On the basis of fourteen focus group discussions in four European countries, our qualitative socio-empirical study examines the perceptions of lay and affected persons regarding the ways organ transplantation shapes and transforms interpersonal relations between donors and recipients. In both cases, the process is frequently described as an interaction characterized by reciprocity. At the same time, there are important differences with regard to the social context. Living donation is usually restricted to the close social spheres of family or friendship, leading to delicate shifts in a pre-existing web of relations. Post-mortem donation constitutes a completely new relationship surrounded by anonymity. Furthermore, there are differences with regard to the point of view of being affected. In the perspective of the donors, notions of self-transcendence and transfer play an important role, e.g. the idea of a reproductive body in the case of living donation and the idea of a continuation of life and personality in the case of post-mortal donation. From the standpoint of the recipient, problems of acceptance and incorporation as well as gratitude, indebtedness or even guilt are in the foreground. We will discuss the implications of these findings with respect to the current ethical debate and political framework conditions of organ transplantation in Europe, problematizing the common rhetoric of altruistic donation as an isolated act and

[*] Corresponding author: Email: Mark.Schweda@medizin.uni-goettingen.de.

a moral one-way street and the dominant anonymity paradigm in post-mortem organ donation.

INTRODUCTION

A new public campaign, intended to raise awareness of and readiness for organ donation among the German population, employs a remarkable strategy. The posters show national celebrities, actors, athletes, and musicians, directly looking at the beholder, combined with the slogan "Du bekommst alles von mir – ich auch von Dir?" ("I'm ready to give you everything – would you do the same for me?") (Wöhlke & Schicktanz, 2011). Against the background of the traditional ideational and legal framework of organ donation, this amounts to a revolutionary, yet at the same time paradoxical turn: Departing from the idea of altruistic, anonymous donation that informs the public discourse and politico-legal organization of post-mortem organ donation in Germany, as well as in most other European countries, the campaign simulates a face to face situation between potential donors and recipients and insinuates mutual bonds and expectations between both sides. Thus, it aims at a relational aspect located at the very heart of the practice of organ donation, but at the same time persistently denied, neglected or distorted in its dominant public representations, political discussions and legal regulations.

As a matter of fact, living organ donation (LOD) and post-mortem organ donation (POD) have become routine procedures in modern biomedicine. At the same time, however, they still have a special status within the scope of biomedical practices: They do not only concern one single patient and the intervention in his or her body, but directly involve at least two different parties – the donor and the recipient –, using organs from the former for the medical treatment of the latter. While the major part of public campaigns, political debates, and the academic ethical discourse traditionally tends to focus either on the selfish or noble motives of (potential) donors or the urgent and desperate needs of (potential) recipients, this procedure has rather far-reaching implications for both sides, touching upon their mutual relations in manifold ways. Since ethics is not least concerned with the moral claims and responsibilities we have in relation to and interaction with each other, this relational aspect of organ transplantation is of high importance for its ethical evaluation and needs increased empirical attention and theoretical reflection.

On the basis of focus group discussions conducted in four different European countries, our qualitative socio-empirical research examines the perceptions of lay and affected persons regarding the ways organ transplantation presupposes, shapes, and transforms interpersonal relations between the donor and the recipient. As we will show, the process is frequently described in terms of reciprocity throughout all group discussions, that is, in the perspective of a moral economy based on mutual and symmetrical relations. At the same time, important differences with regard to the social context of living organ donation and post-mortem organ donation become apparent: While living organ donation is usually legally restricted to the close social spheres of family or friendship, leading to delicate shifts in a pre-existing web of relations, post-mortem organ donation constitutes a completely new and unprecedented type of relationship surrounded and complicated by anonymity. Furthermore, there are differences with regard to the point of view of being affected: In the perspective of the donor, notions of self-transcendence and transfer often play an important role, e.g. the idea of a reproductive body in the case of living organ donation and the idea of a continuation of life and personality in the case of post-mortem organ donation. From the standpoint of the recipient, problems of acceptance and incorporation, as well as gratitude, indebtedness, or even guilt are in the foreground. We will discuss the implications of these findings with respect to the current ethical debate on and political framework conditions of organ transplantation in Europe, problematizing the common rhetoric of altruistic donation as an isolated act and a moral one-way street, as well as the dominant anonymity paradigm in post-mortem organ donation.

BACKGROUND

The persistent discrepancy between the available number of donor organs and the number of people who could be treated by means of organ donation, as well as the repeated failure to increase public willingness to donate, have directed a lot of scientific attention to the individual driving forces behind organ donation. The socio-empirical research conducted in this field is often based on theoretical models of motivation and choice (Horton & Horton, 1991) and on quantitative methods of attitudinal research with opinion surveys (Mocan & Terkin, 2007; Boulware, Troll, Wang, & Powe, 2006; Siminoff, Burant, & Youngner, 2004). In contrast to this focus on attitudes and knowledge of potential donors, our research aims at understanding perspectives and motivations of both donors and recipients. This requires a deeper analysis of public views and attitudes, including their ideational and motivational backgrounds, the subjective meanings they express and the cultural web of ideas and values they are embedded in.

Given the specific direction of our research interest, we used a set of qualitative methods to make this symbolic dimension accessible, and to explore some of its content. In qualitative socio-empirical research, focus groups, moderated group discussions with usually not more than 8-10 participants (Morgan, 1997), are an established tool for investigating common sense beliefs and public topoi on a general level (Barbour, 2011). Our analysis is based on 14 focus groups which were conducted in Cyprus (CY), Germany (DE), the Netherlands (NL), and Sweden (SE) between 2005 and 2009.[i] The selection of countries was guided by an attempt to obtain a rough geographic cross-section of the variety of national regulatory and organizational frameworks of organ donation in Europe (see Abadie & Grey, 2006; Lopp, 2012).

In selecting Germany and the Netherlands, we enlisted two central European countries which are both member states of *Eurotransplant* with quite well-established, but differently regulated transplantation systems. In Germany, the *Transplantation Law* (1997) restricts living organ donation to close relatives and friends and bases post-mortem organ donation on an opt-in solution involving relatives to identify the presumed will of the deceased when no explicit consent was given. A recent amendment requires health insurances to inform citizens in regular intervals and to ask them to make a decision regarding post-mortem organ donation. In the Netherlands, the *Organ Donation Act* (1996) permits living organ donation subject to a number of carefully defined conditions, including the possibility of cross-over donations. For post-mortem organ donation, the Netherlands have established a donor register. Upon reaching the age of 18, all citizens are informed about the register and are requested to either register as potential donors, state that they do not wish to be a donor, or leave the decision up to their relatives. We also included Sweden, one of the northern European countries where organ allocation is organized by *Scandiatransplant*. According to the Swedish *Transplants Act* (1995), consent is required for post-mortem organ donation. If the will of the deceased is unknown, the law takes the position of presumed consent, although the next of kin have a veto right. In Sweden, living organ donation has increased rapidly in recent years, now comprising the majority of all transplants. By selecting Cyprus, we also included a relatively new EU-member state from the Southeast where organ transplantation is not very well established, yet. The country has only one hospital which performs transplantations. The total number of transplanted kidneys per year is about fifty, 60% of which are living organ donations. Many patients are transplanted abroad. Nevertheless, donation of body parts as such constitutes a prominent public and policy issue, as Cyprus has one of Europe's largest bone marrow banks, comprising approximately 100,000 registered donors.

Results

In general, the process of organ donation is frequently described in terms of reciprocity in all focus groups (Schweda, Wöhlke, & Schicktanz, 2009). However, there are important differences due to the social context of living organ donation and post-mortem organ donation. While living organ donation often leads to delicate shifts in a pre-existing web of relations, post-mortem organ donation rather constitutes a completely new and unprecedented kind of relationship. These differences also lead to different forms of being affected: In the donor perspective, notions of self-transcendence and transfer often play an important role, e.g. the idea of a reproductive body in the case of living organ donation and the idea of a continuation of life and personality in the case of post-mortem organ donation (Wöhlke, 2011). In the recipient perspective, problems of acceptance and incorporation as well as gratitude, indebtedness or even guilt are in the foreground.

"[E]very Chain (…) Can Only be as Strong as Its Weakest Link" – Relational Aspects in Living Organ Donation

In many European countries, post-mortem organ donation falls short of the need. Therefore, living organ donation has become the most important alternative. During the last 15 years, many countries have seen an increase in living organ transplantations. For example, Germany recorded an increase from 388 living kidneys in 2001 to 795 in 2011 (Eurotransplant, 2012). Here, living kidneys now account for 22.6% of all transplanted kidneys (Deutsche Stiftung für Organtransplantation, 2011). In general, the donor pool of living organ donation has expanded from genetically related donors to spouses (Terasaki, 1997), friends, acquaintances, and even anonymous donors (Dor et al., 2011). New schemes, such as paired donation, have further increased the complexity of these relationships (ibid., p. 935). Thus, while research has focused on the nuclear family, especially donations between parents and children, donor-recipient relations increasingly comprise other dyads. Besides the parents as the largest group of donors, the number of spouses is on the rise. Siblings are a special case as – apart from the relationship to their parents – theirs is the oldest unchosen familial relationship. Also, living organ donation often not only affects one dyad, but is influenced by other family members as well, in a pattern which can be described as a 'web of relations' (Wöhlke & Motakef, 2013).

As a matter of fact, the one and only factor which is widely considered as providing substantial grounds for living organ donation in our focus groups is a close personal relationship with the recipient. Thus, a German participant states: "If a relative of mine, for example my sister or so, were affected, I would give her my kidney at once. If I knew concretely this and that - yes. (…) Well, I think this wouldn't be difficult for me" (Ms. AK, DE-POD-lay). A closer analysis of the statements by those actually affected by living organ donation shows that it not only affects the donor-recipient-dyad, but also the rest of the family:

> Ms. BC: "(…) but on the other hand, our family was so close that you say, well every chain (…) can only be as strong as its weakest link. She somehow knew that within the small group of our family each one would be ready to do anything for the other" (DE-LOD-aff).

This passage not only illustrates the cohesion within the group but also a resulting motivation to act. This motivation which can grow from an intra-familial sense of obligation is in turn associated with a family ideal which has at its core the close ties between family members. For the family members this means setting aside personal interests and needs for the sake of the sick relative. In this context, a living organ donation often expresses or reinforces already existing constellations, dynamics, or conflicts. Thus, the analysis of our data will first focus on the influence of different relationships on the decision to donate a living organ.

Regarding the *relationship between parent and child*, our results confirm that the original asymmetrical relationship often predetermines how donation is initiated. All speakers confirmed the evident responsibility to donate for their own children. Women especially viewed organ donation as a 'natural expression of their love'. Referring to their reproductive body, some even conceived of their child as part of their own corporeality. They had brought their child into the world, or, rather, had not completely given birth, and now, through living organ donation, belatedly could deliver the healthy organ.

> Ms. AF: "For the mother it really starts with pregnancy. And giving birth. All of that isn't easy, but you still do it. And, well, the organ donation was again. The rest comes later. That's how I (laughs) told my daughter that which I haven't given you then, i've delivered it now" (DE-LOD-aff).

At closer inspection, however, the women's apparently natural and self-evident responsibility to donate an organ is often based on social models of gender roles. Especially in the context of the family, these roles can still be fairly traditional. Consequently, our empirical data show that women in the role of carers for their families do not only feel responsible for the chronically ill child, their role as a mother further leads them to see themselves as the only potential donors (Wöhlke, 2011). In the decision-making process, they do not even consider other options, as, e.g., the child's father. Especially in our focus groups with lay persons in Cyprus, several women asserted that they would even sacrifice themselves for their children: "I would donate my heart to my child" (Ms. CA, CY-POD-lay), or "I would donate both kidneys to my daughter and let myself die" (Ms. PB, CY-POD-lay). When a participant in Cyprus who was on the waiting list for a donor kidney reported how his mother refused to donate one of her kidneys to him and described this as a "traumatic experience" (Mr. MD, CY-POD-aff), the behavior of the mother met a lot of incomprehension and even harsh moral reproach by the other participants. The mother was seen as egoistic and even deemed "not worth living" (Ms. DJ, CY-POD-lay) by one speaker (Schweda & Schicktanz, 2012).

Accepting an organ from a parent usually does not pose a problem for underage children as recipients because of the original relational asymmetry of help and support. Since birth, children have experienced their parents giving more than they received in return from their child. Moreover, our data reflect that the parents mostly made decisions for their underage children. These children who are now adults describe this process as an act of help in which they trusted their parents. By the same token, limits on assuming responsibilities for others' bodies emerged in parent-child relationships when a child wanted to help a parent with a donation – an option our respondents unanimously rejected. The acceptance of others' assuming responsibility for one's body also changes when parents want to donate to their grown-up child. Here, prospective recipients often initiate an intense argument questioning their parents' motivation to donate and their relationship. Only this negotiation makes it possible for the children to accept the donation:

> Ms. FD: "Yes, first we sat in the car saying nothing (laughs) and then, bit by bit, we even talked about (…) that I asked myself, that I felt or wanted to know from her and didn't dare to ask whether she thought that she could set all these things right that had gone wrong with me or with us" (DE-LOD-aff).

After the mother offers a donation, the sick grown-up child challenges her mother's taking responsibility for her body during this argument. She doubts that her mother is only concerned with the responsibility for her body. Thus, several grown-up children conceded that they could never accept an organ from their parents because of their troubled relationship. From the recipient's point of view, the decision for or against an offer does not so much depend on weighing the risks to the parent's health but on their already conflictual relationship which would intensify after the donation. From the perspective of those affected, it becomes clear that recipients limit the process of other's claiming responsibility for their bodies. The grown-up children have emancipated from their parents, their formerly asymmetrical relationship has changed to a symmetrical relationship so that they cannot unconditionally accept a parent's offer of a donation. Rather, in this case, they ask in how far this act of help will change their relationship (Wöhlke & Motakef, 2013).

Finally, the moral obligations within parent-child constellations can also be viewed in the context of genealogical relationships between different generations of a family. From the perspective of the grandparents, a son-in-law is viewed as a 'stranger' in the already existing parent-child relationship – be this genetically, psychologically, or socially. Only the grandchildren whom he fathers are, from this perspective, 'true' blood relations. Consequently, the following quotation does not emphasize the recipient's health but his role towards the grandchildren. The organ recipient's father-in-law justifies his act by drawing on a family ideal in which he puts the cohesion and continuation of the family above maintaining each family member's autonomy: "I only expect him to get well again and that he can then again be a father to his children" (Mr. AB, DE-LOD-aff).

Among the *married couples* in our sample, it was always the healthy partner who suggested living organ donation. Limitations which could affect the relationship, such as possible changes in personality or physical limitations, e.g., in sex life, frequently motivated the donor's offer. As a rule, the sick patients themselves did not ask for a donation because, among other things, they were afraid of being rejected. In most of our cases, the spouse's donation was the only option which puts significant pressure on both the donor and the recipient. Some female recipients moreover state that they felt that their spouse and physicians virtually pressed them to accept the organ. This contrasts with a telling counter example: A married couple who intensively discussed the option of living organ donation and finally "said actually we don't like it because the dependence is really great and she herself said I don't want to be that dependent". Further on during the discussion, the husband addresses the conflict which their joint decision entails:

> Mr. BE: "It's a kind of feeling, you feel relieved, well, I'm not being forced, well, she is not someone who'd go all moral and say ok, so you can make my life easier, actually you should do that for me if you love me. She didn't do that. And if she doesn't do it, then it's a relief, on the one hand, on the other, oh my god, then my love for her cannot be all that great. (…) I have again and again asked her should we not rethink this, shouldn't we go and ask again how this works, but I never insisted. (…) Because it gave me kind of a sense of relief, well, she doesn't insist on this" (DE-LOD-aff).

This is one of the few quotations which shows the ambivalence in the realization of taking on responsibility for the other's body: On the one hand, the relief to be able to maintain one's own bodily integrity and, on the other hand, the emotional bond which engenders an obligation or the responsibility to take action across the boundaries of individual bodies. Thus, for this couple, living organ donation also constitutes a touchstone for their relationship.

Siblings have a life-long relationship which can be characterized by different degrees of intimacy. If they experience their relationship as close, living organ donation seems consistent to both the donor and the recipient. In our study, several recipients reported that they did not want to ask but still received offers from their sisters and brothers. At the same time, because of the complexity of the decision for or against living organ donation, autonomy among siblings cannot be reduced to the sibling dyad. Rather, the whole family structure influences the decision, in fact, both one's own family as well as – in the case of adult siblings – their families.

For donating siblings with a big age gap, reciprocal motives gain prominence. In their relationship, the donation of a younger to an older sibling posed fewer problems if the older recipient had previously been perceived as taking a positive and caring role in the relationship. The underlying motivation here is gratitude and a close emotional relationship. However, conflicts arise when the sick child rejects the older sibling's care and experiences it as limiting their autonomy within the family. These examples illustrate that, on the one hand, symmetrical relationships can be unbalanced due to group dynamics, and, on the other hand, they can contain asymmetrical aspects similar to parent-child relationships (Wöhlke & Motakef, 2013).

In individual cases, lack of communication within the family can lead to automatically singling out one sibling, e.g. a twin, as the best option for a donation.

> Ms. FD: "And then everyone started to pay attention when dialysis began so that then there were these dumb remarks, like my grandma saying: Oh Silvia, so then you will give your kidney that's wonderful. And she went white like a sheet, and she really felt the pressure because she had the feeling that everyone was looking at her and it was also a bit like all the others thought: This doesn't concern me at all because there's the identical twin. (…) I didn't even want everyone saying, I'll donate, I'll donate, I'll donate, but it bugged me that they were all thinking, well, if anyone is qualified, then it's Silvia. Well, that was really, I didn't want to be in her shoes. I would not have wanted to be in her place. i knew how bad she felt" (DE-LOD-aff).

Parents especially take a strong interest in the survival of their sick child. One recipient recounted how his mother broke off the relationship with her son because he did not want to donate a kidney to his brother:

> Mr. EN: "In 2004, during the transplantation, my mother made the emotional cut-off and emotionally distanced herself from my brother. I think she hadn't forgiven him that he had not cared at all about what was happening to his little brother" (DE-LOD-aff).

These examples involving siblings show that obligations towards the family create pressure to act which can affect voluntariness. The service to the family is disproportionate to a family ideal which motivates the supposedly voluntary donation. Here, gender is an important criterion: Although there are not more women than men taking on this responsibility for someone else's body, more women affected by living organ donation state that they expect this from other family members (Wöhlke & Motakef, 2013).

In individualistic and pluralistic societies, *friendships* take on greater significance. However, in the sample we studied, a friend offering to donate was deemed extraordinary. Prospective recipients who had received such an offer from a friend were initially confused and rejected it as they felt overwhelmed by the friend's effort of (bodily) support. If the offer was repeated over the next 6-12 months, the potential recipients started to seriously consider the option.

Specific expectations towards the caring role of women could be responsible for the higher percentage of women donating in the case of donations between friends. One donor explained the reason for her donation was that she did not have any children of her own and could thus help her friend.

> Ms. FB: "(…) because there was this alternative and Maraike said: I have blood group B and I'd be glad to do it, I don't have any children and I won't have any children and I don't want any children and by this I can give life and (…) that's what she'd like to do" (DE-LOD-aff).

The passage shows great ambivalence about responsibility: Friends do not necessarily feel responsible. On the one hand, the altruistic motive of helping is emphasized, but the donation also has to be integrated into the perspective of one's personal fulfillment and life plan.

Donations between non-blood relatives make it clear that the process of taking responsibility across body boundaries is not so much about knowing and understanding the medical intervention including the side-effects of transplantation. Rather, those involved are facing the problem of how donating and receiving the organ will affect their relationship. Taking bodily responsibility for the other, donating an organ can thus be seen as a stabilizing act similar to maintaining and continuing family ideals.

After the donation, too, different typologies can be detected within the relationship. Some donor-recipient pairs openly discuss possible future scenarios. This includes the question of who 'owns' the organ after donation. Is the donor allowed to control the recipient after donation and dictate how they should treat their body (and 'their' organ)? In the second variant, these future scenarios are rather treated as taboos. The majority of respondents saw the acceptance of the organ as a reciprocal act which led to a diffuse sense of gratitude on their part and resulting feelings of guilt which varied according to the relationship with the donor. This 'gratitude', in connection with the desire to 'reciprocate', was least pronounced and problematic in children who received an organ from their parents. This might go back to the already existing asymmetrical relationship in which parents generally give more. A much more direct and pronounced approach to gratitude and feelings of guilt could be observed in symmetrical relationships, as, e.g., among siblings, spouses, and friends. Thus, after the donation, the relationship of a married couple grew imbalanced because of the new-found activity of the sick spouse which the healthy partner had not been used to before. Eventually, their interests drifted apart to such an extent that they separated (Wöhlke, 2013).

> Ms. FA: "(…) which finally made us break up. Just my increasing will to live, and my new lease of life, and just my whole development after the transplantation, when I wanted to live again. Then it just did not work anymore. His state of mind got worse (…), I could not help him with that. I tried all kinds of things to help him, to get him out of this deep depression he was in, but it does not work if the other person does not want it, himself"(DE-LOD-aff).

If such conflicts are not discussed openly, the period after the donation can also give rise to (unexpressed) insecurities and expectations regarding the success of the donation which can create significant pressure. Thus, for example, the donor asking about the recipient's health might already be interpreted as an attempt to control him or her. After the donation, the recipient may feel that their sibling's exaggerated care curtails their autonomy. Conspicuously, after a donation between friends, donors tend to distance themselves from the recipients. Recipients experience this as paradoxical as the donors initially offered the donation. Donors explain that they needed space to (physically) recover. In front of the recipients, they did not want to appear 'vulnerable' because of the operation. This suggests that the donors try to uphold previously defined roles within the relationship (Wöhlke, 2013).

All in all, our results show that relationships play a central role and directly motivate actions in the context of living organ donation. Already existing role expectations and constellations within relationships inform responsibilities and often provide the template for initiating the offer of living organ donation. During the decision-making process for living organ donation, conflictual intra-familial dynamics surface and give rise to or reinforce already existing conflicts. These intra-familial conflicts not only challenge the autonomy and voluntariness of the donors' and recipients' decision, but also the acceptance of this decision within the family which might lead to further conflicts. The question of the relational symmetry is a key issue: On the one hand, asymmetrical relationships, especially those between parents and young children, imply responsibilities and the duty of care which lets living organ donation between them appear natural or even inevitable. On the other hand, conflicts are bound to erupt whenever a clash between individual perspectives and existing asymmetrical role expectations and relationship patterns looms ahead. This especially affects the tension between the traditional caring role ascribed to mothers on the one hand and women's demand for self-determination on the other. Organ donation often requires the prior emancipatory clarification or re-negotiation of the relationship between parents and grown-up children and between siblings of different ages which is aimed at establishing symmetry and reciprocity. If those involved and affected primarily see organ transplantation as a means to resolve already existing conflicts in a relationship, the donation will very likely reinforce these conflicts, asymmetries, and further foster a sense of guilt.

"[B]reathe and Live in Another Body" – Relational Aspects of Post-Mortem Organ Donation

In Europe, post-mortem organ donation is still widely regarded as the primary form of organ transplantation. It is usually centrally coordinated via *Eurotransplant* or other organizations such as *Scandiatransplant*, and performed under the paradigm of anonymous, altruistic and non-directed donations. Therefore, there cannot be any direct personal relationship or moral connection between the donor or his or her family on the one hand and a concrete, personally identified recipient on the other. Nevertheless, public discourses and campaigns frequently seem to try to bridge this gap at least on a symbolic or emotional level by making one of both parties visible. Thus, many campaign posters depict potential post-mortem organ donors in person, mostly as exemplary and praiseworthy characters, at times even in an almost heroic light. Or they lend a face to the potential beneficiaries of post-mortem organ donation by depicting concrete individuals, notably often children and adolescents, who are in need of or have benefited from a donor organ (Wöhlke & Schicktanz, 2012). Both strategies rather appeal to a sense of interpersonal relatedness implying emotional connectivity and moral bonds between the (potential) donor and recipient within a common social context and horizon, be it mankind as such, some band of all-embracing brotherhood, fellow citizenship within a common state or civil society, or solidarity within a concrete social community. Against the background of these presumed relations and alliances, many authors actually postulate a profound moral responsibility to donate organs post-mortem, framed for example as a form of "community obligation" (Fentiman, 1994), a "duty to come to the aid of others", a "moral obligation of humanity and altruism" or even a "duty of love" (National Ethics Council, 2007, p. 35).

For the actual or potential donors and recipients, themselves, this discrepancy between the official ideology, rhetoric and regime of anonymous altruistic donation on the one hand and the relational subtext of many public discourses on the other can create serious moral questions and perplexities. Thus, in one of the German lay focus groups, participants explicitly discuss the degree and range of moral responsibility for post-mortem organ donation in regard to social proximity and commitment. One speaker argues "in a biblical manner", referring "to the commandment to love one's neighbor" in order to support a moral obligation for organ donation:

> Ms. LK: "I would say then that you can't reject it. You can save the life of this person, no question. (…) I would like to interpret it in a way that I say either I give it to him or he will die. And then there is no question about that, and I would give him my kidney. You couldn't say no, could you?" (DE-POD-lay)

The group goes on to discuss the legitimate range of moral responsibility and charity in an 'exegetical' controversy over the biblical commandment to love one's neighbor. Especially the accurate extension of the concept 'neighbor' is the subject matter of some controversy. The aforementioned speaker proposes a rather exclusive interpretation, emphasizing that the commandment is "only about neighbours" and thus restricting responsibility to close personal relationships since "it is not about any children whom I don't know. (…) And it is not about any Tom, Dick or Harry in the Federal Republic, who needs my kidney, but it is about my next of kin" (Ms. LK, DE-POD-lay). However, another speaker insists on a more generous reading, thus formulating a rather expansive understanding of morally significant interpersonal relations and bonds:

> Mr. XA: "What the Bible means by 'neighbor' is something completely different. […] Because the neighbor mentioned in the Bible is for example the person sitting next to me, the next person, no matter how. And when there is a beggar sitting on the floor, he is my neighbor as well" (DE-POD-lay).

Morally relevant interpersonal bonds and responsibilities with regard to post-mortem organ donation are also addressed from the point of view of the (actual or potential) recipients. In general, we frequently find the view that "it is a big responsibility to *receive* an organ, too …" (Mr. LH, SE-POD-aff). This 'recipient responsibility' is not only acknowledged in view of the scarcity of donor organs and the desperate need of other potential recipients, thus appealing to a sense of solidarity among those on the waiting list and constituting a duty to treat the precious gift in a particularly careful and responsible manner:

> Ms. SA: "If you get this organ and someone else has to wait and then you will not take care of your medication – then it is pretty wasted. (…) [T]hey make a huge investment and then they want some back" (SE-POD-aff).

Recipient responsibility is also perceived in terms of something the recipient owes the deceased person who was willing to donate his or her organs so that others could survive. Indeed, many speakers express the idea that organ donation is not simply a moral one-way street, but constitutes a relationship that also implies certain obligations on the side of the recipient. The sense of reciprocity which is implicit in the gift relationship promotes the feeling of indebtedness to the donor. Hence, many recipients in our study spoke of intense feelings of gratitude and even guilt and assumed responsibility to 'give something back' in return of the donor organ. Some of them postulated that post-mortem donation requires a particular attitude on the side of the recipient, he or she "needs to be modest enough to accept (the organ), because he cannot do something in return for the person who donated his liver or his kidney" (Ms. VA, NL-POD-lay). Others even stated they would not accept a donor organ because they deemed themselves unable to "do enough in return" (Mr. RT, NL-POD-lay) and hence feared they would feel guilty for the rest of their lives without any possibility to 'settle their account' (Schweda & Schicktanz, 2009a).

As our study shows, corresponding relational conflicts can actually arise in the aftermath of post-mortem organ donation. Thus, while there obviously cannot be any direct, manifest relation between the donor (or his or her family) and the recipient, many affected speakers in our groups argue that transplantation can indeed create substantial connections in both directions. Especially organ recipients report that for them the transplanted organ establishes a kind of incorporative relation to the deceased donor, "the feeling that the person who died and who donated his liver to me, that he basically is not dead yet. He continues to live on in my body" (Mr. GJ, DE-POD-aff). This perspective even seems to allow conclusions in view of the other side, granting that organ donation can inspire similar feelings of personal continuity on the part of the deceased donor's relatives, as well:

> Mr. GJ: "And I would have the feeling that, if my child dies and an organ can be passed on, I myself would always have the feeling that my child actually continues to live on. Though not the whole body, but a tiny part of it lives on" (DE-POD-aff).

Of course, this sense of personal persistence and transcendence though organ donation can have a merely psychological function for the donor's surviving family members "as a form of coping (…), that you say, ok, then death was not in 'vain', as the saying so nicely goes" (Mr. GN, DE-POD-aff). For some relatives, however, it can also have a much stronger and more literal implication of staying attached to the deceased donor, thus even creating the desire to keep in touch by searching and contacting the organ recipient. As this affected speaker from Cyprus explains: "I would know that a part of my child would breathe and live in another body and I would have a part of my child in life. Apart from saving a life, a part of my child, either an eye or a kidney or whatever, would be alive" (Ms. EI, CY-POD-aff).

Against the background of these ideas of continuity and persistence, many speakers even speculate as to whether concrete personal attributes of the donor "may be transferred to somebody psychosomatically and change a person" (Mr. HA, CY-POD-aff). Although such considerations are often articulated in a slightly facetious manner, they still play a major role in discussions, especially for the affected people. Attributes which are considered to be potentially transferable are e.g. character traits, preferences or aversions, talents or even hobbies, as in this example from a group of affected persons in Cyprus:

> Mr. HA: "I would like to say something I read in a newspaper seven years ago in Canada. A woman received a kidney from a deceased donor. When she went home she wanted to have a beer and a hamburger every day at lunch time, something that she never did in her life. Thus, she wanted to find out who the donor was. She discovered and the donor used to do this every day at lunch time... (Mr. KU, CY-POD-aff) So, these things are transferred" (CY-POD-aff).

On the basis of the notion that the brain is the sole locus of personal identity, several speakers, especially in the groups of lay people, strictly reject any speculations about the possibility of transmitting personality or personal characteristics through transplantation of other organs, since "[p]ersonality does not come with the heart" (Ms. PI, SE-POD-lay) or other organs: "[I]t is a technical organ, I mean, someone's hobbies don't reside in his kidney. Perhaps it resides in your brains, but my kidneys don't indicate that I love sport" (Ms. ZA, NL-POD-lay). A transplant recipient from a Dutch group who declares that he is "not so sensitive to what [he] will disrespectfully call 'ghost stories'", that is, narratives of personality transmission, even offers an alternative, exclusively naturalistic explanation referring to "(...) the physical phenomenon that a tissue has a certain dependence on a certain substance, you know your 'tostis', and that the desire comes with that (...)" (Mr. JD, NL-LOD-aff). Interestingly, in the course of the discussion, the selfsame patient also states that his down-to-earth naturalism might be a coping strategy to avoid emotional stress. This stress could be induced by thinking about 'his' organ donor and "to protect myself from that, also because I'm afraid I would get too carried away" (Mr. JD, NL-LOD-aff) (Schweda & Schicktanz, 2009b).

In analogy to the lay peoples' speculations about reciprocity and guilt, many organ recipients actually express a strong feeling that receiving an organ is not simply an anonymous process, but presumes a personal decision and act on the side of the donor which constitutes, in fact, a relationship associated with notions of reciprocity and mutual exchange, and generating certain responsibilities on the side of the recipient. However, in contrast to the lay peoples' concerns about becoming deeply and irrevocably indebted to the deceased donor, many participants from the groups of affected persons actually seem to have found ways to cope with their feeling of indebtedness by 'repaying' something, e.g. by engaging in self-help groups or public campaigns for organ donation: "I've stayed in this self-help group. And I'm also trying to give back there some of what I've received. That's why I do counseling there every 3 weeks" (DE-POD-aff). It is significant that such societal engagement often seems to concentrate on activities aimed towards increasing the total number of donor organs. This circumstance might be attributable to the notion that the principle of reciprocity not only posits a debt, but also determines the 'currency' of redemption, implying that organs are most appropriately repaid in kind, even if the organs which are offered in return are not one's own (Schweda & Schicktanz, 2009a).

This pronounced notion of reciprocity also plays a central role in the moral evaluation of different models of organ procurement. While many speakers experience the paradigm of altruistic donation as problematic because it blinds out the strong sense of mutuality implied in reciprocal gift-giving, they also unanimously reject a commercialization of organ procurement since its logic of profit maximization undermines the delicate symmetry involved in reciprocal relationships (Schicktanz, Schweda, & Wöhlke, 2010). In contrast to both forms of organ procurement, another mode of exchanging organs and reciprocating donations consequently enjoys great popularity in all groups: The idea that there "should be a connection between donor and receiver" so that "if you do not wish to donate, then you should not receive either" (Ms. GE, SE-POD-lay). This mode of organizing reciprocity of donation on a give-and-take basis actually seems to be favored by a considerable number of participants in all focus groups. Obviously, this model satisfies certain fundamental intuitions regarding justice and fairness which a Dutch participant addresses in the following way: "[Y]ou don't want to give something away, but you do want to receive something, very egoistically, like man is" (Ms. FI, NL-POD-lay).

All in all, our results show how the contradictions between the official regulations of anonymous post-mortem organ donation on the one hand and the relational subtext of many public and political discourses on the other can create serious moral perplexities among those affected. Although any personal relations between the organ donor and his or her family on the one hand and the organ recipient on the other are officially negated and effectively prohibited in the transplantation system, they are at the same time implied in many political and moral discourses and actually experienced by many lay and affected persons themselves. Organ transplantation is embedded in notions of interpersonal relations which can morally motivate persons to donate their organs after death, and can at the same time create notions of enduring indebtedness and guilt on the side of the recipients. This problem becomes particularly manifest in the case of post-mortem organ donation where – due to the anonymity paradigm and the death of the 'addressee' of responsibility – there seems to be no possibility for directly returning anything and thus to fulfill one's responsibility.

CONCLUSION

Contemporary public, political and academic discourses on organ donation often either focus exclusively on the part of the donors in an attempt to understand, qualify and manipulate their motivations, or on the side of the recipients in order to highlight the desolate character of their situation and the legitimacy and urgency of their needs. By contrast, our findings indicate that an appropriate theoretical and practical framework for organ donation has to conceptualize it as a reciprocal social interaction between *both* parties, focusing on the manifold relations existing and evolving between donors *and* recipients before, during and after transplantation. This relational perspective can help to disentangle many of the perplexities and dilemmas implicitly involved in the current practice.

With regard to living organ donation, our findings confirm that families with a member affected by a chronic disease mobilize resources to restore stability. On the one hand, they try to achieve this by emphasizing routines which reinforce family structure. The family adapts to the chronic disease and family support becomes a resource to fall back on. On the other hand, these families tend to uphold or reinforce established roles (Corbin & Strauss, 2004). Like other international findings, these results indicate that organ donation to family members is often regarded as a natural expression of love and belonging (Zeiler, 2011). It is associated with a family ideal based on the notion of mutual support. The imperative of family support is not limited by body boundaries (Wöhlke, 2011; Shim, Russ, & Kaufman, 2007; Motakef, 2011). Furthermore, our findings confirm that the family ideals involved are often gendered, especially with regard to the role of wife and mother (Scheper-Hughes, 2007). Ethics, policy, and law neglect intra-familial processes, especially pressure exerted through emotional dependence within the family. These processes manifest themselves in a stronger sense of obligation towards the family. It is doubtful whether these manifold intra-familial dynamics can be adequately conceptualized so as to ensure voluntariness. Thus, in medical practice, we recommend dealing sensitively with limits to autonomy which can arise from family constellations. That is not to say that there should not be any living donations within families. Rather, greater attention should be paid and professional counseling provided to detect whether donors and recipients might be limited in their autonomy because of already existing relational dynamics (Zeiler, 2009). Moreover, we should raise awareness in individuals considering living donation on whether their desire to donate an organ is based on emotional closeness or stereotypical role expectations which entail certain obligations (Wöhlke, 2011; Wöhlke & Mokatef, 2013).

In the field of post-mortem organ donation, organ transplantation creates a close entanglement of individual fates and new forms of social relations (Hauser-Schäublin, Kalitzkus, Petersen, & Schröder, 2001). At the same time, the legal regulations are aimed at precluding any personal contact between donors and recipients. Hence, the transfer of donor organs is uncoupled from the donor's personal identity and social relations and gains a symbolic dimension (Kalitzkus, 2003). This process can involve intricate feelings of gratitude, indebtedness and guilt on the side of recipients. While they find themselves in the phase of the counter-gift, the anonymization of the whole transaction makes it difficult to identify suitable addressees for returning anything, even on a symbolic level. At the same time, many relatives of deceased donors also criticize that the donation does not receive adequate acknowledgement. In addition, their lasting bonds with the deceased donors can result in a manifest interest in the organs' destination. There are several possibilities of arranging meetings between both sides in order to acknowledge the donors' sacrifice and express gratitude, e.g. public services or other kinds of events. This raises the question why such forms of meetings and exchange cannot be encouraged, supported or even arranged by public institutions, but are left to the voluntary engagement of those personally affected.

It has to be emphasized that our findings cannot claim to be representative in a strict, socio-demographic sense. The samples we used were too small to support strong generalizations and their specific composition may have influenced the outcomes. Thus, we only included persons from particular European countries where organ scarcity is a topic of public concern. Moreover, most of the affected persons we selected were organ recipients. Finally, most of the participants in the groups had experienced successful transplantations and thus were able to tell success stories. However, our research interest was not to make generalizations in view of the total public, but to identify and analyze common sense positions and arguments in an exemplary way. In view of this exploratory purpose, the qualitative methods we employed proved most suitable. The results they produced can be used to reflect the public, political and academic discourse, but also to interpret or instruct broader quantitative studies. Indeed, further research will have to show whether people from other European countries such as France, Spain or Austria, patients on the waiting list, or persons with difficult experiences would express different perspectives.

In view of the academic and biopolitical debate, the consequences of our results amount to a plea to avoid unilateralism in the discussion of transplantation medicine. The protagonists should widen their scope and gain an appreciation of the essentially social nature of organ donation as a reciprocal interaction of two parties with irreducibly different, but – at least prima facie – equally relevant and legitimate perspectives and interests (Schicktanz, Schweda, & Wöhlke, 2010). In concrete terms, this could mean that more theoretical scrutiny should be devoted to the problematic implications of the "tyranny of the gift" (Fox & Swazey, 1992). Psychological counseling for living organ donors and recipients as well as for relatives of cadaveric donors may help in case of unbalanced feelings of gratitude, indebtedness or social expectations. Furthermore, notwithstanding its problems, revisiting the so-called club model that links organ procurement and allocation by making willingness to give a precondition of claims to receive, could accommodate deeply rooted intuitions of justice and solidarity (Biller-Andorno, 2004). Finally, the anonymity paradigm in cadaveric organ allocation should be reconsidered. Although there definitely are good reasons not to immediately abandon the principle of anonymity in post-mortem organ donation (e.g., to ensure just allocation of organs or to protect the relatives' privacy), the exploration of possibilities of expressing public recognition by rewarded gifting or memorial services and plaques might be a step in the right direction (Sharp, 2001).

REFERENCES

Abadie, A. & Gay, S. (2006). The impact of presumed consent legislation on cadaveric organ donation: A cross-country study. *Journal of Health Economics*, *25*, 599-620. doi:10.1016/j.jhealeco.2006.01.003

Biller-Andorno, N. (2004). Between solidarity and self-interest: how fair is the "club model" for organ donation? *American Journal of Bioethics*, *4*, 19-20. doi:10.1080/15265160490911640

Barbour, R. S. (2011). Focus groups. In I. Bourgeault, R. Dingwall, R. de Vries (Eds.), *Qualitative Methods in Health Research* (327-353). London:Sage.

Boulware, L. E., Troll, M. U., Wang, N. Y. & Powe, N. R. (2006). Public attitudes toward incentives for organ donation: A national study of different race/ethnic and income groups. *American Journal of Transplantation*, *6*, 2774-2785. doi:10.1111/j.1600-6143.2006.01532.x

Corbin, J. M. & Strauss, A. L. (2004). *Weiterleben lernen. Verlauf und Bewältigung chronischer Krankheit.* Bern:Hans Huber.

Dor, F. J., Massay, E. K., Frunza, M., Johnson, R., Lennerling A., Lovén C., Weimar, W. (2011). New Classification of ELPAT for Living Organ Donation. *Transplantation*, *91*, 935-938. doi:10.1097/TP.0b013e3182129236

Deutsche Stiftung Organtransplantation. (2011). *Organ Donation and Transplantation in Germany.* Frankfurt am Main:DSO.

Eurotransplant (2012). Retrieved from http://www.eurotransplant.org

Fentiman, L. (1994). Organ donations. The failure of altruism. *Issues in Science and Technology*, *11*, 43-48.

Fox, R. C. & Swazey, J. P. (1992). *Spare Parts. Organ Replacement in American Society.* Oxford:Oxford University Press.

Hauser-Schäublin, B., Kalitzkus, V., Petersen, I. & Schröder, I. (2001). *Der geteilte Leib. Die kulturellen Dimensionen von Organtransplantation und Reproduktionsmedizin in Deutschland.* Frankfurt am Main:Campus.

Horton, R. L. & Horton, P. J. (1991). A model of willingness to become a potential organ donor. *Social Science & Medicine*, *33*, 1037-1051. doi:10.1016/0277-9536(91)90009-2

Kalitzkus, V. (2003). *Leben durch den Tod. Die zwei Seiten der Organtransplantation.* Frankfurt am Main:Campus.

Lopp, L. (2012). Comparative Analysis of European Transplant Laws Regarding Living Organ Donation: An Overview. Retrieved from http://www.eulod.org/Files/Eulod/Content_Files/p2vCMDeliverable.No7.WWUM.Short.Version.pdf .

Mocan, N. & Tekin, E. (2007). The determinants of the willingness to donate an organ among young adults: Evidence from the United States and the European Union. *Social Science & Medicine*, *65*, 2527-2538.

Morgan, D. L. (1997). *Focus Groups as qualitative research.* Thousand Oaks:Sage. doi:10.1016/j.socscimed.2007.07.004

Motakef, M. (2011). *Körper Gabe. Ambivalente Ökonomien der Organspende.* Bielefeld:Transkript.

National Ethics Council (2007). *Die Zahl der Organspenden erhöhen. Zu einem drängenden Problem der Transplantationsmedizin in Deutschland.* Berlin:NEC.

Scheper-Hughes, N. (2007). The tyranny of the gift: sacrificial violence in living donor transplants. *American Journal of Transplantantation*, *7*, 507-511. doi:10.1111/j.1600-6143.2006.01679.x

Schicktanz, S. & Schweda, M. (2012). The diversity of responsibility – the value of explication and pluralization. *Medicine Studies*, *3*, 131-145. doi:10.1007/s12376-011-0070-8

Schicktanz, S. & Schweda, M. (2009). "One man's trash is another man's treasure": exploring economic and moral subtexts of the 'organ shortage' problem in public views on organ donation. *Journal of Medical Ethics*, *35*, 473-476. doi:10.1136/jme.2008.027953

Schicktanz, S., Schweda, M. & Franzen, M. (2008). 'In a completely different light'? – The role of 'being affected' for the epistemic perspectives and moral attitudes of patients, relatives and lay people. *Medicine, Health Care and Philosophy*, *11*, 57-72. doi:10.1007/s11019-007-9074-2

Schicktanz, S., Schweda, M. & Wöhlke, S. (2010). Gender Issues in Living Organ Donation: Medical, Social and Ethical Aspects. In I. Klinge & C. Wiesemann (Eds.), *Sex and Gender in Biomedicine : Theories, Methodologies, Results* (33-55). Göttingen:Göttingen University Press.

Schweda, M. & Schicktanz, S. (2012). Shifting responsibilities of giving and taking organs? Ethical considerations of the public discourse on organ donation and organ trade. In: F. Svenaeus & M. Gunnarson (Eds.), *The Body as Gift, Resource and Commodity. Exchanging Organs, Tissues and Cells in the 21st Century* (235-266). Stockholm: Södertörn University Press.

Schweda, M. & Schicktanz, S. (2009a). Public ideas and values concerning the commercialization of organ donation in four European countries. *Social Science & Medicine*, *68*, 1129-1136. doi:10.1016/j.socscimed.2008.12.026

Schweda, M. & Schicktanz, S. (2009b). The 'spare parts person'? Conceptions of the human body and their implications for public attitudes towards organ donation and organ sale. *Philosophy, Ethics and Humanities in Medicine*, *4*, Art. 4. doi:10.1186/1747-5341-4-4

Schweda, M., Wöhlke, S. & Schicktanz, S. (2009). Understanding Public Skepticism Toward Organ Donation and Its Commercialization: The Important Role of Reciprocity. *Transplantation Proceedings*, *41*, 2509-2511. doi:10.1016/j.transproceed.2009.06.109

Sharp, L. A. (2007). Commodified Kin: Death, Mourning, and Competing Claims on the Bodies of Organ Donors in the United States. *American Anthropologist*, *103*, 112-133.

Shim, J., Russ, A. & Kaufman, S. (2007). Clinical life: expectation and the double edge of medical promise. *Health*, *11*, 245-264. doi:10.1177/1363459307074696

Siminoff, L.A., Burant, C. & Youngner, S. J. (2004). Death and organ procurement: public beliefs and attitudes. *Social Science & Medicine*, *59*, 2325-2334. doi:10.1016/ j.socscimed.2004.03.029

Strathern, M. (2012). Gifts money cannot buy. *Social Anthropology*, *20*, 397-410.

Terasaki, P. I., Cecka, J. M., Gjertson, D. W. & Takemoto, S. (1997). High survival rates of kidney transplants from spousal and living unrelated donors. *New England Journal of Medicine*, *333*, 333-338. doi:10.1056/NEJM199508103330601

Wöhlke, S. (2011). Das Fremde im Eigenen. Geschlechterunterschiede im Körper-Leib-Verständnis bei Lebendorgantransplantierten. In S.Wöhlke, L. Doyé (Eds.), *Damit Du weiterleben kannst. Die geschenkte Niere* (194-210). Hannover:LVH.

Wöhlke, S. (2013). The morality of giving and receiving living kidneys: Empirical findings on opinions of affected patients. In Gurch Randhawa & Silke Schicktanz (Eds.), Public Engagement in Organ Donation and Transplantation. Lengerich: Pabst Science Publisher.

Wöhlke S. & Mokatef, M. (2013). Selbstbestimmung und die Rolle der Familie in der Lebendorganspende. In C. Wiesemann, A. Simon (Eds.), *Patientenautonomie* (396-411) Berlin:Springer.

Wöhlke, S. & Schicktanz, S. (2012). "Vom ‚Geschenk des Lebens' bis zu ‚Du bekommst Alles von mir – ich auch von Dir?' Soziokulturelle Überlegungen und empirische Befunde zur öffentlichen Wahrnehmung der Organspende". *BZgA: Forschung und Praxis der Gesundheitsförderung*, *38*, 23-40.

Zeiler, K. (2009). Just love in live organ donation. *Medicine, Health Care and Philosophy*, *12*, 323-331. doi:10.1007/s11019-008-9151-1

Zeiler, K., Guntram, L. & Lennerling, A. (2010). Moral tales of parental living kidney donation: a parenthood moral imperative and its relevance for decision making. *Medicine, Health Care and Philosophy*, *13*, 225-236. doi:10.1007/s11019-010-9238-3

Endnotes

[i]Our analysis is based on 14 FGs on organ transplantation in Cyprus, Germany, the Netherlands, and Sweden. Eight FGs were recruited, organized, and conducted in 2005, following the guidelines for setting and content of the EU Project Challenges of Biomedicine Contract No. SAS6- CT-2003-510238. Participants (N=166) were lay (abbr. lay) and affected persons (abbr. aff), including patients who were waiting for an organ donation, recipients of donor organs, or persons who had refused to have an organ donation, as well as close relatives of these groups of persons. The two Cypriot FGs (CY-lay and CY-aff) were recruited, organized and conducted by the Department of Clinical Genetics at the Archbishop Makarios III Medical Centre. The two Dutch FGs were recruited, organised and conducted by the Department of Philosophy at the University of Utrecht. The two German FGs (DE-lay and DE-aff) were recruited, organized and conducted by the Research Group Bioethics and Science Communication at the Max-Delbrück-Center for Molecular Medicine Berlin-Buch. The two Dutch FGs (NL-lay and NL-aff) were recruited, organized and conducted by the Institute for Ethics at the University of Utrecht. The two Swedish FGs (SE-lay and SE-aff) were recruited, organized and conducted by the Department of European Ethnology at the University of Lund. For details, see http://www.univie.ac.at/virusss/cobpublication/1050/. Six further FGs were conducted between 2008 and 2009 with persons affected by LOD (N=47). For further details, see: Entscheidungsfindungsprozesse im Rahmen der Lebendnierenspende - Medizinethische und medizinanthropologische Aspekte http://www.egmed.uni-goettingen.de/index.php?id=143. The material presented here is based upon a broad analysis of moral attitudes towards organ donation and commercialization and the involved body conceptions (Schweda and Schicktanz 2009b, Schweda, Schicktanz and Wöhlke 2010), forms of being affected (Schicktanz, Schweda and Franzen 2008) and gender issues (Schicktanz, Schweda and Wöhlke 2010). For a detailed description of the methodology, see Schweda and Schicktanz (2009a).

In: Organ Donation and Transplantation
Editor: Mary Anne Lauri
ISBN: 978-1-62948-257-6

Chapter 11

CRITICAL CONVERSATIONS: ORGAN PROCUREMENT COORDINATORS' INTERPERSONAL COMMUNICATION DURING DONATION REQUESTS

Ashley Anker*
University at Buffalo, The State University of New York, New York, US

ABSTRACT

The conversations that occur between potential donor families, who are often responsible for making a donation decision on behalf of a loved one, and Organ Procurement Coordinators, who must shape requests to educate and influence potential donor families to consent to donation, are the critical juncture in the consent process. Messages communicated by Organ Procurement Coordinators during donation requests stand to influence familial decision-making, and thereby, the lives of those on the national waiting list for transplantation. The current chapter reviews the context of donation requests and introduces readers to four overlying approach philosophies employed by Organ Procurement Coordinators in requesting familial consent to donation: (1) option approach, (2) family-centered care approach, (3) dual advocacy, and (4) presumptive approach. After reviewing the association between Organ Procurement Coordinators' use of communication strategies -- in terms of message source, content, and style -- and donation outcomes, the chapter finds tentative support for use of those communication strategies advocated by the family-centered care approach. Recommendations are offered for improving the study of overlying familial request approach philosophies and determining the mechanisms behind the success of various communication strategies.

INTRODUCTION

Efforts to alleviate the chronic shortage of organs (see United Network for Organ Sharing, 2012) available for transplantation in the United States (U.S.) have often focused on

* Corresponding author: Email: aeanker@gmail.com, aeanker@buffalo.

promoting donor registration and communication of one's donation intentions to next-of-kin. Varied strategies used to educate the public about the need for organs have included worksite campaigns (e.g., Harrison et al., 2011), mass-mediated messages (e.g., Alvaro, Pace Jones, Robles, & Siegel, 2006; Cossé & Weisenberger, 2000), college and school-based programs (e.g., Feeley et al., 2009), and promotions at Department of Motor Vehicle offices (Harrison, Morgan, King, & Williams, 2011). Of late, prominent members of the donation field (Verble & Worth, 2012) have suggested steering attention away from the promotion of donor registration to focus more intently on the interpersonal communication efforts used by Organ Procurement Coordinators in requesting familial consent to deceased organ donation. Although efforts to fill donor registries are important and valuable, only a small proportion of registered donors will ultimately become deceased donors (see Howard & Byrne, 2007). In contrast, the current chapter places emphasis on interpersonal communication during the request process, as any family persuaded to consent to donation of a loved one's organs results in an immediate impact on donation rates.

The current chapter begins with an overview of scholarship and practice surrounding interpersonal communication in the context of donation requests within the United States' donation and transplantation system.[1] Subsequent to reviewing the role of U.S. Organ Procurement Coordinators and outlining the donation request context, the current chapter seeks to demonstrate that: (1) Organ Procurement Organizations' familial request strategies can be tentatively categorized into four overlying approach philosophies, (2) current academic scholarship has focused on testing particular message source, content, and style strategies employed within each of these philosophies, rather than directly comparing models to one another, and thus, (3) although research tentatively supports use of one overlying donation request philosophy, future research should focus on the use of additional methods and measures to more accurately characterize and create effective and appropriate donation requests.

THE U.S. DONATION/TRANSPLANTATION SYSTEM

Since the first recorded transplant from a brain-dead donor in 1963 (Howard, Cornell, & Cochran, 2012), the U.S. donation system has continued to remain heavily reliant on the provision of organs from deceased donors. Of 565,946 transplants completed in the U.S. since 1988, approximately 78.4% [N = 443,575; Organ Procurement and Transplantation Network (OPTN, 2012)] were the result of deceased donors. Deceased donors are a driving force behind the functioning of the U.S. donation/transplantation system for several reasons. First, deceased donors can provide a greater number of organs for transplant than living donors (see OPTN, 2012). Second, deceased donors can donate organs that may only be offered post-mortem (e.g., heart; see Nathan et al., 2003), and finally, transplants from deceased donors have impressive five-year patient survival rates ranging from 47.3% (lung) to 81.8% (kidney; OPTN, 2012). Despite the aforementioned benefits of deceased donation, deceased donor

[1] As countries operate under various laws/regulations, the current chapter focuses on interpersonal communication between Organ Procurement Coordinators and potential donor families in the United States' donation/transplantation system. However, as the consent of next-of-kin to deceased donation plays an important role in the donation process of many other nations (Rosenblum et al., 2011), the findings reported here are potentially relevant to those seeking to increase donation in other countries as well.

transplant cannot be achieved without the penultimate step of obtaining consent to donation from potential donor families.

Unfortunately, the disparity between the magnitude of need for donation and the size of the donor pool (see OPTN, 2012) suggests the U.S. has not yet maximized its potential for organ recovery. As of 2011, the national conversion rate for deceased organ donation stood at 72.9% [Scientific Registry of Transplant Recipients (SRTR), 2012], suggesting that of every 100 potential donor families, approximately 73 families consented to the donation of their loved one's organs *and* these organs were effectively recovered and placed with recipients. Scholars (e.g., Branco et al., 2011) specifically identify lack of familial consent to donation as the leading reason behind less-than-optimal organ recovery rates. Focusing research attention on the interpersonal communication that occurs between Organ Procurement Coordinators and potential donor families toward the end goal of increasing consent to deceased donation is thus both critical and timely.

In the U.S., 58 Organ Procurement Organisations Organizations work with hospitals in their general geographic areas to facilitate the identification and care of deceased donors. When an in-hospital death occurs (or, when prognosis is poor and death appears imminent), hospital personnel are required by law to contact their associated Organ Procurement Organisation Organization (see Siminoff & Mercer, 2001). The Organ Procurement Organisation Organization evaluates the referred case for its donation potential, and in the event of a seemingly eligible case, generally dispatches an Organ Procurement Coordinator[2] to the hospital to request familial consent to organ donation. While practices vary somewhat between one organization and anotherorganizations, Organ Procurement Coordinators may engage in tasks such as informing families about the option of donation, clinically managing a potential donor, providing emotional support, and assisting families with the completion of consent paperwork, such as the donor's medical/social history. Variations in this basic request practice include Organ Procurement Organizations that place in-house coordinators in high-volume trauma hospitals (Shafer et al., 2003), divide the responsibilities of making the donation request, offering family support, and clinically managing the donor between various Organ Procurement Organization staff members (Sade et al., 2002), approach families in conjunction with other supportive individuals (Conti, Jacoby, & Taft, 2001), or occasionally train designated requesters (e.g., physicians, nurses) who are not Organ Procurement Coordinators to speak with families (Williams et al., 2003). Despite practice variations between organizations, all coordinators play an important role in procuring organs for deceased donor transplant. Through their communication efforts, Organ Procurement Coordinators represent the last potential opportunity for persuading families to consent to the donation of a loved one's organs.

---

[2] The authors utilize the term Organ Procurement Coordinator to refer to the individuals who request familial consent to organ donation. Organ Procurement Organisations across the country use a variety of titles (e.g., Requester, Family Advocate, Donation Specialist) to describe this position.

THE DONATION REQUEST CONTEXT

Organ Procurement Coordinators' donation requests cannot be fully understood without first examining the complex context in which coordinators operate. Simply put, donation requests are influenced by a host of familial and environmental factors. Any family approached with a request for deceased donation will likely consider their knowledge (or lack thereof) of the decedent's donation preferences, in addition to their own feelings/beliefs on the topic. Coordinators are then further challenged to shape donation requests while taking into account the emotionally fraught hospital setting, the presence of conflicting media messages about donation, and rules/regulations pertinent to donation. As an Organ Procurement Coordinator approaches a potential donor family, such factors are likely salient, influencing choices in message content and style and potentially facilitating or hindering efforts to obtain consent. Some of the major familial and environmental factors that influence the coordinators' communication choices are highlighted in the next section to provide readers with an adequate understanding of the request context, before delving into Organ Procurement Coordinators' communication efforts.

Familial Factors

Due to the time sensitive nature of organ procurement, requests for deceased donation are presented to families who are still in the hospital environment coping with the recent or impending death of a loved one. Such families may experience a host of emotions ranging from grief and sadness to anger and guilt. Furthermore, as the majority of deceased donors are the result of sudden and/or unexpected causes of death (e.g., intracranial hemorrhage or stroke, blunt injury; OPTN, 2012), potential donor families are often entirely unprepared for the end-of-life decision-making process. In the midst of this emotionally charged context, Organ Procurement Coordinators are tasked with accurately presenting the opportunity for organ donation.

In an ideal request scenario, a potential donor family would be aware of a decedent's inclination toward becoming an organ donor. When such knowledge is available, families routinely implement the decision of their loved one (e.g., Dodd-McCue & Tartaglia, 2007; Rodrigue, Cornell, & Howard, 2006). Cases are complicated, however, when a potential donor family believes their loved one was opposed to donation (see Verble & Worth, 2012) or is unsure of the decedent's donation preferences (Siminoff & Lawrence, 2002). While Verble and Worth (2012) recognize that some decedents may have objected to donation as the result of a well-researched decision-making process – and thus, should be respected by family members -- they also indicate that some statements of unwillingness to participate in donation may be based on inaccurate information or may have been intended as a joke that was mistakenly taken in a serious manner. In cases in which a decedent expresses anti-donation sentiment based on inaccurate information, or when a family simply does not know what the decedent would have intended, it is left to Organ Procurement Coordinators to effectively and appropriately communicate the option of organ donation toward the goal of assisting families in making an educated decision on the topic.

In addition to consideration of the decedent's proclivities toward donation, it is likely that potential donor families also consider their own donation-relevant feelings and beliefs as they undergo the surrogate decision-making process surrounding donation. Although the majority of the public reports positive attitudes toward donation (Gallup, 2005), scholars (Anker & Feeley, 2010; Verble & Worth, 2000a) routinely document familial barriers to the deceased donation process. Organ Procurement Coordinators in Verble and Worth's (2000a) study identified familial concerns about mutilation/disfigurement, bodily wholeness, making a decision for someone else, disregarding a loved one's expressed wishes about donation, and cosmetic appearance of the donor as major barriers to obtaining familial consent. Almost a decade later, Anker and Feeley (2010) documented Organ Procurement Coordinators' frequent reports of familial concerns over bodily disfigurement and wholeness, families' inabilities to understand brain death, concerns about the length of time required to complete the donation process, and familial racial and cultural factors, as leading factors responsible for inhibiting the deceased donation process. As such barriers are harbored by families themselves, they may stand to be modified through the specific content and presentation of information by coordinators during the request process (see e.g., Long, Sque, & Payne, 2006; Verble & Worth, 1999, 2000b).

Environmental Factors

In addition to familial factors, the donation context is also influenced by a number of environmental/structural issues surrounding donation. First, with the prominent role of the media in most American's lives, it must be recognized that majority of families who are approached about organ donation have likely had some prior exposure to the topic. Conflicting media messages about donation range from educational campaigns to promote donor registration (see Feeley & Moon, 2009), to newspaper stories that generally depict altruistic and positively-themed transplant stories (Feeley & Vincent, 2007), to entertainment programming that may foster myths associated with donation (e.g., black market for organs; Morgan, Harrison, Chewning, Davis, & DiCorcia, 2007). As media messages have been found to impact various donation-relevant beliefs and behaviors (see e.g., Cossé & Weisenberger, 2000; Morgan, Harrison, Afifi, Long, & Stephenson, 2008), Organ Procurement Coordinators must recognize that potential donor families enter the request context with information attained from mass mediated and/or interpersonal communications on the topic that may influence perceptions of, and response to, the donation request.

Second, Organ Procurement Coordinators must operate within the hospital environment – a setting in which neither coordinators, nor potential donor families, likely have much control over their surroundings. Specifically, coordinators have documented structural problems with operating in hospitals where hospital staff make uneducated, but well intended, requests for donation without the support and guidance of the Organ Procurement OrganisationOrganization, where poor relations between families and hospital staff can hinder the relationship between coordinators and potential donor families, and where hospitals may pressure coordinators to hasten the donation process (Anker & Feeley, 2010). Within this complicated setting, coordinators must then find a way to communicate support and provide education to an emotionally distraught family, who may be ill-suited to comprehend information (Azoulay et al., 2007) due to the overwhelming nature of the end-of-life context.

Finally, Organ Procurement Coordinators operate in the context of national and statewide rules, regulations, and policies surrounding organ donation. While a complete review of such factors is beyond the scope of this chapter, the practice of using state registries to document preferences for deceased donation in-life is worth mentioning. State registries are of two varieties: (1) *registries of intent* that allow one to declare his/her intentions to become a donor, while still requiring consent from next-of-kin at the time-of-death, and (2) *registries of consent* that allow one to declare his/her legal consent to post-mortem donation. Registries were intended to facilitate familial decision-making at the end-of-life, as families who know their loved one's favorable donation preferences are more apt to consent to deceased donation (see Siminoff et al., 2001). However, with many states transitioning to consent registries (see Institute of Medicine, 2006), Organ Procurement Organizations have started to demonstrate some concern over the role of families in the consent process, in terms of merely being informed of a decedent's donation decision when s/he is on the consent registry, or still being given the responsibility of providing permission for donation to occur (see Christmas et al., 2008). In rare instances of disagreement between a decedent's documented consent to donation and a family's desire to decline donation, Organ Procurement Organizations have demonstrated varied policies about whose wishes should be followed (see Ganikos, 2010; Wendler & Dickert, 2001). The use of donor registries may thus facilitate Organ Procurement Coordinators' requests in situations in which a registered donor's family wishes to proceed with the decedent's expressed wish, or may complicate the request process in more infrequent instances where a documented donor's family expresses disagreement with the decedent's decision.

Recognizing the complexities of the donation request process emphasizes the importance of understanding the nuanced communication that occurs between Organ Procurement Coordinators and potential donor families. Coordinators are tasked with communicating about a topic toward which potential donor families may harbor inaccurate or incomplete knowledge (Verble & Worth, 2000a), may have received information of varied appropriateness from the media (e.g., Feeley & Vincent, 2007; Morgan, 2009), and may not have discussed with loved ones (Siminoff & Lawrence, 2002). Furthermore, organ donation is then discussed at an emotionally trying time, in an uncontrolled setting (Anker & Feeley, 2010), with a family who is likely unprepared to process complex information (Azoulay et al., 2007). Most impressive are the outcomes of this critical conversation surrounding consent to organ donation – the lives of those on the national waiting list for transplant are at stake.

THE OVERLYING DONATION REQUEST PHILOSOPHIES

In response to the complex donation request context, Organ Procurement Organizations have developed general overlying approaches to requesting donation that provide some indication of how Organ Procurement Coordinators should shape the content and style of messages they share with families. Although the approaches have not all been completely explicated in the literature, the current review relies on extant literature and presentations by Organ Procurement Organizations' staff to outline four general overlying approaches used for requesting donation: (1) option approach, (2) family-centered care, (3) dual advocacy, and (4) presumptive approach. Each of these philosophies warrants further description.

Option Approach

Traditionally, Organ Procurement Coordinators requested donation using the option approach. This approach was intended to be value neutral, as coordinators offered families the "option" of participating in organ donation (see Ganikos, 2010). Specifically, the approach focused on identifying familial concerns with donation and providing information to address such opposition (Zink & Wertlieb, 2006). The option approach is considered paternalistic, as coordinators function to protect potential donor families (Mone, 2008). Although Verble and Worth, consultants who have offered extensive training to the Organ Procurement Organization community (see Verble, Worth, & Verble, 2012), have not explicitly noted their use of the option approach, their program has likely historically been built upon it, with the publication of several papers that provide advice on overcoming specific familial objections to organ donation (see Verble & Worth, 1999, 2000b). Providing a concise background on the approach, Zink and Wertlieb (2006) indicate the option approach is passive and non-presumptive; Organ Procurement Coordinators provide information about donation, indicate the family has the option to donate, and offer their support for any donation decision made by the family. Blumenthal (2007) provides evidence that some coordinators may still be of the mindset that donation is most appropriately offered using the option approach, noting "Many donation coordinators in this study emphasized the fact that donation was not the best choice for every family, and that if the family was treated respectfully, given all the information to make a decision, and decided against donation, then it was still considered a positive outcome in their eyes" (p. 16).

Family-Centered Care

The family-centered care approach was initiated by the California Transplant Donor Network and places potential donor families at the forefront of the donation request process. Mone (2008) identifies the approach as evidence-based, developing from the findings of the Breakthrough Collaborative [see Health Resources Services Administration (HRSA), 2003; Shafer et al., 2006], as well as work by other prominent scholars in the donation field (Siminoff et al., 2001). Under the family-centered care approach, donation requests are shaped on the basis of three guiding principles that suggest: (1) excellent family care and optimal request outcomes can occur simultaneously, (2) familial grief and loss should guide the Organ Procurement Organization's intervention at end-of-life, and (3) Organ Procurement Coordinators give families information about donation, rather than taking something from families (see Mone, 2008, slides 12-14). Under the family-centered care approach, attention is given to the timing of events throughout the request process (Liu, 2011), with coordinators ensuring that families are supported, as well as psychologically and cognitively stable (Castro, 2008), prior to initiating the donation request.

Six steps are used to outline the progression of the donation request when operating under the family-centered care approach: (1) information gathering/sharing, (2) beginning family support, (3) discussing brain death, (4) coping with loss, (5) donation discussion, and (6) closure and aftercare (Mone, 2008, slide 19). Although early stages of this approach process emphasize the provision of support, Organ Procurement Coordinators are also taught to incorporate a "preliminary mention" of donation into the stages preceding the actual donation discussion (Castro, 2008). The preliminary mention consists of a brief reference to the concept of organ donation, but does not delve into details or encourage the family to make a decision on the topic (Castro, 2008). Using a team huddle, healthcare providers and the Organ Procurement Coordinator assigned to the cases congregate to determine who should offer the preliminary mention to a family, which is intended to prepare the family for the upcoming, and more extensive, donation discussion (Castro, 2008; Mone, 2008).

In enacting the family-centered care approach, coordinators are encouraged to avoid the use of close-ended questions, such that families do not preemptively decline donation due to their personal grief or lack of information (Castro, 2008). Other behaviors utilized in support of the family-centered care approach's goals include early incorporation and introduction of the Organ Procurement Coordinators to the potential donor family, use of a team huddle, encouraging discussion of the decedent among family members, and provision of information to resolve donation myths and misconceptions (Mone, 2008). Overall, coordinators operating under this approach are trained to ensure that families are fully informed about donation, to re-open the donation conversation if a family initially responds negatively to the suggestion of donation, and to accept and support a family's fully informed final decision (Castro, 2008; Mone, 2008).

Dual Advocacy Approach

The Gift of Life Institute in Philadelphia, Pennsylvania is credited with developing the dual advocacy approach for requesting organ donation (Mone, 2008). Contrary to the option or family-centered care approaches, the dual advocacy approach is considered to be a proactive method for addressing potential donor families (Ganikos, 2010). Mone (2008, slide 7) indicates the dual advocacy approach has three underlying premises: (1) most individuals will save a life if provided with the opportunity to do so, (2) Organ Procurement Coordinators act as dual advocates, supporting both potential donor families and those individuals awaiting organ transplant, and (3) donation is the right thing to do.

Organ Procurement Organizations practicing under the dual advocacy approach indicate that Organ Procurement Coordinators should provide families with information on donation, but suggest that a comprehensive overview of the topic also includes information on the benefits of organ donation to others, as well as the benefit of donation to the grieving family (see Luskin, Glazier, & Delmonico, 2008). In other words, coordinators do not just address any familial concerns about donation, but also proactively discuss donation using terms such as "hero," "legacy," "selflessness" and "act of compassion and kindness" (LifeSource, 2012, p. 43). Specific content included in dual advocacy requests includes the introduction of Organ Procurement Coordinators as members of the healthcare team, the description of donation as an "opportunity," rather than an "option," an emphasis on the need for organ donation, and the sharing of stories about organ recipients (see Mone, 2008). Although Mone (2008, slide 4) indicates that coordinators who operate under the dual advocacy approach still "recogniz[e] and respect each family's right to make their own fully informed decision", dual advocacy is decidedly persuasive in nature with Organ Procurement Coordinators described as being of "value and influence to the process" (LifeSource, 2012, p. 42). In summarizing a recent conference on consent, Metzger et al. (2005) suggested that participants, who consisted mostly of transplant professionals, identified the consent process as "...an opportunity for social persuasion" (p. 382), which is likely in line with the dual advocacy approach to shaping donation requests.

Presumptive Approach

Similar to dual advocacy, the presumptive approach acknowledges that most individuals will want to save a life when provided with the opportunity to do so, and that organ donation is the right thing to do (Zink & Wertlieb, 2006). The approach seems to go a step beyond dual advocacy by noting that requesters "...identi[fy] with organ recipients as much as, or *perhaps more than*, with the grieving families of potential organ donors" (p. 132; emphasis added). In outlining the presumptive approach, Zink and Wertlieb (2006) emphasize that Organ Procurement Coordinators advocate for donation, are introduced as part of the medical care team or as an experts in end-of-life issues/donation, draw similarities between the struggles of those awaiting transplant and potential donor families, explicitly reference recipients, and use presumptive statements and a presumptive "ask" for donation. Requests are thus focused on using open-ended questions to move a family toward donation (see Zink & Wertlieb, 2006). Luskin et al. (2008) indicate that many Organ Procurement Organizations have abandoned the presumptive approach in lieu of the dual advocacy approach.

Effectiveness of Overlying Donation Request Philosophies

Organ Procurement Organizations' overlying approaches to requesting consent to organ donation seem to vary along two dimensions: (1) the *focus of care*, placing various degrees of emphasis on *supporting potential donor families* (e.g., family-centered care approach) or *potential transplant recipients* (e.g., presumptive approach), and (2) the *goal of the approach*, either focusing on the *provision of information* (e.g., option approach) or on *persuading families to consent* to donation (e.g., dual advocacy approach). Within this framework, each overlying approach philosophy seems to emphasize particular practices related to *message source* or the individual(s) who should be responsible for various request aspects, *message content* or statements/information that should be communicated during the request, and *message style* or factors associated with timing, setting, and manner of delivering the request.

To the author's knowledge, there is no empirical work to-date that directly compares overlying approach philosophies to one another. Rather, studies examining the effectiveness of Organ Procurement Coordinators' requests for donation tend to examine specific communication strategies and their association with donation success (e.g., familial consent, Organ Procurement Organizsation consent and conversion rate). The next part of the chapter reviews the extant literature on the effectiveness of various message source, content, and style factors. Findings will be considered in the context of Organ Procurement Organizdations' overlying approach philosophies, making tentative recommendations for the effectiveness of those philosophies.

Message Source

Table 1 provides an overview of study findings characterizing the relationship between donation success and communication factors. With respect to message source, the literature consistently identifies more favorable donation outcomes in association with families who raise the topic of donation themselves (DeJong et al., 1998; Garrison et al., 1991; Linyear & Tartaglia, 1999; Rodrigue, Cornell, & Howard, 2006, 2008b; Siminoff et al., 2001). When a donation request must be communicated to a potential donor family, the bulk of the evidence is in favor of Organ Procurement Coordinators making the request on their own (Rodrigue et al., 2006; Von Pohle, 1996) or accompanied by healthcare professionals (Linyear & Tartaglia, 1999; Siminoff et al., 2001). Presently, routine referral laws (Siminoff & Mercer, 2001) have transferred request responsibility to coordinators, but current practice in the donation community indicates the best source for the approach should be identified following a team huddle of coordinators and healthcare professionals relevant to a case, so that each family's unique circumstances can be taken into consideration (Shafer et al., 2006).

Aside from the professional role of the requester, alternate requester characteristics may also be influential to the consent process. Although not found universally, many studies identify more favorable donation outcomes in response to racially matched requesters (DeJong et al., 1998; Gentry, Brown-Holbert, & Andrews, 1997; Kappel, Whitlock, Parks-Thomas, Hong, & Freedman, 1993). Others indicate the importance of approaching families with an additional source of support (Anker & Feeley, 2011; Conti et al., 2001) or of utilizing a requester with whom the potential donor family is familiar (Rodrigue et al., 2006, 2008b).

Results pertaining to message source characteristics seem to emphasize the importance of operating under an overlying approach philosophy that focuses care on potential donor families. Both the option and family-centered care approaches may be categorized as offering this focus, with the family-centered care model placing the greatest emphasis on familial well-being. As the review of extant literature on message source factors indicates a greater likelihood of consent in association with the specific strategies of providing support (e.g., Anker & Feeley, 2011) and making collaborative requests for organ donation (e.g., Siminoff et al., 2001) – behaviors regularly employed under the family-centered care philosophy - evidence on message source factors seems to tentatively weigh in favor of requesting donation under the family-centered care model.

Message Content

Studies of the messages communicated to potential donor families have often focused on the specific information and types of statements made by requesters. Overwhelmingly, research has shown the importance of providing families with an explanation of brain death (DeJong et al., 1998; Rodrigue et al., 2006), with more favorable donation outcomes occurring when a family has greater knowledge (DeJong et al., 1998) or understanding

(Rodrigue et al., 2008b; Siminoff et al., 2001) of the concept. Other important topics more apt to be discussed with families who consent to donation include the lack of costs, disfigurement, or impact on funeral arrangements associated with donation, as well as the indication that donation can help others and that families may select which organs to donate (Siminoff et al., 2001). In general, DeJong et al. (1998) have suggested that increased likelihood of familial consent is associated with families who believe they have been given enough information to make a donation decision and have received answers to all of their questions about donation.

Of interest, some studies highlight the importance of refraining from communicating particular messages to potential donor families. Siminoff et al. (2001) indicate that a decreased likelihood of familial consent is associated with the requester's statement that he or she is legally required to request donation. Anker and Feeley (2011) indicate that lower conversion rates are associated with Organ Procurement Coordinators' utilization of strategies such as offering to seek any relevant information for a family, discussing the benefits to donation prior to consent in situations in which a family is undecided on donation, emphasizing the need for donation among particular racial/ethnic groups, and querying a decedent's character (e.g., asking if the decedent was a caring/giving person).

Evidence on the effectiveness of message content is inconclusive in terms of providing recommendations for the overlying approach philosophy under which Organ Procurement Organizations may wish to operate. In terms of the goal of the overlying approach philosophy (i.e., informative versus persuasive) – with the option and family-centered care approaches advocating an informative role of Organ Procurement Coordinators, and the dual advocacy and presumptive consent approaches advocating a more persuasive role - the message content literature supports the use of behaviors at both ends of this spectrum. Studies noting the benefits of addressing known familial barriers to donation (e.g., costs; Siminoff et al., 2001) and ensuring a comprehensive understanding of brain death (Rodrigue et al., 2008b) tentatively point toward operating under an approach philosophy with an informative emphasis. However, studies documenting benefits of persuasive statements (e.g., indicating that donation helps others; Siminoff et al., 2001) should not be overlooked (see Anker & Feeley, 2011 for a conflicting finding on persuasive statements).

Message Style

It is also important to consider where, when, and how messages are communicated to potential donor families. In terms of deciding when to intervene with a potential donor family, research indicates that earlier intervention is ideal (Anker & Feeley, 2011). Best practices identified by the Organ Donation Breakthrough Collaborative (HRSA, 2003) cite the importance of hospitals providing early referral (i.e., calling the Organ Procurement Organizsation at early signs of impending brain death), which allows coordinators to begin interacting with potential donor families, establish a presence at the hospital, and prevent a rushed donation request (Shafer et al., 2006). Supporting the importance of early intervention, the implementation of in-house coordinator programs, which place coordinators on-site at busy trauma hospitals, has consistently been associated with increased consent rates (Shafer et al., 2003).

Table 1. Evidence for and against the use of communication strategies in shaping donation requests

Study	Method	Message Source	Message Content	Message Style
Anker & Feeley (2011)	Comparison of strategies endorsed by ORGAN PROCUREMENT COORDINATORSs (N = 102) to OPO-level conversion rates.	Increased conversion rate associated with ORGAN PROCUREMENT COORDINATORSs' use of: • Approaching with additional support No difference in conversion rate associated with ORGAN PROCUREMENT COORDINATORSs' use of: • Shadowing experienced ORGAN PROCUREMENT COORDINATORSs • Attending workshops/conferences • Being introduced to the family by others with an established relationship • Utilizing tactics designed to increase source homophily Decreased conversion rate associated with ORGAN PROCUREMENT COORDINATORSs' use of: • • Engaging in role play as a training strategy	No difference in conversion rate associated with ORGAN PROCUREMENT COORDINATORSs' use of: • Describing donation in clinical terms • Describing the case as a medical examiner's case • Identifying the decedent's donor status • Describing donation as life-saving • Making statements designed to positively frame the donor • Explaining the benefit of donation to the grieving process • Researching the family prior to the request • Re-approaching a family following a decline to non-OPO or OPO staff • Using social proof • Discussing donation as rare Decreased conversion rate associated with ORGAN PROCUREMENT COORDINATORSs' use of: • Seeking relevant information • Discussing the benefits to donation as a persuasive tactic • Querying a patient's character • Emphasizing the need for donation in particular racial/ethnic groups	Increased conversion rate associated with ORGAN PROCUREMENT COORDINATORSs' use of: • Gaining early intervention with a family No difference in conversion rate associated with ORGAN PROCUREMENT COORDINATORS' use of: • Approaching families after the acceptance of death • Observing families for conversation about future events • Being approached by the family • Limiting inclusion in the donation discussion • Approaching for donation in a quiet/private setting • Approaching for donation away from bedside • Changing approach strategy based on presence of estranged family members • Utilizing a 'like' requester of the same racial/ethnic background as the family • Changing nonverbal communication due to the racial/ cultural background of family
Christmas, Mallico, Burris, Bogart,	Comparison of pre-/post-consent rates over a 1.5 year period for a single OPO.		Increased post-intervention consent rate attributed to ORGAN PROCUREMENT OORDINATORSs' use of:	

Study	Method	Message Source	Message Content	Message Style
Norton, & Sing (2008)	Considers change in approach strategy for Department of Motor Vehicle [DMV] registered donors.		• Informing families that decedent is a registered donor and that OPO wishes to "honor the patient's wishes" • Failing to "ask permission" of the family for donation in cases of registered donors	
Conti, Jacoby, & Taft (2001)	Retrospective chart review ($N = 128$) over a two-year time period in area served by a single OPO. Comparison of consent rate for cases with and without additional source of support.	Increased consent rate associated with cases: • Employing the Mothers of Donors program, in which a mother of a prior organ donor is dispatched to the hospital to provide familial support		
DeJong, Franz, Wolfe, Nathan, Payne, Reitsma, et al. (1998)	Interviews with donor and non-donor families previously approached for donation ($N = 164$) by three OPOs	Increased likelihood of familial consent associated with: • First mention of donation by a family member • Request by racially matched requestor No difference in likelihood of familial consent based on: • Prior acquaintance with requestor • Source of donation request (i.e., hospital staff, OPO coordinator, family, other) • Source of brain death explanation	Increased likelihood of familial consent associated with: • Provision of enough information to make an informed donation decision • Provision of donation information in a language understood by family • Family ability to obtain answers to all questions about organ donation from people at hospital • Provision of an explanation of brain death • Familial knowledge of brain death No difference in likelihood of familial consent based on: • Provision of information that patient may not survive for long before s/he died • Perception that brain death was explained in a way that family could understand	Increased likelihood of familial consent associated with: • Family perception of higher quality of care received by decedent (i.e., receipt of care, belief all measures taken to save life, demonstration of caring by staff, provision of answers to family questions) • Timing of donation discussion perceived to be appropriate • Requestor perceived as sensitive • Family comfort with speaking to medical staff about donation • Provision of privacy for making donation decision • Family given enough time to discuss donation • Family given enough time to understand decedent was brain dead

Table 1. (Continued)

Study	Method	Message Source	Message Content	Message Style
			• Familial acknowledgement that decedent was "brain dead"	• Family perception that staff would be, and subsequently was, supportive of any donation decision No difference in consent based on: • Perceived amount of time spent with loved one near or after death • Provision of information that a loved one was deceased prior to first mention of donation • Timing of brain death explanation (i.e., prior, after, during donation discussion)
Dodd-McCue & Tartaglia (2007)	Retrospective review of African-American potential donor cases (*N* = 120) over a 7-year time period in a single medical center			Increased likelihood of familial consent associated with: • Family expression of gratitude or satisfaction in relation to the donation discussion process
Garrison, Bentley, Raque, Polk, Sladek, & Evanisko (1991)	Prospective review (*N* = 155) of potential donor cases during one year referred to a single OPO	Increased likelihood of consent associated with: • First mention of donation by a family member[a] • Source of donation request (i.e., greater proportion consent with chaplain, rather than nurse or physician)[a]		Increased likelihood of consent associated with: • Timing of brain death declaration (i.e., decoupled from donation request)
Gentry, Brown-Holbert, & Andrews (1997)	Retrospective comparison of consent rates over a 9-year time period at a single OPO. Considers change in requestor and public education coordinator.	Increased consent rate associated with: • Use of racially matched African American requestor for African American cases		

Study	Method	Message Source	Message Content	Message Style
		• Use of African American public education coordinator to spearhead community education efforts		
Kappel, Whitlock, Parks-Thomas, Hong, & Freedman (Phase 2; 1993)	Retrospective comparison of consent rates over a 5-year time period at a single OPO. Considers change in requestor.	Increased consent rate associated with: • Use of racially matched African-American requestor for all African-American cases		
Linyear & Tartaglia (1999)	Retrospective comparison of consent rates over a 26-month period at a hospital served by a single OPO. Compares rates after implementation of program.	Increased consent rate associated with: • First mention of donation by a family member • Source of donation request (i.e., request made by ORGAN PROCUREMENT COORDINATORS with hospital-based family communication coordinator or other hospital staff present)		Increased consent rate associated with: • Timing of brain death declaration (i.e., decoupled from donation request) No difference in consent rate based on: • Use of a private setting
Rodrigue, Cornell, & Howard (2008)	Interviews with prior donor and non-donor parents previously approached for pediatric organ donation (*N* = 74) by a single OPO	Increased likelihood of parental consent associated with: • First mention of donation by child's healthcare provider or a family member, rather than ORGAN PROCUREMENT COORDINATORS • Greater familiarity with requestor	Increased likelihood of parental consent associated with: • Greater understanding of brain death	Increased likelihood of parental consent associated with: • Requestor perceived as sensitive to family's needs • Timing of donation discussion perceived as appropriate • Family perception of being given enough time to discuss donation • Greater satisfaction with healthcare team (i.e., child's care before/after death, communication about diagnosis/prognosis, degree of respect shown by medical team)

Table 1. (Continued)

Study	Method	Message Source	Message Content	Message Style
				No difference in parental consent based on: • Requestor perceived as compassionate • Timing of brain death explanation
Rodrigue, Cornell, & Howard (2006)	Interviews with donor and non-donor families previously approached for donation ($N = 285$) by a single OPO	Increased likelihood of familial consent associated with: • First mention of donation by ORGAN PROCUREMENT COORDINATORS or family member • Source of donation request (i.e., OPO personnel more successful that non-OPO personnel) • Prior acquaintance with person requesting donation	Increased likelihood of familial consent associated with: • Provision of an explanation of brain death	Increased likelihood of familial consent associated with: • Requestor perceived as more sensitive and compassionate • Timing of donation discussion perceived as appropriate • Family perception of being given enough time to discuss donation • Greater satisfaction with healthcare team No difference in familial consent based on: • Timing of brain death explanation • Actual amount of time provided for discussing donation
Shafer, Davis, Holtzman, Van Buren, Crafts, & Durand (2003)	Comparison of consent rates over a 9-year period. Considers addition of in-house coordinators to level-one trauma centers.	Increased consent rate as compared to historical performance of same level-one trauma centers associated with: • Introduction of in-house coordinator		
Sade, Kay, Pitzer, Drake, Baliga, &	Comparison of consent rates over a 5-year period at a single OPO.	Increased consent rate associated with: • Division of procurement role into five separate positions,		

Study	Method	Message Source	Message Content	Message Style
Haines (2002)		including a family support counselor who offers the donation option and provides emotional support to families		
Siminoff, Gordon, Hewlett, & Arnold (2001)	Retrospective recall of healthcare provider, OPO staff, and family experiences during the donation request ($N = 420$ cases), accompanied by chart review. Data collected over five years at nine trauma hospitals.	Increased likelihood of familial consent associated with: • First mention of donation by a family member • Source of donation request (i.e., request by non-physician hospital-based healthcare provider followed by an approach by an ORGAN PROCUREMENT COORDINATORS superior to all other sources) No difference in likelihood of familial consent associated with: • Healthcare providers' demographic characteristics (i.e., age, sex, ethnicity, religious affiliation, professional role) • Initial source of donation request (i.e., physician, nurse, social worker, OPO staff member)	Increased likelihood of familial consent associated with: • Discussion of the lack of costs associated with donation • Discussion of the impact of donation on funeral arrangements • Discussion of lack of disfigurement to the body • Indication that family may choose which organs to donate • Indication that donation can help others • Greater number of conversations about donation • Discussion of a greater number of topics of familial concern • Provision of more answers to familial questions • Greater understanding of brain death Decreased likelihood of familial consent associated with: • Indication that requestor is required to ask about donation • First person to request donation was identified as the most important requestor	Increased likelihood of familial consent associated with: • Healthcare providers' personal comfort with answering familial questions about organ donation • Speaking with an ORGAN PROCUREMENT COORDINATORS before being asked to make a donation decision • Speaking with an ORGAN PROCUREMENT COORDINATORS for a longer period of time No difference in likelihood of consent based on: • Satisfaction with hospital care • Timing of donation request (i.e., prior to notification of death, after notification of death, at same time as notification of death) Decreased likelihood of familial consent associated with: • Family surprise at the donation request • Family report of being harassed or pressured during the donation request • Family report of interacting with one or more healthcare providers who seem uncaring or unconcerned

Table 1. (Continued)

Study	Method	Message Source	Message Content	Message Style
Von Pohle (1996)	Retrospective chart review over a two-year time period of deaths by neurological criteria (N = 157) at a single medical center served by one OPO. Considers use of decoupling and requestor from OPO.	Increased consent rate associated with: • Request for donation by ORGAN PROCUREMENT COORDINATORS		Increased consent rate associated with: • Timing of brain death explanation (i.e., prior to request for organ donation)
Anker & Feeley (2011)	Comparison of strategies endorsed by OPCs (N = 102) to OPO-level conversion rates.	Increased conversion rate associated with OPCs' use of: • Approaching with additional support No difference in conversion rate associated with OPCs' use of: • Shadowing experienced OPCs • Attending workshops/conferences • Being introduced to the family by others with an established relationship • Utilizing tactics designed to increase source homophily Decreased conversion rate associated with OPCs' use of: • Engaging in role play as a training strategy	No difference in conversion rate associated with OPCs' use of: • Describing donation in clinical terms • Describing the case as a medical examiner's case • Identifying the decedent's donor status • Describing donation as life-saving • Making statements designed to positively frame the donor • Explaining the benefit of donation to the grieving process • Researching the family prior to the request • Re-approaching a family following a decline to non-OPO or OPO staff • Using social proof • Discussing donation as rare Decreased conversion rate associated with OPCs' use of: • Seeking relevant information	Increased conversion rate associated with OPCs' use of: • Gaining early intervention with a family No difference in conversion rate associated with OPCs' use of: • Approaching families after the acceptance of death • Observing families for conversation about future events • Being approached by the family • Limiting inclusion in the donation discussion • Approaching for donation in a quiet/private setting • Approaching for donation away from bedside • Changing approach strategy based on presence of estranged family members • Utilizing a 'like' requester of the same racial/ethnic background as the family

Study	Method	Message Source	Message Content	Message Style
			• Discussing the benefits to donation as a persuasive tactic • Querying a patient's character • Emphasizing the need for donation in particular racial/ethnic groups	• Changing nonverbal communication due to the racial/cultural background of family
Christmas, Mallico, Burris, Bogart, Norton, & Sing (2008)	Comparison of pre-/post-consent rates over a 1.5 year period for a single OPO. Considers change in approach strategy for registered donors.		Increased post-intervention consent rate attributed to OPCs' use of: • Informing families that decedent is a registered donor and that OPO wishes to "honor the patient's wishes" • Failing to "ask permission" of the family for donation in cases of registered donors	
Conti, Jacoby, & Taft (2001)	Retrospective chart review ($N = 128$) over a two-year time period in area served by a single OPO. Comparison of consent rate for cases with and without additional source of support.	Increased consent rate associated with cases: • Employing the Mothers of Donors program, in which a mother of a prior organ donor is dispatched to the hospital to provide familial support		
DeJong, Franz, Wolfe, Nathan, Payne, Reitsma, et al. (1998)	Interviews with donor and non-donor families previously approached for donation ($N = 164$) by three OPOs.	Increased likelihood of familial consent associated with: • First mention of donation by a family member • Request by racially matched requestoer No difference in likelihood of familial consent based on: • Prior acquaintance with requesteor • Source of donation request (i.e., hospital staff, OPO coordinator, family, other)	Increased likelihood of familial consent associated with: • Provision of enough information to make an informed donation decision • Provision of donation information in a language understood by family • Family ability to obtain answers to all questions about organ donation from people at hospital • Provision of an explanation of brain death • Familial knowledge of brain death	Increased likelihood of familial consent associated with: • Family perception of higher quality of care received by decedent (i.e., receipt of care, belief all measures taken to save life, demonstration of caring by staff, provision of answers to family questions) • Timing of donation discussion perceived to be appropriate • Requeste or perceived as sensitive • Family comfort with speaking to medical staff about donation.

Table 1. (Continued)

Study	Method	Message Source	Message Content	Message Style
		• Source of brain death explanation	No difference in likelihood of familial consent based on: • Provision of information that patient may not survive for long before s/he died • Perception that brain death was explained in a way that family could understand • Familial acknowledgement that decedent was "brain dead"	to medical staff about donation • Provision of privacy for making donation decision • Family given enough time to discuss donation • Family given enough time to understand decedent was brain dead • Family perception that staff would be, and subsequently was, supportive of any donation decision No difference in consent based on: • Perceived amount of time spent with loved one near or after death • Provision of information that a loved one was deceased prior to first mention of donation • Timing of brain death explanation (i.e., prior, after, during donation discussion)
Dodd-McCue & Tartaglia (2007)	Retrospective review of African-American potential donor cases ($N = 120$) over a 7-year time period in a single medical center.			Increased likelihood of familial consent associated with: • Family expression of gratitude or satisfaction in relation to the donation discussion process
Garrison, Bentley, Raque, Polk, Sladek, & Evanisko (1991)	Prospective review ($N = 155$) of potential donor cases during one year referred to a single OPO.	Increased likelihood of consent associated with: • First mention of donation by a family membera • Source of donation request (i.e., greater proportion consent with chaplain, rather than nurse or physician)a		Increased likelihood of consent associated with: • Timing of brain death declaration (i.e., decoupled from donation request)

Study	Method	Message Source	Message Content	Message Style
Gentry, Brown-Holbert, & Andrews (1997)	Retrospective comparison of consent rates over a 9-year time period at a single OPO. Considers change in requesteor and public education coordinator.	Increased consent rate associated with: • Use of racially matched African American requesteor for African American cases • Use of African American public education coordinator to spearhead community education efforts		
Kappel, Whitlock, Parks-Thomas, Hong, & Freedman (Phase 2; 1993)	Retrospective comparison of consent rates over a 5-year time period at a single OPO. Considers change in requesteor.	Increased consent rate associated with: • Use of racially matched African-American requesteor for all African-American cases		
Linyear & Tartaglia (1999)	Retrospective comparison of consent rates over a 26-month period at a hospital served by a single OPO. Compares rates after implementation of program.	Increased consent rate associated with: • First mention of donation by a family member • Source of donation request (i.e., request made by OPC with hospital-based family communication coordinator or other hospital staff present)		Increased consent rate associated with: • Timing of brain death declaration (i.e., decoupled from donation request) No difference in consent rate based on: • Use of a private setting
Rodrigue, Cornell, & Howard (2008b)	Interviews with prior donor and non-donor parents previously approached for pediatric organ donation (*N* = 74) by a single OPO.	Increased likelihood of parental consent associated with: • First mention of donation by child's healthcare provider or a family member, rather than OPC • Greater familiarity with requesteor	Increased likelihood of parental consent associated with: • Greater understanding of brain death	Increased likelihood of parental consent associated with: • Requesteor perceived as sensitive to family's needs • Timing of donation discussion perceived as appropriate • Family perception of being given enough time to discuss donation • Greater satisfaction with

Table 1. (Continued)

Study	Method	Message Source	Message Content	Message Style
				healthcare team (i.e., child's care before/after death, communication about diagnosis/prognosis, degree of respect shown by medical team) No difference in parental consent based on: • Requesteor perceived as compassionate • Timing of brain death explanation
Rodrigue, Cornell, & Howard (2006)	Interviews with donor and non-donor families previously approached for donation ($N = 285$) by a single OPO	Increased likelihood of familial consent associated with: • First mention of donation by OPC or family member • Source of donation request (i.e., OPO personnel more successful that non-OPO personnel) • Prior acquaintance with person requesting donation	Increased likelihood of familial consent associated with: • Provision of an explanation of brain death	Increased likelihood of familial consent associated with: • Requesteor perceived as more sensitive and compassionate • Timing of donation discussion perceived as appropriate • Family perception of being given enough time to discuss donation • Greater satisfaction with healthcare team No difference in familial consent based on: • Timing of brain death explanation • Actual amount of time provided for discussing donation
Shafer, Davis, Holtzman, Van Buren, Crafts, &	Comparison of consent rates over a 9-year period. Considers addition of in-house coordinators to level-one trauma centers.	Increased consent rate as compared to historical performance of same level-one trauma centers associated with:		

Study	**Method**	**Message Source**	**Message Content**	**Message Style**
Durand (2003)		• Introduction of in-house coordinator		
Sade, Kay, Pitzer, Drake, Baliga, & Haines (2002)	Comparison of consent rates over a 5-year period at a single OPO.	Increased consent rate associated with: • Division of procurement role into five separate positions, including a family support counselor who offers the donation option and provides emotional support to families		
Siminoff, Gordon, Hewlett, & Arnold (2001)	Retrospective recall of healthcare provider, OPO staff, and family experiences during the donation request ($N = 420$ cases), accompanied by chart review. Data collected over five years at nine trauma hospitals.	Increased likelihood of familial consent associated with: • First mention of donation by a family member • Source of donation request (i.e., request by non-physician hospital-based healthcare provider followed by an approach by an OPC superior to all other sources) No difference in likelihood of familial consent associated with: • Healthcare providers' demographic characteristics (i.e., age, sex, ethnicity, religious affiliation, professional role) • Initial source of donation request (i.e., physician, nurse, social worker, OPO staff member)	Increased likelihood of familial consent associated with: • Discussion of the lack of costs associated with donation • Discussion of the impact of donation on funeral arrangements • Discussion of lack of disfigurement to the body • Indication that family may choose which organs to donate • Indication that donation can help others • Greater number of conversations about donation • Discussion of a greater number of topics of familial concern • Provision of more answers to familial questions • Greater understanding of brain death Decreased likelihood of familial consent associated with: • Indication that requesteor is required to ask about donation	

Table 1. (Continued)

Study	Method	Message Source	Message Content	Message Style
				Increased likelihood of familial consent associated with: • Healthcare providers' personal comfort with answering familial questions about organ donation • Speaking with an OPC before being asked to make a donation decision • Speaking with an OPC for a longer period of time No difference in likelihood of consent based on: • Satisfaction with hospital care • Timing of donation request (i.e., prior to notification of death, after notification of death, at same time as notification of death) Decreased likelihood of familial consent associated with: • Family surprise at the donation request • Family report of being harassed or pressured during the donation request • Family report of interacting
Von Pohle (1996)	Retrospective chart review over a two-year time period of deaths by neurological criteria (N = 157) at a single medical center served by one OPO. Considers use of decoupling and requesteor from OPO.	Increased consent rate associated with: • Request for donation by OPC		Increased consent rate associated with: • Timing of brain death explanation (i.e., prior to request for organ donation)

Notes: The following abbreviations are employed in Table 1: OPO = Organ Procurement Organization; OPC = Organ Procurement Coordinator; [a] Note that statistical significance tests were not conducted in this study

A second important aspect of message style is the timing associated with presenting information to potential donor families. Much research has focused on when the donation request should be made, particularly in relation to the declaration of brain death. Many studies support the use of "decoupling" or ensuring the brain death declaration and the donation request are separated in time (Garrison et al., 1991; Linyear & Tartaglia, 1999; Von Pohle, 1996). Alternate studies have failed to find evidence that actual timing of the brain death declaration influences consent (e.g., Siminoff et al., 2001), but rather, suggest that familial perception of the brain death discussion as occurring at an appropriate time is the more critical factor in achieving familial consent (see e.g., DeJong et al., 1998; Rodrigue et al., 2006, 2008b).

Timing has also been noted as important in relation to familial perceptions of being given enough time to discuss donation (DeJong et al., 1998; Rodrigue et al., 2006). Some studies note that actual amount of time provided for the donation discussion fails to distinguish donor from non-donor families (Rodrigue et al., 2006), but others indicate that speaking with an Organ Procurement Coordinator for a longer period of time (Siminoff et al., 2001) is associated with a greater likelihood of consent. In general, it appears that familial perceptions take precedence; families who feel pressured are less likely to donate (Siminoff et al., 2001), and thus, assessing familial readiness and progress throughout the donation request process is advisable.

Additional evidence on message style indicates that requesters should aim to communicate in a manner that is perceived by families as sensitive (DeJong et al., 1999; Rodrigue et al., 2008) and compassionate (Rodrigue et al., 2006), as those families who perceive at least one member of the healthcare team as uncaring or unconcerned are less apt to donate (see Siminoff et al., 2001). In addition, research also indicates that familial satisfaction with the decedent's care (DeJong et al., 1998), the healthcare team (Rodrigue et al., 2006, 2008) and the donation discussion (Dodd-McCue & Tartaglia, 2007), are associated with an increased likelihood of consent.

Evidence on message style seems to again point to the benefit of operating under an overlying approach philosophy that places an emphasis on focusing care on potential donor families. Specific message style elements noted as beneficial in the current review – such as early intervention (Anker & Feeley, 2011), closely monitoring the timing of events (e.g., brain death discussion; Garrison et al., 1991), and utilizing sensitive and compassionate requesters (DeJong et al., 1999; Rodrigue et al., 2006) are all consistent with the family-centered care model's focus on providing families with early intervention, support, and appropriately timed information. Thus, based on message style, evidence again seems to weigh in favor of operating under the family-centered care approach.

Limitations and Recommendations for Future Research

Results of the current review seem most supportive of those specific message source, content, and style factors that are advocated within a family-centered care approach to obtaining familial consent to organ donation. Although the current review should not be seen as conclusive, it does provide a comprehensive summary of knowledge surrounding consent practices to-date. Given the promise shown by the family-centered care approach in the current review, the chapter concludes by providing recommendations for further study of this particular request philosophy, as well as offering general recommendations for the improvement of methods and measures in the study of donation consent.

Future Study of the Family-Centered Care Approach

Future research should aim to determine *why* the dimensions underlying the family-centered care approach (i.e., focus on provision of information, focus on potential donor families) may be most effective for obtaining familial consent to organ donation. One potential reason for the effectiveness of this philosophy may be that strategies contained within the approach are not perceived as manipulative by potential donor families. Anker and Feeley (2011) suggest that some messages utilized by Organ Procurement Coordinators may induce psychological reactance (i.e., anger and negative cognition; see Dillard & Shen, 2005), as potential donor families perceive they are being directed toward a particular donation decision. Such strategies could feature more prominently in other overlying donation request philosophies - particularly, those with a greater focus on organ potential transplant recipients - limiting their effectiveness. Commenting on the presumptive approach, for example, Truog (2008) expressed concerns that coordinators may employ statements that are "…clearly misleading or manipulative" (p. 1210). As families are less likely to consent to donation when they feel pressured (see Siminoff et al., 2001) and as a proportion of families have reported traumatic memories of the donation request when organ-focused behaviors (i.e., requests focused on procurement, rather than familial well-being) are used (see Kesselring, Kainz, & Kiss, 2007), the focus of the family-centered care approach on familial well-being and unconditional acceptance of an informed donation decision may benefit consent rates and familial psychological outcomes.

An alternative explanation for the effectiveness of the family-centered care approach may be the approach is particularly good at building trust between potential donor families and Organ Procurement Coordinators. HRSA (2003) notes the consent process involves, "…carefully conveyed communications, all within a context of trust" (p. 591). The family-centered care approach seems to devote an extensive amount of time to the interaction between coordinators and potential donor families. Under this approach, coordinators are encouraged to learn about a family prior to their approach, intervene early, provide support, and give information on donation. Due to the level of devotion shown by Organ Procurement Coordinators to potential donor families under the family-centered care model, the development of extensive trusting relationships between coordinators and families may be anticipated. Anecdotal evidence from data collected by Anker and Feeley (2011) support this notion, with Organ Procurement Coordinators in their study describing obviously trusting relationships in which coordinators attended the funerals of potential donors or maintained contact with families for years following a donation request.

Future research should examine both trust and psychological reactance as potential mediators in the relationship between coordinators' use of communication strategies and measures of donation success. Extant literature indicates that many families regret declining the opportunity for donation (Rodrigue et al., 2008a). Similarly, Sanner (2007) suggests that potential donor families may view declining donation as a default or "non-decision" on the topic. Given that familial decline to donation may be unintended (i.e., a "non-decision") or regrettable, it is important that Organ Procurement Coordinators develop a trusting relationship with families in which the donation information they aim to present is understood to the best of a family's capabilities and not hindered by any unintended emotions (i.e., psychological reactance) stemming from the phrasing of the request.

Despite the tentative evidence pointing toward the beneficial nature of communication strategies employed by the family-centered care approach, this chapter should not be viewed as conclusive and is far from the final word on request effectiveness. Quantitative methods (i.e., meta-analysis) were not utilized to examine the association of strategy use with donation success, and the methods of many of the studies reviewed herein suffer from a number of flaws. To conclude, the chapter highlights problems with extant methods and measures of interpersonal communication between Organ Procurement Coordinators and potential donor families, before identifying some potential future areas for research.

Limitations of Current Methods and Measures

One common method of studying communication surrounding the consent process is to compare families' or coordinators' recollections of the request process (see e.g., Rodrigue et al., 2006; Siminoff et al., 2001) to familial decisions to consent to (or decline) donation. Such studies are reliant on retrospective recall and aim to contact participants in relative proximity to the donation request. However, such methods are flawed in that participants' recall of events can be incomplete (Reimer & Matthes, 2007) or may be open to response bias in the form of social desirability. Furthermore, families or requesters may be unable to recall portions of the request process, neglect to mention important behaviors that occurred during the request, or be unable to adequately explain a critical aspect of the process.

Other studies in the current review rely on tracking measures of donation success over time (e.g., consent rate) to consider changes associated with altered consent processes (e.g., Christmas et al., 2007). Without a control group, such studies open themselves up to a variety of threats to internal validity that may offer alternative accounts for pre- to post-test changes in donation success. Additionally, as some studies implement programs consisting of multiple simultaneous changes to the consent process, it can be difficult to conclusively determine which specific communication strategies are most effective at influencing consent rates.

Finally, many studies are flawed by their reliance on samples referencing only one (e.g., Rodrigue et al., 2006) or a handful (e.g., DeJong et al., 1998) of Organ Procurement Organizations, thereby calling into question the generalizability of the study findings (see Anker & Feeley, 2011 for an exception). Such studies limit knowledge of the request process to those practices that are likely facilitated within participating organizations, rather than exploring the diversity of approaches and strategies that are present across the donation field.

Recommendations for Future Research

To improve upon existing research, scholars may wish to consider whether they can obtain detailed records of actual donation requests made by Organ Procurement Coordinators to potential donor families. Studies in the domain of tissue donation (Siminoff, Traino, & Gordon, 2010) have recently started to analyze audio-recorded telephone conversations between tissue requesters and potential donor family members, leading to detailed analyses of conversational patterns (see e.g., Weathersbee & Maynard, 2009). Although the donation conversation is incredibly sensitive, non-intrusive recordings of other difficult end-of-life discussions (i.e., family conferences on the withdrawal of patient care; Curtis et al., 2002) have been conducted in an ethical and appropriate manner, and would be incredibly valuable in the context of organ donation. By obtaining in-depth documentation (e.g., audio-recordings, video-recordings) of the donation request process, researchers could overcome the methodological flaws inherent to studies that are reliant on families' and Organ Procurement Coordinators' retrospective self-reports of behavior during the request process (e.g., Siminoff et al., 2001). Recordings of donation requests might lend themselves to analyses of behaviors that are difficult to self-report (e.g., nonverbal communication) or may provide insight as to how to appropriately situate topics within the consent discussion.

Second, scholars may wish to conduct more extensive research to consider whether coordinators' use of message source, content, and style factors is consistent with the overlying donation request philosophy to which an Organ Procurement Organization wishes to adhere. As coordinators have experienced conflicts with organization administration surrounding the use of particular strategies (i.e., unconditionally supporting fully informed familial decline to donation; see Blumenthal, 2007), it is possible that coordinators may not always be loyal to the recommendations of an organization's overlying donation request philosophy. In addition, with the variety of message source, content, and style strategies available, coordinators may have become favorable toward strategies stemming from various philosophies, potentially presenting potential donor families with messages that were not intended to supplement one another.

In considering the functioning of overlying donation request philosophies, it is unlikely that scholars will be able to avoid further use of the quasi-experimental designs (e.g., single group pre-/post-test) inherent in the donation consent literature to-date. To provide more support to extant literature, however, scholars might test overlying philosophy and strategy effectiveness using a variety of research methods. For example, Organ Procurement Organizations could be matched based upon baseline consent rate, geographic location (e.g., urban, rural), or demographic composition of their donor pool, with an organization from each pair then assigned to implement an approach philosophy or a series of particular message source, content, and style characteristics toward the goal of comparing changes in consent over time. Alternatively, coordinators within a single large organization could be randomly assigned to either provide standard request processes or implement an alternate change in consent. Finding alternative methods of testing the effectiveness of communication strategies will reinforce those findings highlighted in the literature to-date.

Finally, scholars should seek to study consent using a national sample of Organ Procurement Organizations. With many studies involving only one, or a handful, of organizations, it is possible that many tests of communication strategy use have not involved coordinators who employ strategies representing the full spectrum of donation request philosophies. For example, if the bulk of published literature has been reliant on samples of Organ Procurement Coordinators from a family-centered care background, it would not be surprising to find little support in the literature for strategies stemming from other donation request approach philosophies. Undertaking large-scale, national tests of communication strategy effectiveness can ensure the variety of strategies used by coordinators across the field are both accurately described and extensively tested.

Conclusion

Organ Procurement Coordinators play a key role in maintaining the functioning of the U.S. donation and transplantation system based upon their crucial role in requesting consent to donation from potential donor families. There are few settings in which the stake of a conversation is as high as that faced by a coordinator, who ultimately assists in saving the lives of those awaiting transplant by communicating donation requests. Based on a review of the literature, the current chapter tentatively points to the benefits of shaping such requests under a family-centered care approach. Before adhering to this approach, however, scholars and practitioners must work together to more extensively examine donation requests, using national samples of Organ Procurement Organizations, and operating under various research designs. Upon such replication and extension, the field should advance its knowledge of the request process and have solid recommendations for how to best request consent to donation from families.

References

Alvaro, E. M., Pace Jones, S., Robles, A. S. M. & Siegel, J. (2006). Hispanic organ donation: Impact of a Spanish-language organ donation campaign. *Journal of the National Medical Association, 98*(1), 28-35.

Anker, A. E. & Feeley, T. H. (2010). Why families decline donation: The perspective of Organ Procurement Coordinators. *Progress in Transplantation*, *20*(3), 239-246.

Anker, A. E., & Feeley, T. H. (2011). Asking the difficult questions: Message strategies utilized by Organ Procurement Coordinators in requesting familial consent to organ donation. *Journal of Health Communication*. *16*(6), 643-659.

Azoulay, E., Chevret, S., Leleu, G., Pochard, F., Barboteu, M., Adrie, C., Canoui, P., Le Gall, J. R. & Schlemmer, B. (2000). Half the families of intensive care unit patients experience inadequate communication with physicians. *Critical Care Medicine, 28*(8), 3044-3049.

Blumenthal, P. A. (2007). “It’s not a job; it’s a lifestyle:” The experience of being a donation coordinator. *Progress in Transplantation, 17*(1), 8-22.

Branco, B. C., Inaba, K., Lam, L., Salim, A., Barmparas, G., Teixeira, P. G. R., et al. (2011). Donor conversion and procurement failure: The fate of our potential organ donors. *World Journal of Surgery, 35*, 440-445.

Castro, J. (2008, September). *Preliminary mention and re-opening the donation discussion*. Presentation at the annual meeting of the Association for Multicultural Affairs, Minneapolis, Minnesota. Presentation retrieved August 24, 2012 from: http://www.asmhtp.org/events.aspx.

Christmas, A. B., Mallico, E. J., Burris, G. W., Bogart, T. A., Norton, H. J. & Sing, R. F. (2008). A paradigm shift in the approach to families for organ donation: Honoring patients’ wishes versus request for permission in patients with Department of Motor Vehicles donor designations. *The Journal of Trauma Injury, Infection, and Critical Care, 65*(5), 1507-1510.

Conti, D., Jacoby, L. & Taft, F. (2001). A novel volunteer intervention to increase organ donation. *Transplantation Proceedings*, *33*, 966-967.

Cossé, T. J. & Weisenberger, T. M. (2000). Words versus actions about organ donation: A four-year tracking study of attitudes and self-reported behavior. *Journal of Business Research*, *50*, 297-303.

Curtis, J. R., Engelberg, R. A., Wenrich, M. D., Nielsen, E. L., Shannon, S. E., Treece, P. D., Tonelli, M. R., Patrick, D. L,. Robins, L. S,. McGrath, B. B. & Rubenfeld, G. D. (2002). Studying communication about end-of-life care during the ICU family conference: Development of a framework. *Journal of Critical Care*, *17*, 147-160.

DeJong, W., Franz, H. G., Wolfe, S. M., Nathan, H., Payne, D., Reitsma, W., et al. (1998). Requesting organ donation: An interview study of donor and nondonor families. *American Journal of Critical Care*, *7*(1), 13-23.

Dillard, J. P. & Shen, L. (2005). On the nature of reactance and its role in persuasive health communication. *Communication Monographs*, *72*, 144-168.

Dodd-McCue, D. & Tartaglia, A. (2007). African American consent and nonconsent cases: Are there significant differences? *Progress in Transplantation*, *17*(3), 215-219.

Feeley, T. H., Anker, A. E., Watkins, B., Rivera, J., Tag, N. & Volpe, L. (2009). A peer-to-peer campaign to promote organ donation among racially diverse college students in New York City. *Journal of the National Medical Association*, *101*(11), 1154-1162.

Feeley, T. H. & Moon, S. (2009). A meta-analytic review of communication campaigns to promote organ donation. *Communication Reports*, *22*(2), 63-73.

Feeley, T. H. & Vincent, D. (2007). How organ donation is represented in newspaper articles in the United States. *Health Communication*, *21*(2), 125-131.

Gallup Organization. (2005). *2005 National survey of organ and tissue donation attitudes.* Retrieved from: ftp://ftp.hrsa.gov/organdonor/survey2005.pdf

Ganikos, M. (2010). Organ donation: An overview of the field. (13-39). In E. Alvaro & J. Siegel (Eds.). *Understanding Organ Donation: Applied Behavioral Science Perspectives.* West Sussex, UK: Wiley-Blackwell.

Garrison, R. N., Bentley, F. R., Raque, G. H., Polk, H. C., Sladek, L. C., & Evanisko, M. J. (1991). There is an answer to the shortage of organ donors. *Surgery, Gynecology, & Obstetrics*, *173*, 391-396.

Gentry, D., Brown-Holbert, J. & Andrews, C. (1997). Racial impact: Increasing minority consent rate by altering the racial mix of an organ procurement organization. *Transplantation Proceedings*, *29*, 3758-3759.

Harrison, T. R., Morgan, S. E., Chewning, L. V., Williams, E. A., Barbour, J. B., DiCorcia, M. & Davis, L. A. (2011). Revisiting the worksite in worksite health campaigns: Evidence from a multisite organ donation campaign. *Journal of Communication*, *61*, 535-555.

Harrison, T. R., Morgan, S. E., King, A. J. & Williams, E. A. (2011). Saving lives branch by branch: The effectiveness of driver licensing bureau campaigns to promote organ donor registry sign-ups to African Americans in Michigan. *Journal of Health Communication*, *16*(8), 805-819.

Health Resources Services Administration. (2003). The organ donation breakthrough collaborative: Best practices final report (September 2003). *Nephrology Nursing Journal*, *30*(5), 529-591.

Howard, D. H. & Byrne, M. M. (2007). Should we promote organ donor registries when so few registrants will end up being donors? *Medical Decision Making*, *27*, 243-249.

Howard, R. J., Cornell, D. L. & Cochran, L. (2012). History of deceased organ donation, transplantation, and organ procurement organizations. *Progress in Transplantation*, *22*(1), 6-17.

Institute of Medicine. (2006). *Organ Donation: Opportunities for Action.* Washington, DC: The National Academies Press.

Kappel, D. F., Whitlock, M. E., Parks-Thomas, T. D., Hong, B. A. & Freedman, B. K. (1993). Increasing African American organ donation: The St Louis experience. *Transplantation Proceedings*, *25*(4), 2489-2490.

Kesselring, A., Kainz, M. & Kiss, A. (2007). Traumatic memories of relatives regarding brain death, request for organ donation and interactions with professionals in the ICU. *American Journal of Transplantation*, *7*, 211-217.

LifeSource. (2012). *Certified Designated Requestor training manual. Dual advocacy: A value-centered approach to organ, tissue, and eye donation.* (5th ed.). Retrieved August 21, 2012 from: http://www.life-source.org/partners/hospital-professionals/cdrs/.

Linyear, A. S. & Tartaglia, A. (1999). Family communication coordination: A program to increase organ donation. *Journal of Transplant Coordination*, *9*(3), 165-174.

Liu, A. (2011, October). *Improving family-centered care through standardized brain death diagnosis.* Presentation at the Organ Donation and Transplantation Symposium. Retrieved August 21, 2012 from: http://www.onelegacy.org/site/professionals/20111011_odtsymposium.html.

Long, T., Sque, M. & Payne, S. (2006). Information sharing: Its impact on donor and nondonor families' experiences in the hospital. *Progress in Transplantation*, *16*(2), 144-149.

Luskin, R. S., Glazier, A. K. & Delmonico, F. L. (2008). Organ donation and dual advocacy. *The New England Journal of Medicine*, *358*(12), 1297-1298.

Metzger, R. A., Taylor, G. J., McGaw, L. J., Delmonico, F. L. & Prottas, J. M. for the UNOS Research to Practice Steering Committee (2005). Research to practice: A national consensus conference. *Progress in Transplantation*, *15*(4), 379-384.

Mone, T. (2008). *The evolution of family care, approach, and consent for donation.* Presentation at the National Organ Donation Summit, Adelaide, Australia. Retrieved August 21, 2012 from: http://www.sahealth.sa.gov.au/wps/wcm/ connect/fec2f68044bd08e8baaabed3777922da/NODS+1+2+Dual+Advocacy+and+Family+Approach+Mone.pdf?MOD=AJPERES&CACHEID=fec2f68044bd08e8baaabed3777922da&CACHE=NONE.

Morgan, S. E. (2009). The intersection of conversation, cognitions, and campaigns: The social representation of organ donation. *Communication Theory*, *19*(1), 29-48.

Morgan, S. E., Harrison, T. R., Afifi, W. A., Long, S. D. & Stephenson, M. T. (2008). In their own words: The reasons why people will (not) sign an organ donor card. *Health Communication*, *23*, 23-33.

Morgan, S. E., Harrison, T. R., Chewning, L., Davis, L. & DiCorcia, M. (2007). Entertainment (mis)education: The framing of organ donation in entertainment television. *Health Communication*, *22*(2), 143-151.

Nathan, H. M., Conrad, S. L., Held, P. J., McCullough, K. P., Pietroski, R. E., Siminoff, L. A. & Ojo, A. O. (2003). Organ donation in the United States. *American Journal of Transplantation*, *3*(Supp 4), 29-40.

Organ Procurement and Transplantation Network. (2012). *Data.* [Database on the Internet]. Retrieved August 20, 2012 from: http://optn.transplant.hrsa.gov/data/.

Reimer, M. & Matthes, B. (2007). Collecting event histories with TrueTales: Techniques to improve autobiographical recall problems in standardized interviews. *Quality & Quantity*, *41*, 711-735.

Rodrigue, J. R., Cornell, D. L. & Howard, R. J. (2006). Organ donation decision: Comparison of donor and nondonor families. *American Journal of Transplantation*, *6*, 190-198.

Rodrigue, J. R., Cornell, D. L. & Howard, R. J. (2008a). The instability of organ donation decisions by next-of-kin and factors that predict it. *American Journal of Transplantation*, *8*, 2661-2667.

Rodrigue, J. R., Cornell, D. L. & Howard, R. J. (2008b). Pediatric organ donation: What factors most influence parents' donation decisions? *Pediatric Critical Care Medicine*, *9*(2), 180-185.

Rosenblum, A. M., Horvat, L. D., Siminoff, L. A., Prakash, V., Beitel, J. & Garg, A. X. (2011). The authority of next-of-kin in explicit and presumed consent systems for deceased organ donation: An analysis of 54 nations. *Nephrology Dialysis Transplantation*. Advance online publication. doi:10.1093/ndt/gfr619.

Sade, R. M., Kay, N., Pitzer, S., Drake, P., Baliga, P. & Haines, S. (2002). Increasing organ donation: A successful new concept. *Transplantation*, *74*(8), 1142-1146.

Sanner, M. A. (2007). Two perspectives on organ donation: Experiences of potential donor families and intensive care physicians of the same event. *Journal of Critical Care*, *22*, 296-304.

Scientific Registry of Transplant Recipients. (2012). *Transplant and OPO specific reports* [database on the Internet]. Retrieved August 26, 2012 from: http://www.srtr.org/opo/Default.aspx.

Shafer, T. J., Davis, K. D., Holtzman, S. M., Van Buren, C. T., Crafts, N. J. & Durand, R. (2003). Location of in-house organ procurement organization staff in level I trauma centers increases conversion of potential donors to actual donors. *Transplantation*, *75*(8), 1330-1335.

Shafer, T. J., Wagner, D., Chessare, J., Zampiello, F. A., McBride, V. & Perdue, J. (2006). Organ donation breakthrough collaborative: Increasing organ donation through system redesign. *Critical Care Nurse*, *26*(2), 33-49.

Siminoff, L. A., Gordon, N., Hewlett, J. & Arnold, R. M. (2001). Factors influencing families' consent for donation of solid organs for transplantation. *Journal of the American Medical Association*, *286*(1), 71-77.

Siminoff, L. A., & Lawrence, R. H. (2002). Knowing patients' preferences about organ donation: Does it make a difference? *Journal of Trauma Injury, Infection, and Critical Care, 53*(4), 754-760.

Siminoff, L. A. & Mercer, M. B. (2001). Public policy, public opinion, and consent for organ donation. *Cambridge Quarterly of Healthcare Ethics*, *10*, 377-386.

Siminoff, L. A., Traino, H. M. & Gordon, N. (2010). Determinants of family consent to tissue donation. *The Journal of Trauma Injury, Infection, and Critical Care*, *69*(4), 956-963.

Truog, R. D. (2008). Consent for organ donation – Balancing conflicting ethical obligations. *The New England Journal of Medicine*, *358*(12), 1209-1211.

United Network for Organ Sharing. (2012). *Transplant trends.* Retrieved August 21, 2012 from: www.unos.org.

Verble, M. & Worth, J. (1999). Dealing with the fear of mutilation in the donation discussion. *Journal of Transplant Coordination*, *9*(1), 54-56.

Verble, M. & Worth, J. (2000a). Fears and concerns expressed by families in the donation discussion. *Progress in Transplantation*, *10*(1), 48-55.

Verble, M. & Worth, J. (2000b). Overcoming families' fears and concerns in the donation discussion. *Progress in Transplantation*, *10*(3), 155-160.

Verble, M. & Worth, J. (2012). Addressing the unintended adverse consequences of first-person consent and donor registries. *Progress in Transplantation*, *22*(1), 25-32.

Verble, M., Worth, J., & Verble, D. (2012). *Verble, Worth, & Verble.* Retrieved August 20, 2012 from: http://www.verbleworthverble.com/.

Von Pohle, W. R. (1996). Obtaining organ donation: Who should ask? *Heart & Lung*, *25*(4), 304-309.

Weathersbee, T. E. & Maynard, D. W. (2009). Dialing for donations: Practices and actions in the telephone solicitation of human tissues. *Sociology of Health & Illness*, *31*(6), 803-816.

Wendler, D. & Dickert, N. (2001). The consent process for cadaveric organ procurement: How does it work? How can it be improved? *Journal of the American Medical Association*, *285*, 329-333.

Whiting, J. F., Kiberd, B., Kalo, Z., Keown, P., Roels, L. & Kjerulf, M. (2004). Cost-effectiveness of organ donation: Evaluating investment into Donor Action and other donor initiatives. *American Journal of Transplantation*, *4*, 569-573.

Williams, M. A., Lipsett, P. A., Rushton, C. H., Grochowski, E. C., Berkowitz, I. D., Mann, S. L., Shatzer, J. H., Short, P. & Genel, M. (2003). The physician's role in discussing organ donation with families. *Critical Care Medicine*, *31*(5), 1568-1573.

Zink, S. & Wertlieb, S. (2006). A study of the presumptive approach to consent for organ donation: A new solution to an old problem. *Critical Care Nursing*, *26*(2), 129-136.

In: Organ Donation and Transplantation
Editor: Mary Anne Lauri

ISBN: 978-1-62948-257-6

Chapter 12

ORGAN DONATION IN THE NETHERLANDS: THE SHORTAGE OF DONORS AND A NEW WAY TO IMPROVE THE DONATION RATE

*Nichon E. Jansen, PhD**
Dutch Transplant Foundation, Leiden, The Netherlands

ABSTRACT

Organ donation and transplantation have a long history in the Netherlands. Within the 47 years since the first kidney transplantation new ways of donation have been developed. These include multi-organ donation from brain dead donors and donors who died after circulatory death, and living organ donation. Despite the increase of alternative ways of donation the waiting list for organ transplantation in the Netherlands remains long, and patients die whilst waiting. As long as there is a shortage of suitable organs for transplantation, the need to identify bottlenecks in the organ donation process is crucial for further improvement of donation rates. The main reason for potential organ donor losses appeared to be objection to donation by relatives. Approaching family members of a potential organ and/or tissue donor, and to request donation under emotional circumstances, is not an easy task for health care professionals. Therefore, the Dutch Transplant Foundation developed a training 'Communication about Donation'. This training turned out to be effective, not only in facilitating professionals in broaching the subject of donation, but also by positively influencing the family consent rate.

INTRODUCTION

Organ transplantation is a well-accepted form of medicine, which began in the Netherlands as early as 1966 with the first kidney transplantation in the University Hospital of Leiden. Professor J. Van Rood played an important role in this new development, not only because of his knowledge of the HLA-system but also as one of the founding fathers of the

* n.jansen@transplantatiestichting.nl.

first European organ exchange organisation, better known as Eurotransplant International Foundation (Kootstra, 1998). Due to the new Dutch Organ and Tissue Donation act, which aims to regulate organ donation and allocation in the Netherlands, the Dutch Transplant Foundation was established 1997. The two key tasks are to function as an organ procurement organisation and to facilitate organ and tissue donation in hospitals (Dutch Transplant Foundation, 2011). The Dutch Donation Act, based on the opting-in system, established a national Donor Register to improve the transparency of the donation process. Dutch citizens older than 12 years may register their preferences about organ or tissue donation in the Donor Register. The Donor Register provides four options:

- Yes, I give permission (including the possibility to give permission for only some organs or tissues
- No, I do not give permission
- My next of kin will decide
- A specific person will decide

Within the 47 years since the first kidney transplantation new ways of post-mortem donation have been developed. These include kidney donation from a brain death donor to 'multi-organ donation', defined as a donor from whom at least 2 different organs are transplanted. Additionally, since the beginning of the 1980s kidneys of donors who died after circulatory death have been transplanted (Kootstra, Wijnen, Van Hooff, & Van der Linden, 1991; Oomen, Daemen, & Kootstra, 2000). It is now also possible to conduct multi-organ donation from these type of donors. Despite the increase of this alternative way of post-mortem donation and the rise of numbers of organs available from one donor, the waiting list for organ transplantation in the Netherlands remains long, and patients die whilst waiting. As long as there is a shortage of suitable organs for transplantation, the need to identify bottlenecks in the organ donation process is crucial for further improvement of donation rates.

This chapter focuses on the problem of the shortage of deceased organ donors. After an overview of the donation figures, it focuses on identifying the main bottleneck in the organ donation process. The chapter finishes with a new way to increase the number of organ donors in the Netherlands.

ORGAN DONOR SHORTAGE

Post-Mortem Organ Donors

The problem of post-mortem organ donor shortage in the Netherlands is visible in Figure 1, which shows that the number of donors and organs transplanted is far below the number of patients on the waiting list. For patients with end-stage renal failure there is an alternative therapy while waiting for kidney transplantation - dialysis can largely take over the renal function for a number of years. Patients requiring a transplant of another organ have almost no medical alternatives, which can lead to death of potential recipients on the waiting list. Also patients with end-stage renal failure who have to wait too long for a kidney transplant die while waiting.

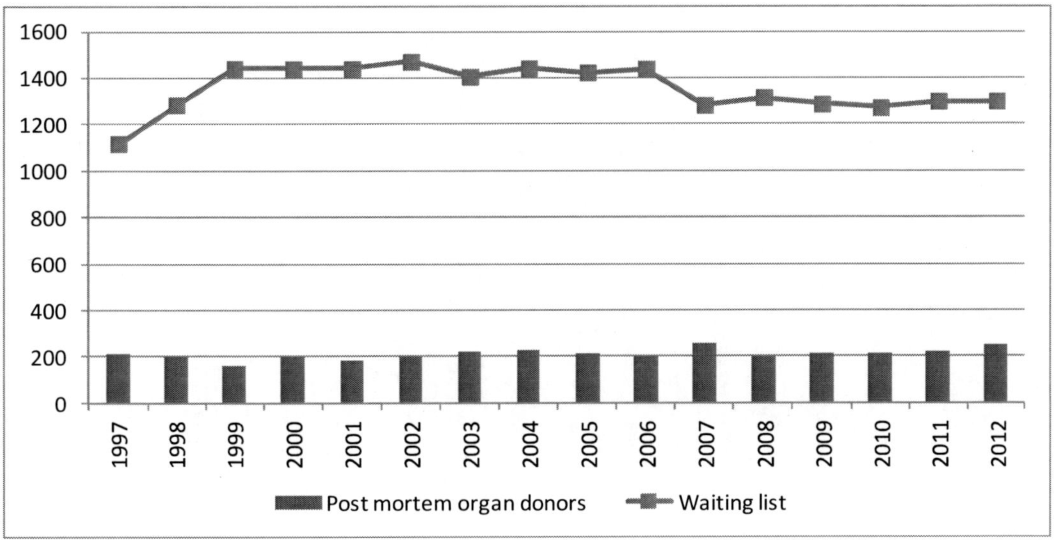

* The number of patients on the waiting list covers only those who are transplantable on December 31 of the years 1997-2012.

Figure 1. Number of post-mortem organ donors and the number of patients on the active waiting list (for kidneys, livers, lungs, hearts, pancreas, small bowel, or combinations) per year in the Netherlands.

Types of Organ Donors

Post-mortem organ donation can be divided into two different types - donation after brain death (DBD) and donation after circulatory death (DCD). Donation after brain death can be performed when the death of a patient is established by diagnosing brain death, in a situation where the patient is admitted to an intensive care unit, is mechanical ventilated, and suffering from irreversible loss of brain functions. The organs which can be donated are the heart, lungs, liver, kidneys, pancreas, and since 2002 also the small bowel. Donation after circulatory death can take place when the medical condition is considered irreversible and treatment is futile. This can be in a situation on the intensive care unit where the patient is mechanically ventilated. Treatment will be withdrawn and ventilation switched off, awaiting the cardiac and circulatory arrest. Another situation is where treatment will be stopped in case of a sudden cardiac arrest, which can also occur outside the intensive care unit (mainly in the emergency room). When cardiopulmonary resuscitation is unsuccessful organs can be removed after five minutes of 'no-touch', after five minutes without circulation of the brain death can be declared. The transplantable organs are kidneys, liver (since 2001), lungs and pancreas (since 2005). In summary there are four categories of donation after circulatory death donors (Kootstra, 1997);

- Dead on arrival, DCD donor category 1
- Unsuccessful resuscitation, DCD donor category 2
- Awaiting cardiac arrest, DCD donor category 3
- Cardiac arrest while brain dead, DCD donor category 4

Figure 2 shows that the total number of deceased organ donors fluctuated around 200 donors per year, but the number of DCD donors increased from 1997 until 2005.

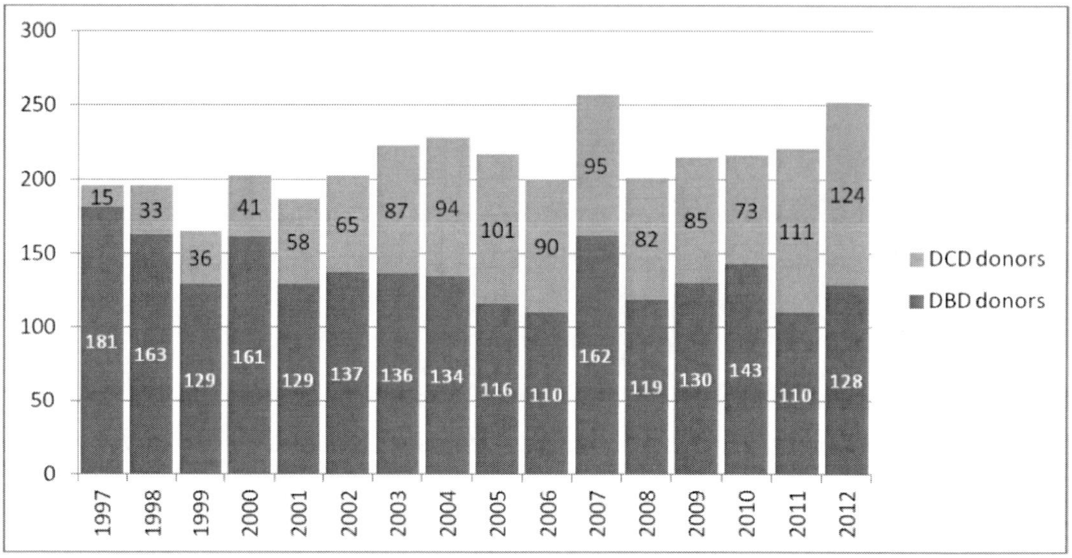

*Multi-organ donation in DCD donors since 2001.

Figure 2. Numbers of brain death donors (DBD) and donation after circulatory death donors (DCD) donors per year in the Netherlands* .

Living Organ Donation

The additional number of donations after circulatory death is still not sufficient to decrease the number of patients on the waiting list. Another alternative is living organ donation. This type of donation is not new in the Netherlands, however there has been a substantial increase in recent years (Figure 3). Especially when looking at the number of 'living unrelated donors (LUR)', including anonymous donors, a steep line is visible. Since 2008 the number of kidney transplants from living donors exceeds the number of transplants from post-mortem donors.

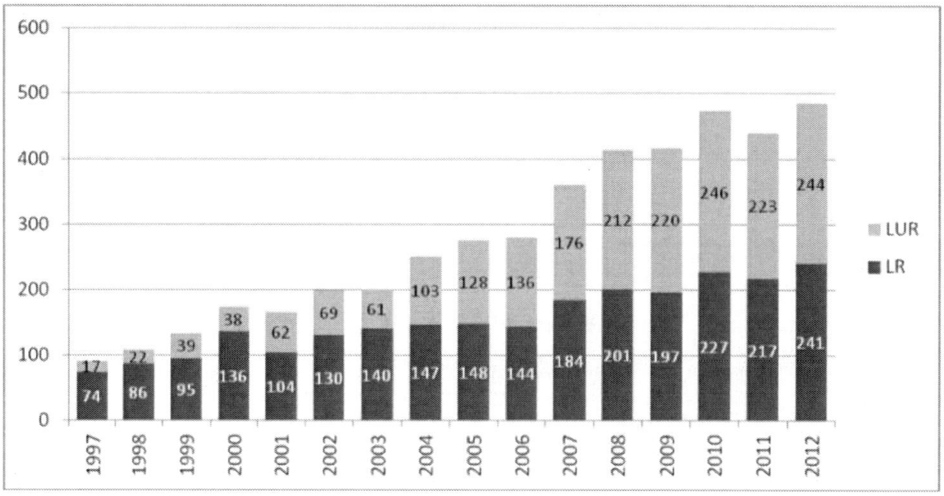

Figure 3. Number of living organ donors; living related (LR) and living unrelated (LUR) per year in the Netherlands.

Although the number of living donors has increased, this is only a solution for kidney recipients. In addition, since 2004 approximately 3 donors per year donate a part of their liver (19 in total from 2002-2010). Given this number of living liver donors this has a small effect on the waiting list. Patients waiting for a heart, pancreas, lung or small bowel, do not benefit from this kind of organ donation. Considering the total numbers of transplants from post-mortem and living donors, the effect is that the waiting list has only slightly decreased during the last years. This is almost entirely in favour of kidney recipients.

EUROPEAN DONOR RATES

Number of Donors Per Million Population

The post-mortem donation performance of the Netherlands, 13.7 organ donors per million population (p.m.p.), is low compared to other European countries (Council of Europe, 2011). For example, Belgium has 20.5 donors, Malta 22.5, France 23.8, and on the top of the list is Spain with 32.0 donors p.m.p. These figures express that donation rates can be much higher in the Netherlands. To make a valid comparison, the number of organ donors p.m.p. should be divided into donation after brain death and donation after circulatory death donors. Then the Netherlands has one of the highest number of donation after circulatory death donors p.m.p (Dominguez-Gil, Delmonico, Shaheen, Matesanz, O'Connor, Minina, & Noël, 2011). In addition, our country has the highest number of living kidney donors in Europe. Here there seems to be a correlation; in general, countries with lower deceased donation rates have higher living donation rates (Kranenburg, Zuidema, Weimar, Hilhorst, IJzermans, Passchier, & Busschbach, 2009).

Identifying the Pool of Potential Organ Donors

Comparing numbers of organ donors per million population does not give insight into the number of potential organ donors of countries. Therefore, many studies in various countries reviewed medical records of patients who died in intensive care units (ICUs) to identify the pool of potential donors. For example, two large studies have been conducted by Sheehy and colleagues, and Barber, reviewing ICU deaths in a large number of hospitals in the USA and UK (Barber, Falvey, Hamilton, Collett, & Rudge, 2006; Sheehy, Conrad, Brigham, Luskin, Weber, Eadkin, … Hunsicker, 2003). However, potential organ donors could also be located outside the ICU, for example in the Emergency Department. The outcome of reviewing medical charts provides insight into the pool of potential organ donors, the reason for the loss of potential donors, the reasons for non-procurement, and finally the number of actual donors. This provides important information about the main bottlenecks in the organ donation process as areas for improvement. The conversion rate, the number of actual organ donors divided by the number of potential donors, can be determined from the potential donor pool. This rate is an indicator of the effectiveness of the donation performances.

In the Netherlands a study was conducted by reviewing medical records of deceased patients in ICUs of 64 hospitals (Jansen, Van Leiden, Haase-Kromwijk, & Hoitsma, 2010).

This represents almost two-thirds of all hospitals in the Netherlands. Data of these hospitals were collected from the years 2005-2008, in total 23508 charts were reviewed. The percentage of all potential organ donors out of the total number of deaths' decreased from 8.2% in 2005 to 7.1% in 2008. Donor detection increased from 96% in 2005 to 99% in 2008. The overall conversion rate (the number of actual donors divided by the number of potential donors) was low with an average of 30% in these years. From this study we could conclude that the maximum number of potential organ donors DBD and DCD is three times higher than the number of actual organ donors. The main reason for potential organ donor losses was objection to donation by families (approximately 60% of all donor losses during the study period). Therefore, all our improvements should focus on decreasing the high family refusal rates.

Family Refusal

Approaching Families of Potential Donors

Approaching family members of a potential organ and/or tissue donor, to request donation under emotional circumstances, is not an easy task for health care professionals (Roels, Spaight, Smits, & Cohen, 2010; Siminoff, Arnold, & Caplan, 1995). Especially in situations where the potential donor did not register his/her donation preferences in the Donor Register (62% of the Dutch population did not register). Bearing in mind that this request is not frequently asked, it is conceivable that it is difficult for professionals to become skilful in these kinds of conversations. Siminoff and colleagues studied factors influencing families' consent for donation and concluded that the way families are approached by health-care practitioners is crucial (Siminoff, Gordon, Hewlett, & Arnold, 2001). De Jong and colleagues analysed from an interview study of donor and non-donor families that the request for donation should be made in a way that meets the families' informational and emotional needs (De Jong, Franz, Wolfe, Nathan, Payne, Reitsma, & Beasley, 1998). The Dutch Transplant Foundation started a project to improve the decision making process. With the financial help of the Dutch Ministry of Health, a new training programme 'Communication about Donation' was developed for all professionals who approach families to request for organ and/or tissue donation. This training follows after many years of experience with the European Donor Hospital Education Programme (EDHEP) (Blok, Van Dalen, Jager, Ryan, Wijnen, Wight, … Cohen, 1999). Reasons for a new training were not inspired by a lack of quality of this former training, but due to the persisting high family refusal rate in the Netherlands and the need to train as many professionals as possible. The present training is an 'in hospital' training of maximum 4 hours. According to the latest educational insights it is a blended-learning training, including an e-learning module, to follow at home or at work, and a practical module.

Improving Organ Donation

We performed a multi-centre study between December 2007 and December 2009 to assess the effect of the 'Communication about Donation' training on the family consent rate

(Jansen, Van Leiden, Haase-Kromwijk, Van der Meer, Van der Lely, Van Zon, … Hoitsma, 2011). Three hospitals participated in the study, on the basis of average hospital size and expected numbers of organ and tissue donors. None of these hospitals had a transplant program. In an intervention hospital a special group of part-time or former ICU nurses was trained according to the 'Communication about Donation' program. We named them 'trained donation practitioners' (TDP), and their role was to guide the family throughout the time in the ICU until a decision regarding organ and/or tissue donation had been reached. A first control hospital had no special professionals for family care and donation was requested by the physician without any extra trained support. A second control hospital had 'hostesses' for family support, but without any special training related to donation. The primary outcome measurement was the consent rate, and secondly the experiences of families were measured by use of a questionnaire. The results showed that the family consent rate was significantly higher in the intervention hospital (57.6%) compared to both control hospitals (1st control hospital 34.6% and 2d control hospital 39.4%, intervention hospital versus 1st control hospital *P*=0.003, intervention hospital versus 2d control hospital *P*=0.022) (Figure 4).

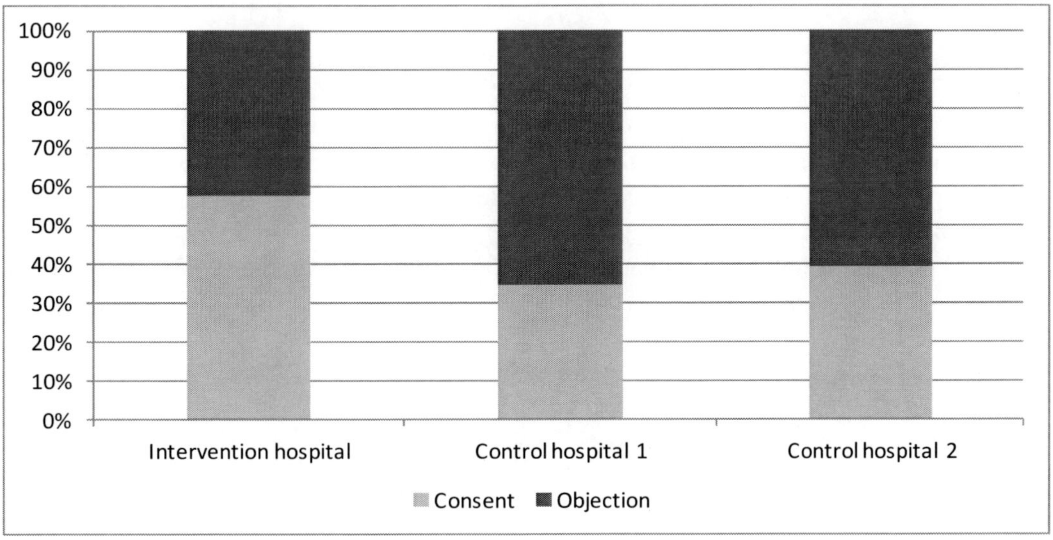

Figure 4. Percentage of consent and objection of families requested for organ and/or tissue donation per participating hospital.

Even after excluding potential donors with 'consent' registered in the Donor Register, the family consent rate in the intervention hospital was significantly higher than in the control hospitals. The number of families who responded to the questionnaire was high (69%). We did not find confounding variables that could have influenced this increased consent rate. Therefore, we concluded that in the donation decision-making process the implementation of TDPs, who were highly dedicated to guide families from admittance to the ICU, lead to higher family consent rates.

The study on the effect of the 'Communication about Donation' training is unique within our Dutch system. Thus far, no study has proven a positive effect on the family consent rate. Compared to other countries, the Netherlands nowadays has no experience with the standard availability of a transplant coordinator for collaborative requesting (physician together with a transplant coordinator). For example in Spain, intensivists combine their own profession with the profession of transplant coordinator (Matesanz, 2003), in the US and UK organ procurement staff is involved in the organ donation request (Siminoff Mercer, Graham, & Burant, 2007; Verble & Worth, 2000; Simpkin, Robertson, Barber, & Young, 2009). The strength of our study is a special training in combination with the support of families from the moment of admittance to the intensive care unit. This addresses the conversation about donation as the natural completion of a complete guidance. The positive effect of training on the family consent rate is suggested in a study of Siminoff and colleagues (Siminoff, Marshall, Dumenci, Bowen, Swaminathan, & Gordon, 2009). In addition, the importance of emotional and informational support of families is consistent with outcomes of other studies (Jacoby & Jaccard, 2010; Sque, Long, & Payne, 2005).

After our pilot study the training was implemented in another 40 hospitals (without a special team for family guidance) and is well accepted throughout the country. Our aim is to implement the training in many more hospitals *including* the concept of family guidance throughout the period of admittance in the ICU. Appointing TDP does not only improve the family consent rate, but has a significant impact on the quality of care in the ICU.

Conclusion

The persisting shortage of donor organs for patients on the waiting list for transplantation asks for new ways to improve donor rates. After identifying the main bottleneck in the organ donation process, being the family refusal rate, we focussed on reducing this rate. The training 'Communication about Donation' turned out to be effective, not only in facilitating professionals in broaching the subject of donation, but also by positively influencing the family consent rate.

References

Barber, K., Falvey, S., Hamilton, C., Collett, D. & Rudge, C. (2006). Potential for organ donation in the United Kingdom: audit of intensive care records. *BMJ, 332,* 1124-1127.

Blok, G. A., van Dalen, J., Jager, K. J., Ryan, M., Wijnen, R. M., Wight, C., … Cohen, B. (1999). The European Donor Hospital Education Programme (EDHEP): addressing the training needs of doctors and nurses who break bad news, care for the bereaved, and request donation. *Transpl Int, 12,* 161-167.

Council of Europe. International figures on organ donation and transplantation – 2010. *Transplant Newsletter* 2011; 16: 1.

De Jong, W., Franz, H. G., Wolfe, S. M., Nathan, H., Payne, D., Reitsma, W., & Beasley, C. (1998). Requesting organ donation: an interview study of donor and nondonor families. *Am J Crit Care, 7,* 13-23.

Dominguez-Gil, B., Delmonico, F.L., Shaheen, F. A. M., Matesanz, R., O'Connor, K., Minina, M. & Noël, L. (2011). The critical pathway for deceased donation: reportable uniformity in the approach of deceased donation. *Transplant International, 24,* 373-378.

Dutch Transplant Foundation. *Annual report 2010.* Leiden, The Netherlands 2011; in Dutch.

Jacoby, L, & Jaccard, J. (2010). Perceived support among families deciding about organ donation for their loved ones: donor vs nondonor next of kin. *Am J Crit Care, 19,* 52-61.

Jansen, N. E., Van Leiden, H. A., Haase-Kromwijk, B. J. J. M, & Hoitsma, A. J. (2010). Organ donation performance in the Netherlands 2005-2008; Medical Record Review in 64 hospitals. *Nephrol. Dial. Transplant, 25,* 1992-1997.

Jansen, N. E., Van Leiden, H. A., Haase-Kromwijk, B. J. J. M, Van der Meer, J. M, Van der Lely, N., Van Zon, H., … Hoitsma, A. J. (2011). Appointing 'trained donation practitioners' results in a higher family consent rate in the Netherlands; a multicenter study. *Transpl Int, 24,* 1189-1197.

Kootstra, G., Wijnen, R., Van Hooff, J. P., & Van der Linden, C. J. (1991). Twenty percent more kidneys through a non-heart-beating program. *Transplant Proc, 23,* 910-911.

Kootstra, G. (1997). The asystolic, or non-heartbeating, donor. *Transplantation, 7,* 917-921.

Kootstra, G. (1998). History of organ transplantation.In H. B. M. van Wezel, M. J. H. Slooff & H. van Goor (Eds.), *Organ donation: organisational, legal, ethical and medical technical aspects of organ and tissue donation* (pp 1-6). Houten, The Netherlands: Bohn Stafleu Van Loghum.

Kranenburg, L., Zuidema, W., Weimar, W., Hilhorst, M., IJzermans, J., Passchier, J., & Busschbach, J,. (2009). Strategies to advance living kidney donation: a single center's experience. *Prog Transplant, 19,* 71-75.

Matesanz, R. (2003) Factors influencing the adaptation of the Spanish model of organ donation. Transpl Int, *16*:736-741.

Oomen, A. P. A, Daemen, J. H. C., & Kootstra, G. (2000). The value of non heart beating donors for developing countries. *Journal of Nephrology Urology and Transplantation, 1,* 55-61.

Roels, L., Spaight, C., Smits, J., & Cohen, B. (2010). Critical Care staffs' attitudes, confidence levels and educational needs correlate with countries' donation rates: data from the Donor Action database. *Transpl Int, 23,* 842-850.

Sheehy, E., Conrad, S.L., Brigham, L.E., Luskin, R., Weber, P., Eadkin, M., … Hunsicker, L. (2003). Estimating the number of potential organ donors in the United States. *N Engl J Med, 349*, 667-674.

Siminoff, L. A., Arnold, R. M., & Caplan, A. L. (1995). Health care professional attitudes toward donation: effect on practice and procurement. *J Trauma, 39,* 553-559.

Siminoff, L. A., Gordon, N, Hewlett, J, & Arnold, R. M. (2001). Factors influencing families' consent for donation of solid organs for transplantation. *JAMA,* 286, 71—77.

Siminoff, L., Mercer, M. B., Graham, G., & Burant, C. (2007). The reasons families donate organs for transplantation: implications for policy and practice. *J Trauma, 62,* 969–978.

Siminoff, L. A, Marshall, H. M, Dumenci, L., Bowen, G.,,Swaminathan, A., & Gordon, N. (2009). Communicating effectively about donation: an educational intervention to increase consent to donation. *Prog Transplant, 19,* 35-43.

Simpkin, A. L., Robertson, L. C., Barber, V. S., & Young, J. D. (2009). Modifiable factors influencing relatives' decision to offer organ donation: systematic review. *BMJ,* 21, 338:b991.

Sque, M., Long, T., & Payne, S. (2005). Organ donation: key factors influencing families' decision-making. *Transplant Proc, 37,* 543-546.

Verble, M., & Worth, J. (2000). Overcoming families' fears and concerns in the donation discussion. *Prog Transplant, 10*, 155-160.

In: Organ Donation and Transplantation
Editor: Mary Anne Lauri
ISBN: 978-1-62948-257-6

Chapter 13

METAPHORS OF ORGAN DONATION, SOCIAL REPRESENTATIONS OF THE BODY AND THE OPT-OUT SYSTEM

*Mary Anne Lauri**
University of Malta, Malta

ABSTRACT

Organ donation is the only available treatment for end-stage failure of organs such as liver, lung and heart and therefore increasing the number of organ donors is a priority for most countries.

One measure that could be taken by a country to increase the number of organ transplants is to introduce the opt-out system of organ donation. Public opinion is divided on this issue and policy-makers need to tread with caution before introducing legislation. This paper proposes that understanding the social representations the public has of organ donation is important in taking the right policy decisions.

We propose here that an in-depth study of the views held by people on the issue is essential in this regard and that this can best be done by investigating the metaphors people use to describe organ donation, interpreted within the theory of social representation.

In this study the social representations of organ donation were investigated through five focus groups with 57 participants living in Malta. Analysis of the transcriptions of these focus groups yielded pertinent issues related to organ donation. Moreover, metaphors of organ donations and how these were related to social representations of the body and attitudes toward the opt-out system are discussed. It is being suggested that these findings could be of relevance to the present discussion on the opt-out system in the United Kingdom and in other countries.

---

* E-mail: mary-anne.lauri@um.edu.mt.

Introduction

In Britain there are more than 8,000 patients waiting for an organ transplant and more than 1000 a year die without receiving the organ that could save their lives (EU Consultation Document on Organ Donation, 2006). Organ transplantation is now the most cost-effective treatment for end-stage renal failure. It is also the only available treatment for end-stage failure of organs such as liver, lung and heart (ibid).

On January 13, 2008, several news agencies discussed the controversy stirred up by what the British Prime Minister Gordon Brown wrote in The Telegraph. The Prime Minister wrote in favour of the opt-out system of organ donation and said that parliament was considering legislation to enable doctors to remove organs from dead patients without permission of their next of kin. This policy of "opting-out" or "presumed consent" means that, unless people opted out of the donor register, hospitals would be allowed to take their organs for transplants without the need of the relatives' consent. (Brown, 2008). There was a strong reaction to his statement. On one side, the lobby groups for patients' rights claimed that the state does not own the body of a dead person and the decision whether or not to donate one's organs after death should be a private decision. On the other hand, England's chief medical officer, Sir Liam Donaldson as well as The British Medical Association supported the opt-out system. Donaldson said that the current uncoordinated practice vis-a-vis organ transplantation was poor, with many distressed relatives rejecting requests to donate organs of their dead relatives (Wintor, 2008).

This difference in opinion on whether or not to introduce the opt-out system exists among the general public as well as the professionals and authorities. A quick look at the online comments posted on January 14th by readers of the Times (Webster, 2008) shows that some readers did believe that in the context of long waiting lists for organ transplants, legislation should intervene in order to save the lives of people waiting for a transplant. However, many of the readers' letters showed how talk about the opt-out system can revive the fears surrounding organ donation. Readers wrote about "mutilated", "violated" and "incomplete" bodies. One reader exclaimed "Over my dead body," describing the system as "corpse robbing" and used the terms "evil", "ungodly" and "repugnant".

But perhaps of more concern are the objections raised by those who, in principle, are in favour of organ donation. One such person wrote that "If people want to give the gift of life, that is their right, but it must be something that is voluntary." Another insisted that organ donation should be an "active choice" and another wrote that, instead of forcing the issue through legislation, the Prime Minister should be "educating people and using a campaign to donate organs." (Webster, 2008).

The e-debate on the Telegraph raged even more widely. By 18th April, Mr Brown's article had provoked 693 online postings by readers of the Telegraph, ranging from complete agreement with the introduction of the opt-out system to threats by donor card holders that they would tear up their card if the system were to be introduced.

A similar public discussion on organ donation and the opt-out system took place in Malta when a national communication campaign was launched to create greater awareness about organ donation in 1996. Several issues emerged from the research conducted to inform the campaign and the evaluative research carried out to evaluate its short term and long term effects. These issues are reported in detail in Lauri (2001) and Lauri (2008). This paper will focus on one aspect of these findings which has greatest relevance to the situation in the UK today, that is, the reasons why there are such different positions among the public regarding the introduction of the opt-out system. It will be argued that one's opinion on whether the legislator has a right to introduce "presumed consent" depends on various factors, two major ones being: (i) how one looks upon organ donation and (ii) how one looks upon one's own body.

In order to understand people's views on a complex issue like organ donation, the researchers involved in the design of the campaign decided that is was important to tap into the roots of the social representations people had on organ donation. The theory of social representations was used to inform the design of the campaign. This is because this theory helps the researcher understand how people make sense of such a complex issue by giving their own lay interpretation of the views and opinions directed at them by experts such as medical practitioners, political leaders and the church, and how different ways of elaborating these views lead to different public opinions. The decision to have the theory of social representations as the main theoretical underpinning of the campaign could arguably account for its success. The main slogan of the campaign made use of the actual words which participants used in the focus groups to describe organ donation "Give a new life." This slogan was consistently used throughout the campaign in all radio, television and print media.

One indication of the success of the campaign was the number of organ transplants carried out. In the year before the campaign there were 12 transplants. In the year following the campaign the number of transplants increased to 32 and in the next year to 30. It is of course impossible to claim that the increase in the number of transplanted organs was solely the result of the campaign but it is reasonable to suppose that the campaign was a main instigator of the increase in the number of organ transplants.

In the next section we shall describe some aspects of the theory of social representations which are most relevant to this research. In the following sections we shall use this theory to analyse the focus groups carried out before the campaign. Finally, we shall discuss how this experience in Malta might be relevant to the present public discussion in the U.K.

Social Representations and Metaphors

In his book "La psychoanalyse, son image et son public" published in 1961, Moscovici described what psychoanalyses meant to French people (Moscovici, 1961). He described how psychoanalytic concepts, normally discussed in the "reified universe" of psychologists and psychiatrists, proliferated among different groups of French society and transformed themselves into lay theories which formed the bulwark of everyday discourse and commonsense (ibid). This seminal work was the beginning of an area of study which has today become one of the most researched areas in social psychology and one of the most important tools to study public opinion.

Social representations are not simply opinions or attitudes. They are lay theories about issues, concepts or events, which feature in everyday conversations. They are systems of values, ideas and practices which enable people to understand and make sense of various aspects of their material and social world and enable them to master this world (Moscovici, p. xiii in his forward to Herzlich, 1973). Ultimately, "the purpose of all representations is to make something unfamiliar, or unfamiliarity itself, familiar" (p.24 Moscovici, 1984). Jovchelovitch (2007) points out that the work of representation "relates to the construction of worldviews, to the establishment of systems of everyday knowledge that not only seek to propose a framework to guide communication... but also actively express projects and identities of social actors and the interrelations between them" (p12).

The notion of social representations is therefore of paramount importance to policy makers who need public support for their reforms such as that being suggested regarding the donation of organs. The facts as presented to the policy maker by the experts in the field, Moscovici's "reified universe", might very well indicate that it is reasonable to expect that the reform should meet with wide public support. But the lay theories on which public opinion is based could be quite different from those held by the experts.

But how are these "worldviews" constructed? How is the unfamiliar made familiar? Moscovici (1984) posits the two closely linked processes of "anchoring" and "objectification" as the means through which a novel concept is introduced into everyday discourse. These processes assimilate and accommodate the new concept "to already familiar concepts that are socially shared and culturally available" (Augoustinos and Penny, 2001, p.4.4). Anchoring is the "assimilation of unfamiliar phenomenon to pre-existing representations, thereby 'converting' an external object into a mental content" (Wagner, Elejabarrietta and Lahnsteiner, 1995, p.672).

One key element often involved in the process of objectification is the metaphor. According to Wagner and Hayes (2005), social representations are related to thinking in terms of images, icons and metaphors. "The concrete form that content-rational knowledge and social representations adopts in the heads of its bearers can best be compared with images and metaphors" (p. 170). Wagner, Elejabarrietta and Lahnsteiner (1995) describe images, metaphors and symbols as "objectification 'devices', i.e. 'tools' by which the end of understanding through objectification is achieved" (p.673).

So how are metaphors in the context of the theory of social representations defined? To answer this question we shall mostly follow the work by Wagner and Hayes (2005) (see also Wagner, Elejabarrietta and Lahnsteiner, 1995). Essentially a metaphor is a mapping between a source domain and a target domain. The source domain is the familiar domain, close to personal experience and easily comprehensible. The target domain is the unfamiliar domain, farther away from personal experience, and more difficult to understand. The mapping is an association between elements of the source domain and the target domain. But such a mapping is not simply the attaching of familiar labels to unfamiliar concepts. The mapping "defines a structural correlation" between the source and the target domain and "establishes relevant structural similarities between target and source" (Wagner and Hayes, 2005, p.171). It projects relationships between elements in the familiar source domain into analogous relationships between elements in the target domain. We shall use the term "homomorphism" to describe a mapping with this property. In Wagner, Elejabarietta and Lahnsteiner, 1995, for example, this homomorphic character of metaphors is very well illustrated. In this paper subjects compared the sperm and the ovum in process of fertilization with sexual and sex-role behaviour where the roles of men and women were projected upon sperms and ovum, respectively, implying that sperms are seen as more active, harder, stronger and more dominant than the ovum.

We shall argue in a later section how the metaphors identified from the analysis of our focus groups have this homomorphic property. This characteristic of metaphors can help the researcher understand how and why people have different views on the opt-out system and how these can be addressed to effect change and reduce resistance to changes in policy.

As Wagner and Hayes (2005) point out, the mapping which constitutes the metaphor "is the result of a constructive effort in communication and discourse" (p.171). Metaphors and social representations are societal creations. One way of discovering these metaphors is by listening to people talking in informal settings. These informal conversations guide the researcher to discover the lay theories which the public have and use to argue and form opinions. One method which simulates this process in a relatively controlled setting is the focus group. The focus group is the thinking society in miniature (Farr, Trutkowski and Holzl, 1996) and therefore it is ideal for bringing out the social representations held by participants on complex issues such as organ donation.

METHODOLOGY

Before designing the campaign it was important to study public opinion, attitudes and representations the Maltese people had of organ donation. Three data collecting tools were used. These were surveys, interviews and focus groups. One survey, the interviews and the focus groups were carried out before the campaign, in order to inform its design and conduct. The survey was also repeated three times after the campaign over a ten-year period in order to assess its short-term and long-term effectiveness. In this paper we will consider only the data elicited in the focus group discussions. For a more detailed discussion of the findings from the interviews and the surveys one can refer to Lauri (2001), Lauri and Lauri (2005) and Lauri (2006).

Five focus group discussions were organized with a volunteer sample of 57 persons recruited from 14 different towns and villages in Malta, an island in the Mediterranean with a population of about 400,000 people. The participants were recruited from supermarkets in different geographic regions of Malta. They were evenly distributed between women and men, between young and middle-aged persons and had different levels of education. Sixteen participants dropped out and did not attend the focus groups. Only two participants were donor card holders.

Focus group discussions lasted between 60 and 90 minutes and were recorded with the permission of the participants. Each recorded session was transcribed fully. These transcriptions were the primary texts for the subsequent analysis. Appendix A gives information about the composition of the focus groups.

A FIRST ANALYSIS OF THE DATA: CATEGORIES, THEMES AND KEYWORDS

The transcripts of the focus group discussions were analysed using ATLAS/ti. The analysis of the focus group discussions yielded themes which were grouped under the headings (i) normative context, (ii) decision-making, (iii) death and body image, (iv) ethical issues and (iv) medical issues. These categories and the associated themes and keywords are shown in Table 1.

Table 1. Classification of Keywords from Focus Group Discussions

CATEGORIES	THEMES	KEYWORDS	
(i).Normative context	a. Lack of information	Lack of awareness Lack of information	New concept Not on public agenda
	b. Social influence	Church teachings Influence of church Interpersonal influence Media influence	Significant others Group decision Conformity
	c. Motivations	A good deed Charity Help others Altruistic act Recycling	Love thy neighbour Part of person lives on Violation of body Saves lives
	d. Fears	Taking risks Fear of mutilation Not really dead Will not save my life	No chance for miracle Revive from coma Predetermined life-span Superstition
(ii). Decision making	a. Decision to sign a donor card	Card, form of will Laws My body is my property	Futility of donor card Honouring wish of deceased
	b. Decision to donate organs of relative	Attitude of deceased Difficult decision	Family decision Time of crisis
(iii). Death and body image	a. Death anxiety	Death Discomfort	Existential questions
	b. Body image	Body image Last impression Eyes	Heart Kidneys Whole body
	c. Afterlife	Eternal life Heaven	Resurrection Missing organs
	d. Sacredness of body	Untouched cadaver Sense of void Body integrity	Respect towards body Cremation Burial
	e. Miracles	Miracles	
(iv). Ethical issues	a. Declaration of death	Brain death Coma	Beating heart
	b. Choice of recipient	Criteria of choice Who chooses recipient Bribes	Right of donor family to decide
	c. Abuses and exploitation	What happens abroad Children's farms Rumours	Satanism Stealing of organs Selling and buying of organs
	d. Opt-out system	Opt-out	
(v). Medical issues	a. Faith in doctors	Expertise Faith in doctors	Method of approach Organ procurement
	b. Experimentation and research	Research and advancement of science Xenotransplantation	Tampering with nature Autopsy

We shall briefly discuss these five categories which will provide the insight for extracting the metaphors and representations presented in the next section.

(i) Normative Context

The Catholic Church is a powerful influence in Malta, and this was reflected by the importance many participants gave to what the Church says when expressing normative views on organ donation. Many of the reasons which participants gave for wanting to donate organs were related to altruism. As in the findings of Morgan and Miller (2002), many felt that organ donation is good because it helps someone live. Organ donation was also seen as a concrete way of practising one's religion which places a lot of emphasis on helping others. It was looked upon as an act of altruism based on the commandment "love your neighbour as yourself".

Whereas some considered organ donation as a moral duty, something that all people should do, others looked upon it as an act of charity, something, over and above what is expected of a person. One participant said that saving a person's life is a chance to do something heroic. Another reason given for donating one's organs was that of the recycling of resources. A few participants felt that it is a waste to let good organs rot away when they can be used to help other people lead a normal life. These images are discussed in more detail in the next section.

(ii) Decision-Making

Many participants saw the signing of the donor card as the result of a decision taken freely in one's own time, sometimes spontaneously and at other times after deliberate thought. It is a pledge which, at the time of signing, seems distant and improbable. On the other hand the decision to donate the organs of a close family member occurs at a time of crisis when the family is still trying to come to terms with the death of a loved one. It is a situation laden with emotions. Similar to the findings of Calvo et al. (2002) and Perkins (1987), participants said that knowing the wishes of the deceased about organ donation would help them in taking a decision.

Connected with this issue, and very relevant to the question of the opt-out system, is the discussion of who owns the cadaver and consequently who should decide about whether or not to donate organs. The belief in the individual's right of choice was virtually shared by everyone, even by those who were in favour of organ donation.

(iii) Death and Body Image

Different participants had different conceptions of their body. Some saw their body in the light of the teaching of the Catholic Church as belonging to God and that it was theirs "on loan". Others saw the body more as a treasured possession, something dear that belonged to them. There were other participants who made no distinction between the physical, the psychological and the spiritual aspects of the body. Similar findings were found by Sanner (1994).

The question of what would happen to the organs in the afterlife was a frequent theme of discussion. Since the Church teaches resurrection of the body as well as of the soul, some participants believed that if they gave some of their organs away, the process of resurrection would be hindered.

(iv) Bio-Ethical Issues

There are many ethical issues involved in organ donation. One major issue discussed by the participants was the choice of the recipient. There were two major questions related to this issue, one concerning the criteria of choice, the other related to who should make the final choice.

Regarding the criteria of choice, all participants agreed that the person who is most in need of the organ should get the transplant. Some participants felt that young people and young mothers who have children should be given preference over older people. Others expressed the opinion that it should be on a first come first served basis, irrespective of age, sex and urgency. This way, they claimed, there would be no abuses.

Another issue was whether the donor family has a right to dccidc to whom to give the organs. The official criteria do not make provisions for the donor family members to decide to donate an organ to somebody they know or even to a relative in need of a transplant. It was argued that whereas the cadaver is considered to be the property of the family, the same family cannot decide to give the organs to some other relative in need.

Participants were divided on the issue of the opt-out system. The few participants who were strongly in favour of organ donation were also in favour of the opt-out system, but others were more hesitant. Participants believed that the opt-out system could give rise to a situation where the organs of the dead person are removed when he or she would not have wanted to be an organ donor. Some considered the opt-out system as an infringement of one's human rights.

(v) Medical Issues

Doctors are respected for their technical skills, trusted on a professional level but still open to criticism and suspicion as a professional class. Many feared that if they carried a donor card, doctors would not try to save their life if they are involved in an accident or if they are critically ill.

They also feared that doctors will certify them dead, when in actual fact they are not, so that they can give the organs to friends and clients. McIntyre et al. (1987) similarly found that non-donors were afraid that if they carried a donor card, doctors could declare death prematurely for the purpose of obtaining their organs.

Some of the participants voiced their concern about the breakthroughs in science and technology. They were of the opinion that perhaps we should not be tampering with nature and that when our time is up on this earth, we should accept our faith and go with dignity.

A FURTHER ELABORATION OF THE DATA: METAPHORS OF ORGAN DONATION

In the previous section we briefly presented the data extracted from the focus group discussions classifying it into themes and then categories. In this section we shall use the insight gained from this analysis in order to understand how the participants were trying to make sense of the concept of organ donation through the use of metaphors, how these metaphors were linked to social representations which participants had of the body, and how these social representations could be related to their attitudes towards the opt-out system. A similar study was carried out by Molony and Walker, (2002) in Australia. These researchers found that the social representation of organ donation and transplantation could be best understood as a representational field organized around two diametrically 'opposed' images – the gift of life and the mechanistic removal and replacement of body parts. These images were also found in our study however, as we shall see below, the results in the Maltese study indicated a more complex scenario involving more representations and inter-relationships between them. In the rest of this section we shall illustrate the way these metaphors were expressed by means of quotes taken from the focus group discussion transcripts.

Metaphors of Organ Donation Resulting from the Focus Group Discussions

The concept of organ donation was not so familiar among the general public when these focus groups were held. Therefore participants in the focus groups had to express their ideas by comparing organ donation with more familiar concepts and phenomena. The words and metaphors used in the discussions were in themselves indications of the ideas they borrowed to understand this new concept. Table 2 presents the twelve metaphors and images which participants used to describe organ donation. The connotations associated with each metaphor explain in some more detail the nuances expressed by the participants using the metaphors.

(i) Giving a gift. The donation of organs was compared to giving a gift. It was believed that just like the decision to give a gift is completely in the hands of the giver, so should the decision whether or not to give the organs of the dead person, be taken by family of the dead person. Moreover participants argued that as one chooses to whom to give gifts so should the family of the dead person have a right to decide to whom to give the organs of their loved one and that this decision should not be taken by the hospital authorities.

> I think that, as in everything else, if your body belongs to you, then you have the right to determine who receives what. If there's a member of the family who needs an organ, then I should have the right to decide. (*Participant 30, male, 32 years*)

> I don't agree that doctors can take the organs without permission first. I think it would be immoral to do so. (*Participant 41, female, 25 years*)

(ii) Giving charity. Organ donation was seen by many participants as giving charity. These participants believed that just like a person can give money or other possessions to people in need without knowing exactly who is going to benefit from their donations, so can a

person decide to give his or her organs or those of a relative to patients who are in need of an organ transplant without knowing the names of the recipients.

> Organ donation is the greatest act of charity you can think of *(Participant 1, female, 32years)*

> I think organ donation is an act of brotherly love. You should love your neighbour as yourself and therefore be willing to help by giving your organs when you die. *(Participant 12, male, 25 years)*

(iii) Doing one's duty. A number of participants believed that it is one's duty to donate organs after one's death. These participants believed that not doing so implies lack of certain principals and values just like for example not taking care of the environment.

> Today, amongst the Maltese it might sound a bit hard at the beginning, but eventually this, yes, would become a duty. (*Participant 19, male, 56 years*)

> If I am alive God would want me to continue living, so I would not be able to give the organs to you. After death, however, it is my duty that I give away my organs. Otherwise I will not be practising what I believe in. (*Participant 19, male, 56 years*)

(iv) Giving life. Most of the participants believed in God. These believed that as God gave them life, then it was 'expected' that after their death they help give "a new life" to those who need an organ to survive. They believed that giving back life to a person who is on the point of dying is a heroic act.

> I first heard about it in a film and it looked like a heroic act to me - to give an organ to save someone else's life. It's your chance to be great. (*Participant 32, female, 40 years*)

(v) Recycling of organs. Some participants compared their body to a machine and organ donation to the recycling of spare parts. Just as engineers replace parts from a machine into another machine to make it work again, so should doctors use organs of dead people to cure living ones.

> First of all I think recycling is a good thing - nothing is wasted. Secondly it's all for a good cause. I don't like wasting anything - not even a piece of paper - imagine organs, which can be so useful to others. They can give them a new lease of life. (*Participant 7, female, 39 years*)

(vi) Taking out an insurance policy. There were participants who believed that organs should be donated to those who are willing to donate their own organs and who are willing to carry a donor card. One participant believed that persons whose names appear on the organ donor register should be given preference over others, should they need an organ transplant.

> I think that if your name is on the donor register there should be a policy that if a family member or friend need a kidney, they should have first preference. The doctor should not come and tell you, we are giving the kidney to X or to Y. (*Participant 41, female, 25 years*)

(vii) Living on after dying. Some participants saw organ donation as a chance to keep the memory of the dead relative alive by actually having his or her organs living in another person. These people believed that the blow of loosing a close relative is made easier by knowing that the deceased has helped another person live on.

> Let's suppose it's your son or daughter who dies, God forbid! The thought that a part of him or her is living in another person is a great consolation. (*Participant 22, female, 55 years)*

> When the girl Claudette from Dingli died I was very moved. I heard her mother saying that she wished she knew who received the organs because she feels her daughter is still alive. And she really impressed me. *(Participant 10, female,49 years)*

(viii) Desecrating the human body. Some participants claimed that according to their religious believes it was wrong to cut up the body of the dead person after death. They believed that the body is sacred and should be respected by being buried intact.

> That's why I asked you earlier about the position of the Church. Because the Church has always taught us to respect corpses. As a matter of fact there was a belief that you shouldn't touch a corpse or wash it before an hour passed over the person's death. *(Participant 30, male, 32 years)*

> You feel you are removing a part of the person you loved, taking it out. You feel you are committing an act of violence against the dead person, whose absence is already causing pain. How can you not bury him or her intact? *(Participant 18, male, 32 years)*

(ix) Dismembering the body. Others had this vivid picture of a dismembered body. They believed that when organs are taken from the dead body, the cadaver is left in a pitiful state with limbs and other organs lying about.

> One of the reasons is the one mentioned by "X". When my father died I thought about it, but the fear of them butchering him up and leaving him in an unsightly mess…! Probably I believe they would say why bother to tidy up the bits and pieces? I don't like it. *(Participant 39, female, 38 years)*

(x) Destroying a person's chance of an afterlife. Many participants believed in an afterlife. They had different opinions of what forms the body would take but some argued that donating some organs of the dead person's body would destroy their chance of a second life.

> As far as I know, St. Paul had said these words, "Let the last trumpet play when the dead will rise without spoil." Because, I start to think "without spoil"—does it mean we shall be resurrected as we are now? So if they will take away my kidneys, will I be resurrected with them missing? Then I say, I do not want to think about these things. *(Participant 23, male, 67 years)*

> You die, and then the soul rejoins the body, and you go to heaven .... That's the image we have. If you donate a kidney, then in the future you will have a kidney less. *(Participant 30, male, 32years)*

(xi) Destroying a person's identity. For some participants, the image of the body was intimately related to the person's identity. These participants believed that if doctors removed organs from the dead person, they were destroying the identity of the person and his or her uniqueness. They also voiced the concern about the identity of the recipients.

> What I want to know is where science is leading us to, with all these transplants. The kidneys are all right. But the heart, the eyes, then we'll have the brain, so with your memory. Who will the person who receives the heart or the brain of the other be, himself or the other person? *(Participant 35, male, 50 years)*

(xii) Playing God. Some believed that God creates us and has a plan for us. No one, according to these participants, can take the role of God and decide when a person lives and when a person dies. In this context, organ donation was seen as "playing God".

Table 2. Metaphors used to describe organ donation

METAPHORS	CONNOTATIONS
Giving a gift	Donation of organs compared to giving a gift. Just like the decision to give a gift is in the hands of the giver who decides to whom to give a gift, so should the decision to give organs be in the hands of donor or donor family who should also decide to whom to give organs.
Giving charity	Just like a person can give charity to people in need without knowing the beneficiaries, so can a person decide to donate organs without knowing who will receive them.
Doing one's duty	Donating organs is a duty similar to for example taking care of the environment.
Giving life	God gives life. It is expected for one to give back life to others by donating organs.
Recycling of organs	Just like engineers replace parts from a machine into another to make it work, so should doctors use organs of dead people to cure living ones in need of an organ transplant.
Taking out an insurance policy	People should carry donor cards. If in need of an organ, those who have card should be given first preference when waiting for an organ. It's like having an insurance policy.
Living on after dying	Organ donation was seen as a chance of keeping the organs and the memories of the dead relative alive in the recipient.
Desecrating the body	Dead body should be buried intact.
Dismembering the body	Organ donation is seen as cutting up a person.
Destroying a person's chance of an afterlife	A person cannot go to heaven or have a second life if organs from the body are missing
Destroying a person's identity	Removing organs from the body is destroying the identity of the person.
Playing God	God creates the body and He has a plan for how long the person should live. Organ donation interferes with this plan.

No, if you're about to go, you should go, and that's it. You shouldn't try to prolong life. Your time is up. You shouldn't make it longer. From experience I know that those who received an organ kept coming in and out of hospital. Something always goes wrong. *(Participant 20, male, 40 years)*

The metaphors discussed in this section are summarised in Table 2.

METAPHORS OF ORGAN DONATION AND REPRESENTATIONS OF THE HUMAN BODY

Table 3 below describes how positive and negative views towards organ donation were rooted in the metaphors which the participants used to describe organ donation. These, in turn, were dependent on the images they had of the body, again expressed through metaphors. We have classified these images within three major social representations of the body: the body as belonging to God or a Higher Being, the body as a personal possession and the body as self. The table also shows how attitudes towards the opt-out system were related to how metaphors on organ donation and representations of the body were interlinked. Table 3 is followed by a discussion which amplifies the information given in the table and the interrelationships between its different elements. We structure this discussion around the three representations of the body.

My body belongs to God. A very popular belief among participants was that one's body belonged to God or a Higher Being who created it. These participants claimed that their religion teaches that the body is a sacred temple where God dwells. God lives in each and every person. The body is created by God and belongs to God and hence everyone must take care of one's body both physically and spiritually.

Some of these people believed the above strongly and believed it literally. They therefore believed that the person had no right to decide to give away parts of the body both before and after death. Giving away organs, for these participants, meant destroying God's temple. It was an act of total disrespect towards the person and towards God. They argued that since it was God who created the person, only God could decide whether a person lived or died. If God wanted a person to live, He could perform a miracle and heal him or her. He did not need some other person's organs. The fact that a person was sick and was going to die meant that it was God's plan for him or her. Organ donation would mean interfering with God's plans and with nature. It was like playing God. Only God can give life. It was not the doctor's role to interfere with a person's predetermined lifespan. They argued that doctors could help people get better with "natural" means but if this were not possible then they should not meddle with nature. Organ donation was not considered "normal medicine". People holding these beliefs were against the opt-out system because they saw organ donation as going beyond the limits set by nature and, if practised, would create confusion and chaos.

Others believed the symbolic meaning of this claim. They believed that God created their bodies and hence their bodies were a gift from God. Because it was a gift, they believed that one must treasure it and could not do things with it which would go against God's wishes. Among these participants, there were those who saw organ donation as going against God's plan. These people saw organ donation as the desecration of the human body.

Table 3. Metaphors for Organ Donation and Representations of the Body

Social Representations of the body	Metaphors used to describe the body	Implications	Attitudes towards organ donation	Metaphors used to describe organ donation	Attitudes towards opt-out
Body belongs to God	body is a sacred temple	cannot touch the body	negative	Desecration playing God	negative
	body is a gift from God	must take care of it	negative	Desecration butchery	negative
			positive	giving a gift doing one's duty charity giving life	Positive
	body is a tool in God's hands	must use it well	positive	doing one's duty giving life	Positive
I own my body	body is a machine	can replace parts	positive	Recycling	Positive
	body is a treasured possession	can give it to someone dear	positive	a gift	Negative
	body is a commodity	can exchange it for money or in kind	positive	insurance policy	Negative
I am my body	body is whole	cannot be divided into parts	negative	butchery desecration	Negative
	body is unique	parts do not fit in with another body	negative	destruction of person's identity	Negative
	body is eternal	the body lives on	negative	destruction of person's immortality	Negative
			positive	living on in another person	Positive

Others, on the other hand, saw it in a positive light. These people claimed that if it is God's wish that a person helps others by donating one's organs then it was right to do so. It was an altruistic act, worthy of praise. It was like giving a gift of love. Some even saw it as a ticket to heaven. If one did such a noble act then God would reward him or her by accepting them in heaven.

Others still, saw their body as a tool in God's hands. These people saw themselves as channels or means by which and through which, God showed His love for humankind. Giving back life to a person who was at the point of death, was like performing a miracle. In this case, the donor was in a "partnership" with God to save the person's life, an accomplice in this great act of love. These people saw the opt-out system as helping God save more lives.

I own my body. Another image of the body was that a person owned his or her body and therefore the person was responsible for it. He or she had to take care of it, keep it healthy, and enjoy it. If something went wrong, one had the duty to do all that is humanly possible to make it right. These people's relationships with their body were various. Some looked upon it as a machine - a complex mechanism which enabled the person to live and enjoy a healthy life. Others looked upon it in a more emotional way, more as a treasured possession, maybe their most treasured possession. They took care of it and shared it only with people they cared about or loved. Others still looked upon it as a commodity, something they could trade or negotiate.

Those who saw their bodies as a machine, looked upon the organs as spare parts. If a part was not functioning well, then it had to be repaired. If that failed it had to be replaced. Since organs cannot be manufactured, the only way of obtaining them was through the process of organ transplantation. To these people, recycling of body parts made sense and they looked upon organ donation and transplantation as a wise use of human physical resources. For them not doing so would be a shameful waste. These participants were generally in favour of the opt-out system.

Some people looked upon their bodies as a treasured possession, something which could not be given a financial value. It was like a gift given to you by someone you loved. You could not just give it away to anybody. Like a keepsake, you could give it to somebody who was very dear to you, somebody who you knew was going to take care of it and treasure it. These people, while accepting the idea of organ donation, could not accept that the donor or donor family had no right to decide to give these precious organs to relatives or dear friends in need. Moreover, some organs, like the eyes or the heart had a deeper significance for these people. Hence these people believed that it should be possible to choose the person to whom to give the organs and to be able to give one organ but not another if the person so desires. These participants also believed that donating one's organ should be a completely voluntary decision and were against the opt-out system.

Those who looked upon their body as a commodity, saw organs as having a value and an exchange value. They were for one's service but unlike those who looked upon their bodies as a machine, these participants believed that they could use their body to gain affection, acquire material possessions, or even sell their body for financial gain. Hence these people believed that organ donation in such cases should be rewarded either financially or in kind. Some of these people saw organ donation as an instrument or insurance policy. They believed that people who pledged their organs should be given preference if they or their families were ever in need of an organ. They also believed that organs should be stored in banks and that it should become possible to buy or exchange organs. These participants too were against the opt-out system. They believed that since they own their body, it is them and not the State who should decide what to do with it.

I am my body. Whereas some people had a dualistic view of the human being others did not distinguish between their physical bodies and their spiritual and psychological selves. They had a monistic view of the human person and did not separate the body from the spirit. The body was seen to be at the core of the identity of the individual. The body was the self.

Almost all participants who had this representation of the body were against the opt-out system.

Some of these people looked upon the body as something whole, not made up of parts. They also saw the body as sacred and therefore could not be tampered with. Giving permission to doctors to take some organs was to them the same as allowing somebody to destroy a person, to destroy his or her identity and to tarnish his or her memory. This was seen as an insult to the sacredness of the human person and was an act of disrespect towards the person who died.

Some of these participants pointed out that persons were unique beings, one different from the other. Some people who had this view of the human person could not conceive of parts of one person being transferred into another. This created dissonance for them because a person was one whole being and not made up of parts. The body had one identity and each organ contributed to that identity. If the heart was contributing to the identity of a person, then when the heart was given to somebody else, they asked, who would the recipient be, a receptacle for the person's heart? What would happen to the identity of the donor and to that of the recipient?

Some people could not accept organ donation on the premise that it would interfere with the resurrection of the body after death. These people believed that the body lived on after it died. Because they viewed the body as something whole, they looked upon a body with missing organs as incomplete. Organ donation, they believed, would interfere with God's plan to resurrect the body. Some of these people believed that in the afterlife we would have the same body, with the difference that nothing could go wrong with it.

Whereas some people looked upon organ donation as destroying a person's chance of immortality, others looked upon it as a way of gaining a kind of immortality by living on in the other person. These believed that since a person's organs were still living in other people, then the person who had given his or her organs was not dead but was living in the recipients. These people were mostly in favour of opt-out.

Discussion

The Metaphors as Homomorphisms

We have already said that the explanatory power of the metaphor for the researcher studying how people view an issue derives from the way metaphors project familiar relationships onto the novel concepts. Amongst those who saw the body as belonging to God, two of the metaphors used to describe organ donation (Table 3) were desecration of the body and doing one's duty. It is not surprising that these participants differed in their attitudes towards the opt-out system. The metaphors used by these participants to describe the body give a more interesting picture. Some participants described the body as a sacred temple. Sacred temples are known to be inviolable, therefore it is natural that these participants would be against organ donation. At the other extreme, some participants saw their body as a tool in God's hands. These people therefore did not find it difficult to let go of their rights to this tool which did not belong to them, and were therefore in favour of organ donation. A more complex picture is presented by those who saw their body as a gift from God. Some participants reasoned that when somebody presents you with a gift, it is the norm not to give it to somebody else unless the second recipient is very dear. These participants therefore opposed the opt-out system. But some, perhaps thinking in terms of the parable of the talents as narrated in the New Testament (Matthew 25, verse 14), considered a gift from God to imply the responsibility to use the gift wisely. These people, although using the same metaphor to describe their body, were therefore in favour of the opt-out system.

This analysis of the metaphors and what meanings they project onto the concepts of the body and organ donation runs through Table 3 and helps to explain the different views held by the participants within the same social representation of the body. It is perhaps not surprising, for example, that amongst the category of participants who identified themselves with their body, most would be against both organ donation and the opt-out system. But a few of these participants described the body as eternal and organ donation as living on, in another person. These images suggested immortality and therefore led these particular participants to be in favour of both organ donation and the opt-out system.

Implications for Changing Attitudes towards the Opt-Out System

Changing the attitudes of people towards organ donation through public communication campaigns helps to increase the number of people who are willing to donate their organs after their death (Kopfman et al., 2006; Lauri, 2008). But changing attitudes on such a complex issue as organ donation requires that the change agents understand the deeply rooted views held by the general public. People's beliefs towards organ donation are often shrouded in fears which are rooted in religious beliefs, death and the afterlife, pain, the way people look at their own body and many other complex issues. Often, change agents need to be guided by experts who advise them on how to address people's concerns. This is certainly an essential component in the process of preparing a communication campaign. Ignoring the lay theories which the public creates to explain the issue in question could risk having a campaign talking at cross purposes with the public it is supposed to address. The theory of social representations seems to be the ideal theoretical tool to help avoid this from happening.

The Organ Donation Campaign held in Malta in 1996 was perhaps unique in that all its major components were designed around the social representations which were gleaned from the pre-campaign formative research. This included the content of the messages and the manner in which these messages were delivered. Extensive use was made of the very words uttered by the participants in the focus groups. Social representations were also the basis upon which the target population was segmented (Lauri, 2001; Lauri, 2008).

As a result of the formative research carried out before the campaign, the researchers involved in its design decided not to try to change the public's strongly held social representations of the body, but instead to design campaign messages which would resonate with the metaphors associated with organ donation and exploit the fact that within every one of the three representations there was a nucleus of people who were in favour of the opt-out system. Moreover, the results of the national survey had indicated that while attitudes towards organ donation in general were very positive, the views towards the opt-out system were very mixed, even amongst those who were in favour of organ donation and who carried a donor card. It was therefore felt that a campaign coming out heavily in favour of the opt-out system might create resistance and the effort would backfire. The final decision on this matter was that the campaign should not try to push hard for the opt-out system.

Conclusion

In countries where many people on the waiting list for an organ transplant are dying, introducing legislation on the opt-out system might be the only way to save lives. But to minimise resistance to change, legislation must be accompanied by campaigns based on knowledge of the public's beliefs about organ donation. The lesson drawn from the results presented in this paper is that knowing how views towards organ donation are embedded within social representations of the body informs the campaign's messages to greater effect. The above discussion has shown that within all three major social representations of the body there were attitudes for and against the opt-out system. Campaign messages which try to change people's social representations of the body are doomed to failure, since these representations are deeply rooted. But messages designed to change attitudes towards the opt-out system within the same social representation of the body might be more effective. These messages should exploit and resonate with the different metaphors about organ donation expressed by persons whose views of the body are located within the three major social representations presented in Table 3. This point of view can offer a radically different way of segmenting the target population in a public communication campaign and the designing of the appropriate message for each segment (Lauri, 2001; Lauri 2008).

Of course, the Maltese context presents a different scenario from the British one. The Maltese population is smaller, more homogeneous and greatly influenced by the Catholic Church. This sometimes had an important influence on the way the campaign proceeded. For example, all the pre-campaign research showed that one major misconception which many Maltese participants shared was that the Catholic Church was against organ donation. After a discussion between the researchers designing the campaign and the Church authorities, the Maltese bishops issued a pastoral letter in favour of organ donation. This immediately addressed most people's religious doubts about organ donation. Such an event may not be so easily available to a change agent in a country like the UK.

We believe that the findings presented in this paper can be relevant to policy makers, practitioners and academics in other countries. A cursory look at the online objections to Mr. Brown's article, referred to in the introduction indicates that objections raised by the British readers are congruent with the attitudes of the participants in the focus groups carried out in Malta. It would not be surprising if images of the body would still feature prominently if similar research is carried out in the UK. However, it is very probable that, in the context of a country where attitudes to religion are so heterogeneous, this might not be the only or indeed the main factor, and any such analysis would have to include other important issues. Although specific details may be different, the use of social representations anchored in the metaphors people use to describe organ donation would still be a powerful tool in order to understand how people view organ donation and related issues such as the opt-out system.

In their article, "Social marketing and communication in health promotion", Hastings and Haywood (1991) quote from the book "To Kill a Mocking Bird" (Lee, 1960). The character Atticus Finch says "you never really understand a person until you consider things from his point of view—until you climb into his skin and walk around in it." This is what policy makers should do and the best way to do it is perhaps to understand the social representations related to the changes in policies being advocating.

This chapter also appeared in the British Journal of Health Psychology, 2009, Vol 14, 647-666.

REFERENCES

Augoustinos, M. and Penny, S. L. (2001). Reconciliation: The genesis of a new social representation. *Papers on Social Representations,* 10, 4.1- 4.18. http:/www.swp.uni-linz.ac.at/psr.htm

Brown, G. (2008, January 13). Organ donations help us make a difference. The Telegraph, 13 January 2008. Retrieved on 13 January 2008 from http://www.telegraph.co.uk/ news/main.jhtml?xml=/news/2008/01/13/norgans213.xml

Calvo, B. R., Blanca , M. J., and de Frutos, M. A. (2002) Decision making about organ donation in the Andalusian population. *Psicothema,* 14(2), 300-309.

EU Consultation Document on Organ donation. (2006). Organ donation and transplantation policy options at EU level. Retrieved August 14, 2006, from http://ec.europa.eu/ health

Farr, R. M., Trutkowski, C., and Holzl, E. (1996). Public opinion, group discussion and theory of social representations. (Research Papers in Psychology No. 9602). London School of Economics.

Hastings, G. and Haywood, A. (1991). Social Marketing and communication in health promotion. *Health Promotion International*, 6(2), 135-145.

Jovchelovitch, S. (2007). Knowledge in context. Representations, Community and Cculture. Sussex: Routledge.

Kopfman, J. E. and Smith, S. W. (1996). Understanding the audiences of a health communication campaign: A discriminant analysis of potential organ donors based on intent to donate. *Journal of Applied Communication Research,* 24, 22-49.

Lauri, M. A. (2001). The social psychology of social marketing: Promoting organ donation in Malta. Unpublished PhD dissertation. University of London.

Lauri, M. A. and Lauri, J. (2005). Social representations of organ donors and non-donors. *Journal of Community and Applied Social Psychology,* 15, 108-119.

Lauri, M. A. (2006). Attitudes towards organ donation in the last decade. *Malta Medical Journal,* 18(4), 27-31.

Lauri, M. A. (2008). Changing Public Opinion Towards Organ Donation. A social psychological approach to social marketing. In L. O. Pietrieff and R. V. Miller. Public Opinion Research Focus. Nova Science Publishers, 9-36.

Lee, H. (1960). To Kill a Mockingbird. Penguin Bks.

Molony, G. and Walker, I. (2002). Talking about transplants: Social Representations and the dialectic, dilemmatic nature of organ donation and transplantation. *British Journal of Social Psychology,* 41, 299-230.

McIntyre, P., Barnett, M. A., Harris, R. J., Shanteau, J., Skowronski, J.and Klassen, M. (1987). Psychological factors influencing decisions to donate organs. Advances in Consumer Research, XIV, 331-334.

Morgan, S. and Miller, J. K. (2002). Communications about gifts of life; the effect of knowledge, attitudes and altruism on behavioural intentions regarding organ donation. *Journal of Applied Communications Research,* 30(2), 163-178.

Moscovici, S. (1961). La Psychanalyse: Son image et son public. Etude sur la representation sociale de la psychanalyse. Paris: Presses Universitaires de France.

Moscovici, S. (1973). Forward, in C. Herzlich, Health and Illness: A social psychological analysis. London: Academic Press.

Moscovici, S. (1984). The phenomenon of social representations. In R. M. Farr and S. Moscovici (Eds.), Social Representations (pp.3-69). Cambridge: Cambridge University Press.

Perkins, K. (1987). The shortage of cadaveric donor organs for transplantation: Can psychology help? *American Psychologist,* 42(10), 921-30.

Sanner, M. (1994). Attitudes toward organ donation and transplantation. A model for understanding reactions to medical procedures after death. *Social Science Medicine,* 38(8), 1141–1152.

Wagner, W., Elejabarrieta, F. and Lahnsteiner, I. (1995). How the sperm dominates the ovum - Objectification by metaphor in the social representation of conception. *European Journal of Social Psychology,* 25, 671-688.

Wagner, W. and Hayes, N. (2005). Everyday Dscourse and Common Sense – The theory of social representations. Basingstoke: Palgrave-Macmillan.

Webster, P.(2008, January 14). Gordon Brown seeks to make everyone an organ donor - with opt-out. Retrieved on 14 January 2008 from http://www.timesonline.co.uk/tol/news/politics

Wintor, P. (2008, January 14) Brown backs opt-out system to boost organ transplants. Retrieved on 14 January 2008 from http://www.guardian

APPENDIX A

	Group 1	Group 2	Group 3	Group 4	Group 5
No. of participants	9	8	10	6	8
Males	4	1	7	1	5
Females	5	7	3	5	3
Age range	19-50 yrs	20-49 yrs	20-67 yrs	19-44 yrs	19-43 yrs
Participant number	1-9	10-17	18-27	28-33	34-41

In: Organ Donation and Transplantation
Editor: Mary Anne Lauri
ISBN: 978-1-62948-257-6

Chapter 14

ORGAN DONATION MEDIA CAMPAIGNS: KEY CONSIDERATIONS FOR IMPROVING CAMPAIGN EFFECTIVENESS

Eusebio M. Alvaro, Ph.D., M.P.H.*
Claremont Graduate University, California, US

ABSTRACT

Drawing on theory and research across multiple behavioral science domains, this chapter addresses how the mass media can be used to educate the public about organ donation and motivate donation-related behavior. Both non-living and living organ donation are examined. A key proposition is that, organ donation is well-suited for mass media interventions—especially given media's ability to increase issue salience. A second central proposition is that research on organ donation mass media campaigns must move beyond basic "something versus nothing" approaches and embrace a more complex and richer messaging perspective. To explicate both propositions, the chapter reviews broad theories of mass media effects, summarizes theory and research on a message perspective relative to mass media, and considers the implications of this body of knowledge for furthering applied research on nonliving and living organ donation campaigns.

INTRODUCTION

"Half the money I spend on advertising is wasted; the trouble is I don't know which half"
John Wannamaker (1838 - 1922)

An alternate quotation by Disraeli was also considered as a lead-in to this chapter—I paraphrase here: knowing what you don't know is a huge step towards knowing. With this in mind, this chapter may be viewed as a reflection on, in general terms, what is known about

* E-mail: eusebio.alvaro@cgu.edu.

organ donation campaigns and what we have still to know. The musings herein hopefully address what we do know while also offering some suggestions for how we may endeavour to know more.

This chapter will draw on theory and research in the domains of Communication, Psychology, and Marketing to address how the mass media can be used to educate the public about organ donation and motivate donation-related behavior. Both non-living and living organ donation will be examined as, while both are amenable to mass media interventions subject to general campaign principles, their uniqueness leads to different messaging considerations.

Organ donation, whether non-living or living, may be very well-suited for mass media interventions. Nonliving donation is a low-vested and low-salience issue. Registration as an organ donor is a behavior that seemingly has little direct impact on one's life and is also one that may be seemingly delayed—there is no urgent need to register as a donor. In fact, one can avoid enacting the behavior entirely and leave the decision up to loved ones following death. In the case of living donation, while patients in need of organs are highly vested—it is their life after all—potential donors may be largely unaware and uninformed about living donation and transplantation. In both instances, while media campaigns may not directly motivate organ donation registration or actual donation, they are an excellent means by which to introduce new ideas and enhance their salience among a target audience.

A key consideration guiding this chapter is that research on organ donation mass media campaigns must move beyond basic "something versus nothing" approaches and embrace a more complex and richer messaging perspective. Asking whether mass media campaigns are effective in either encouraging donor registration or actual living donations is not nearly as valuable as understanding the types of campaigns and, more specifically, the ads within campaigns, that are most effective. Moreover, what does effective mean? What are appropriate outcomes for organ donation media campaigns?

Organ donation campaigns—addressing either nonliving or living donation—should have a key goal of increasing organ donation discussion. Discussion has long been a staple outcome of organ donation education efforts and it is an outcome that is highly relevant to mass media campaign impact. A long-noted strength of the mass media is the fostering of interpersonal communication about issues portrayed in the media. Of course, much remains to be learned about how campaigns can maximize this outcome.

The messaging perspective advocated by this chapter takes into account the relative impact of both the content and executional elements of organ donation messages. A focus on content addresses the nature of the information provided as well as the type of persuasive appeal being utilized while a focus on executional elements would examine how the content is delivered. To begin then, some familiarity of scholarly reflections on mass media impact is an essential starting point.

Mass Media Theory

While a more detailed description of the intersection of mass media theory and organ donation is provided in a recent volume addressing behavioral science approaches to organ donation (Alvaro and Siegel, 2010), a brief overview of scholarly thinking on what one may reasonably expect from the mass media is necessary prior to a more specific focus on particular campaign messages. Quite simply, most of us are unable to recognize an effective media campaign when we see one. Moreover, there is no need to rely on intuition or post-hoc explanations of evaluation findings when perfectly reasonable, applicable—and arguably most important—research-supported, theoretical approaches exist. Admittedly, their existence is mostly a lonely one. They largely languish in actual or metaphorically dusty tomes on library shelves/databases the world over; only to be occasionally taken out for fresh air by interested media scholars. Media theories stipulate the nature of media effects that one may reasonably anticipate—a key piece of information to guide both the development and evaluation of campaigns.

While it still rears its head in populist musings regarding mass media impact, the initial "hypodermic needle"or the "Silver Bullet" model (Schramm, 1982), whereby powerful mass media simply 'inject' a message into a passive audience too powerless to resist, has been rejected by serious scholars for some time. Understanding of mass media effects is much more complex than it was at the start of the prior century. As early as the 1940's the notion that mass media had direct and powerful effects was rejected with the introduction of the Two-Step Flow model (Lazarsfeld, Berelson, and Gaudet, 1948) positing that mass media messages influence opinion leaders who then influence others in their social group via direct contact. This perspective views interpersonal communication about mediated messages as more important to attitude formation and change than the specific nature of the messages themselves—at least for the broader audience. Support for this view, or at least for the proposition that mass and interpersonal communication act in concert to attain persuasion goals, has been found in a number of health contexts (Durkin and Wakefield, 2006; Gunther, Bolt, Borzekowski, Liebhart, and Dillard, 2006; Hafstad and Aaro, 1997, and Morton and Duck, 2001).

The Two-Step Flow model proposes that the mass media have limited effects and that these effects are largely indirect. The Agenda-setting model (McCombs and Shaw, 1972) returns to a view of mass media as powerful, although the nature of that power is indirect. At the most basic level, the model conceptualizes mass media as setting the order of importance for social issues and also setting the context in which these issues are debated. In the language of the model, the mass media is a tool for telling audiences what to think *about*, not what to *think*. Issue salience, not persuasion, is the key outcome. While most of the supporting research was conducted in the context of news programs, more recently, the model has garnered attention in the health behavior domain.

Combining the Agenda-setting and Two-Step Flow models (see Alvaro and Siegel, 2010), one could propose that mass media campaigns may be ideally suited to introduce new ideas to a targeted population where a social context may be created to foster discussion about those ideas. The goal of mass media campaigns then becomes to use messages to attract the attention of opinion leaders so as to stimulate campaign-related discussion in order to make the issue one of import; garnering further attention and consideration. In this view, media influence can take some time and it may be felt more at a level broader than the individual.

Gerbner's (1969, 1980) Cultivation Analysis model of mass media influence takes such a broad perspective; the approach focuses on cumulative exposure to mass media messages and the resultant gradual shifts in societal perceptions. Again, mass media have powerful effects but those effects are indirect and more subtle than simple direct change. In fact, mass media influence our sense of reality by "cultivating" or reinforcing particular values, beliefs, and perceptions, in targeted audiences. Through a variety of psychological processes, the 'reality' depicted in the mass media is socialized and, ultimately influences individual behavior.

One more model of media effects that deserves consideration reminds us that, despite the broad societal impact that mass media may have, individuals still have a role to play. The Uses and Gratification approach (Bauer, 1964) proposes that audiences do not just consume media; they are active, purposive, and goal-directed. People actively seek out media messages that will satisfy their needs and, ultimately, help them achieve desired goals. Some needs identified in the research (McQuail, 1971) include surveillance, personal identity, personal relationships, and diversion/entertainment. Audiences have well-formed expectations for mass media and these expectations must be taken into account when developing campaigns.

In summary then, mass media may have powerful and broad effects that impact audiences both individually and collectively. Moreover, active audiences seek out media and their reactions may be based on their particular needs and goals. Regardless, the collective impact of mass media may be mediated/moderated by interpersonal conversation about media depictions of social issues, with such conversations both impacting, and being impacted by, broader social perceptions of issue importance and how an issue is contextualized. Regardless of any particular mass media model or combinations of models one draws on, mass media can most decidedly be a powerful tool to raise awareness, provide information, increase discussion, enhance perceived importance, and, ultimately change attitudes and behaviors relevant to organ donation. However, while necessary, a familiarity with general models of mass media influence is insufficient to develop an effective media campaign.

Messaging Approach

Communication theorists have long proposed basic models sharing core features to describe communication processes—whether enacted at the mass-media or interpersonal level, or any points in between. These models generally conceptualize communication as a process whereby a *source* sends a *message* through a particular *channel* that then impacts a *receiver*. It is illustrative to consider the example of a televised presidential speech: the president (source) delivers a speech (message) via television (channel) that is attended to by a TV audience (receivers). Following this view of the communication process, theorists and researchers have staked out areas of inquiry devoted one element or another or, even interactions among elements. While admittedly lacking in theoretical sophistication, and arguably even elegance, the aforementioned model nonetheless provides for a much more nuanced view of the communication process than that often supplied by published reports of organ donation campaigns. Of course, it should be mentioned that campaigns in other health domains, reported in decades-long accumulations of scientific literature, have suffered from a similar ignominy. Regardless, as Crano has so elegantly noted (Crano, 2010), there is every reason to avoid repeating this sad state of affairs in the relatively new domain of organ donation research.

One prescription is to forgo campaigns and related evaluations that feature comparisons between "the campaign" and its absence. It may be conceded that "something" is more often than not better than "nothing"; albeit one must always bear in mind the possibility of iatrogenic effects with any campaign attempting to influence an audience (Burgoon, Alvaro,

Grandpre, and Voloudakis, 2003; Crano, Siegel, and Alvaro, 2012). Regardless, a "something vs. nothing" approach will be unable to provide an explanatory mechanism for either positive or iatrogenic outcomes. A message perspective is one antidote. As proposed in a recent review of organ donation mass media campaigns, not all messages are created equal (Alvaro and Siegel, 2010). Maximizing campaign effects depends partly on creating campaign messages based on behavioral science theory and research; without such a basis, no knowledge of *why* a particular campaign succeeds or fails is attained. Moreover, campaigns using varied messages should be pitted against each other—as well as no-campaign comparisons—in order to determine relative campaign effects. It is only via the systematic variation of theory- and research-based messages that effective campaign approaches can be determined, and perhaps more importantly--understood. Lacking a comprehensive explanation and understanding of campaign effects, one is left, in the best case, with a successful campaign without any knowledge as to why success was obtained and whether or not it may be obtained in other contexts with different audiences.

In a rush to intervention development and implementation, much-needed efficacy trials assessing relative message impact are rarely undertaken and, to the extent that they exist, are apparently relegated to the sidelines. In such a context, no collective knowledge will accumulate, "failed" campaigns will be little- or misunderstood while successes will be blindly touted as panaceas—only to be met with despair, confusion, wailing, and gnashing of teeth when not replicated elsewhere. A scientific understanding of organ donation campaigns will never be attained by simply reporting multiple instances where a particular campaign—perhaps even based on high quality formative research—successfully outshone its absence. At best, one may surmise that, when it comes to organ donation outcomes X and Y, mass media campaigns may work. Now what?

Of course, any nascent domain of inquiry may needfully be initially subjected to gross level questions such as "Do mass media campaigns lead to improved organ donation registration outcomes?" My co-authors and I have certainly felt the need to establish such facts (Alvaro, Siegel, Robles, and Pace Jones, 2006; Alvaro, Siegel, Crano, and Dominick, 2010) and have noted that the increasing methodological sophistication being brought to bear on this question appears to be providing an affirmative response—at least in the context of nonliving donation (Alvaro and Siegel, 2010). However, in order to develop a complete understanding of how mass media campaigns may have a positive impact on organ donation behavior, we must go beyond improvements in methodology and concern ourselves with theory and research-based guidance in the development of actual campaign messages. One appropriate question is: "What mass media message types are best able to achieve desired organ donation outcomes?"

The communication and social influence literature highlights the importance of understanding the relation between message features and desired outcomes, as well as the interaction of message features with audience characteristics (Crano, 2000, 2001; Crano and Prislin, 2008; McGuire, 1978, 1985). Many of the modest effect sizes observed in mass media campaigns designed to change health behaviors may be partly due to a failure to consider these relationships—focusing instead on the impact of a campaign relative to the absence of a campaign. For example, it is axiomatic that communication occurs on both the relational and the content level (Anderson and Guerrero, 1998; Crano and Prislin, 2006; Foley and Duck, 2006; Selnow and Crano, 1987; Watzlawick, Beavin, and Jackson, 1967). Relational features refer to non-content aspects of messages that indicate the nature of the relationship between the source and the receiver—*how* something is said. Content features refer to the factual information being conveyed in a message—*what* is said. Content and relational features may interact; thus, the same relational approach may work with one type of message content but not another (Crano, Siegel, Alvaro, and Patel, 2007; Lee and Aaker, 2004), or with one type of audience (e.g., adults) and not another (adolescents). Owing to their impact on the social influence process, both relational and content features must be considered in proper message design.

Relational message features may affect message acceptance by their very nature, or they may serve as immediate barriers to persuasion by activating resistance via selective exposure, negative affective message-directed responses, and unfavorable cognitive responses (Anderson, Levin and Lorch, 1977; Petty, Cacioppo and Schumann, 1983). The latter two mechanisms have long been suggested as being of special importance in social influence (Chaiken, 1980; Crano and Prislin, 2006; Hovland, Janis, and Kelly, 1953; McGuire and Papageorgis, 1962; Petty and Cacioppo, 1986). The content of a message will matter little if the message is rejected prior to its processing. How then, may one forestall message rejection?

Future organ donation campaigns should be based upon a solid messaging theory/research base and stringently evaluated. At a minimum, more efficacy studies are needed wherein relative message impact is assessed in a controlled and largely inexpensive context. Data from these studies would then inform message development for a larger study assessing the impact of a mass media campaign implemented in a less controlled but real world context; an effectiveness study. Alternatively, multiple campaign messages may be implemented in different mass media campaigns targeting varied communities.

Regardless of the approach taken, a serious consideration of message types is sorely needed. Such consideration may start with an extensive audience and context analysis wherein descriptive data is collected to provide a full understanding of the human and social environment in which a campaign is to be implemented. Once the context is described, behavioral science theories relevant to the issues raised may be selected in order to provide a substrate upon which specific campaign messages can be built. Care must be taken to craft messages that accurately operationalize theoretical constructs while being sensitive to specific contextual factors such as dialects, jargon, and culturally appropriate terms and imagery. Theory and research should ideally inform both the content of a message and its relational attributes. These ideas are explored below in the contexts of both nonliving and living organ donation. What would a messaging perspective on organ donation look like?

A Messaging Approach to Nonliving Organ Donation

Over the past few decades, nonliving organ donation has received a fair bit of attention world-wide via a number of media campaigns and, while there have been deficits in design rigor and a general lack of theory to guide these efforts, there is growing evidence that such campaigns can work (Alvaro and Siegel, 2010). What is needed henceforth is an improved understanding of how to maximize organ donation campaign effectiveness. Is there a research base from which one may draw conclusions about potentially successful nonliving organ donation campaign messages? What would a message perspective on nonliving organ donation—complete with applied test of the relative impact of messages—look like?

Research on Message Effects in Nonliving Organ Donation

Just as some scholars (Siminoff, Traino, and Gordon, 2011; Anker and Feeley, 2011a,b) have examined "messages" used by requestors approaching families for organ donation consent following the passing of a loved one, some effort has been made at a descriptive level to examine extant nonliving organ donation advertisements to identify message themes and strategies (Tian, 2010; Reinhart and Anker, 2012). Oddly, given decades of campaigns, such descriptive research has recent origins. While such descriptive information has some value for the development of future nonliving organ donation campaigns, a more appropriate emphasis would be on theory-derived messages developed a priori.

While seemingly existing in a realm distant from the senses of campaign developers, a message variation approach has typified a sadly underdeveloped and under-appreciated body of research conducted—with a few exceptions—in controlled contexts. Mystifyingly, the insights gained by these efficacy studies seemingly rarely influence larger applied effectiveness trials conducted with life-size campaigns in the real world. While not large, this largely high-quality research does exist—apparently published at the rate of small handful of studies per decade. One of the earliest of these studies was conducted by Winkel (1984) in the early 80's. Drawing on communication theory, he compared organ donation messages utilizing either one-sided or refutational messages—discovering that addressing both positive and negative behavioral outcomes of nonliving organ donation is superior to addressing only positive outcomes.

Winkel's (1984) early findings were built on by Smith and colleagues (Ford and Smith, 1991; Smith, Morrison, Kopfman, and Ford, 1994) – initiating an admirable program of lab-based efficacy studies examining the relative impact of theory-based nonliving organ donation messages. A study comparing the use of narrative and statistical content soon followed (Kopfman, Smith, Yun, and Hodges, 1998) and a new message emphasis grew (Feeley, Marshall, and Reinhart, 2006; Weber, Martin, Members of COMM 401, and Corrigan, 2006). Message framing has threatened to become yet another emphasis area. The few extant studies examine the relative impact of creating messages that emphasize either the positive outcomes to be gained or lost by becoming/not becoming an organ donor (Reinhart, Marshall, Feeley, and Tutzauer, 2007; Cohen, 2010). Lastly, a number of one-off studies examine message aspects such as: variation in narrative content (Lindsey and Yun, 2005), normative and referent information (Marshall and Feeley, 2006), compliance gaining and reactance (La Vail, Anker, Reinhart, and Feeley,2010), and counterargumentation, affective, motivating action, and dissonance (Siegel, Alvaro, Pace Jones, Crano, Lac, and Ting 2008).

Example of a Messaging Approach to Nonliving Organ Donation

A more detailed examination of Siegel and colleagues' (Siegel et al., 2008) study serves to highlight the particulars of a messaging approach to nonliving organ donation. The study is an effectiveness trial of a print message campaign utilizing a rigorous counterbalanced quasi-experimental design featuring the rotation of four theory-derived message approaches, executed in four different poster styles and implemented in four different examples of four different location types (i.e. hospitals, libraries, universities, and community colleges).

Formative pre-campaign research indicated that registering to be a nonliving organ donor was perceived as something that: a) could be put off nearly indefinitely (in fact one's family could make the decision upon one's death), b) was a behavior that many were not eligible to do, c) was positively viewed yet seldom done, and d) was an issue often addressed via emotional stories of those in need or no longer alive due to an organ shortage. Behavioral science theory and research was reviewed for perspectives addressing each of these issues and subsequently guided a message development process including both behavioral scientists and professional staff from a local organ procurement agency.

A key feature of this study was the use of multiple exemplars for each theory-based message. For example, one message type involved forestalling counter-argumentation by addressing common reasons people gave for not registering to be a donor (i.e. too old, too sick, not eligible).

Four specific poster variations or exemplars were created—all featuring the same content but each using a different format to convey the content. In one case, content was delivered via comic-book style dialogue bubbles. In another, the same content was delivered via a mock "quiz". This multiple exemplar approach is important in allowing one to determine if a particular theory-based message approach is effective; rather than any impact being due to a particular execution of that approach. If one message type performs better than another, regardless of how the message is specifically executed, one may have reasonable confidence in the superiority of the message approach itself.

The resultant messages were tested in the field with posters placed above computer kiosks in order to enable collection of actual organ donor registration data. The posters drew members of the general public to the kiosks whereby they could officially register on the newly created registry. Results of the study readily revealed the benefits of the messaging approach.

The counterargument message was responsible for nearly 50% more registrations than would be expected by chance alone. Moreover, it garnered almost twice as many registrations as the least effective message. Out of 419 unique registrations collected over the course of the study, 151 could be attributed to the counterargument message. The success of this message type was evident across all message exemplars and locations where, at worst, the appeal was equally effective and, at best, it was significantly more effective, than the other three appeals.

The messaging approach taken, tested via a rigorous design, provides solid evidence for the superiority of one particular message—a highly desirable outcome that is unfortunately far too uncommon in organ donation research.

SUMMARY

There are a number of noteworthy aspects of the handful of studies largely comprising the experimental examination of nonliving organ donation messages. First, the bulk of the above studies were conducted in the controlled experimental confines of a university using a student sample. Only rarely (i.e. Lindsey and Yun, 2005; Siegel et al., 2008) is research implemented in applied contexts where factors such as audience attention to message materials and audience homogeneity are not the norm. Given the limited number of studies on a little-studied domain, more controlled efficacy studies are expected and even desired; nonetheless, future efforts could extent beyond the academy to include participants from all walks of life.

A second observation that may be made by even the least cognitively complex among us is that the bulk of the research on nonliving organ donation messaging approaches is conducted in a somewhat programmatic manner under the influence of a few key individuals. Even a cursory perusal of the citations above readily reveals that Smith and Feeley have maintained a commendable level of activity and involvement in this important work.

A final observation is that behavioral outcomes are exceedingly rare; Siegel et al (2008) being one exception. Given the ready availability of either printed donor registry forms or online links to donor registries, a creative research team may certainly devise ways to incorporate actual organ donor registration into their studies.

A Messaging Approach to Living Organ Donation

While nonliving organ donation has received some worldwide attention in the form of mass media campaigns (Alvaro and Siegel, 2010), similar campaigns addressing living organ donation are largely absent. In fact, with rare exceptions (i.e. McGregor, Ferguson, and O' Carroll, 2012), while the messaging literature on organ donation is small, similar research addressing living donation is nearly non-existent.

While there are disagreements as to whether living organ donation should be publicized and encouraged, there may be room for agreement on, at minimum, increasing public awareness of, and education about, this issue. In the absence of any concerted mass educational effort, living organ donation is an issue subject to ignorance, misinformation, and very low salience.

As has been argued in this chapter, mass media campaigns are highly suitable for addressing these specific deficits. In the US, the government has acknowledged the need for some form of living donation education and, indeed, does fund such efforts through the Department of Health and Human Services (see Ganikos, 2010)—recently taking a firm stance on supporting only those projects focused on education rather than persuasion. While commendable, it is unfortunate that, to date, projects funded via this program have overwhelmingly focused only on dialysis patients and, in some cases, their families. Public education campaigns targeting the general population or specific demographic segments thereof, rather than non-patients and/or families, are largely absent.

The need for such public education campaigns is high and is highest among the population segments most at risk for health conditions placing individuals in need or living organ transplants – liver, and most commonly, kidney disease. In the USA, minority populations that more adversely impacted by kidney disease would appear to be a good starting point for public education campaigns addressing living kidney donation and transplantation.

In fact, minority receptivity to health information delivered via the mass media, further serves to highlight the usefulness of well-designed living donation campaigns. Moreover, public education would have the additional benefit of circumventing information processing biases associated with renal disease patients that may be suffering from the co-morbidity of depression—as was the case in a recent study of Latinos (Gonzalez, Siegel, Alvaro, and O'Brien, in press)

In the USA, African-Americans and Latinos are two minority populations at high risk for kidney failure. Fortunately, at least for the purposes of this chapter, there exists formative research as well as an example of a public education campaign addressing living organ donation—at least in regard to the Latino population in the USA.

Example of a Living Organ Donation Campaign

Prior to our own research program (Alvaro, Siegel, Crano, and Dominick, 2010, Alvaro et al, 2008, Siegel, Alvaro, and Maurer, 2011, Siegel, Alvaro, Lac, Crano, and Dominick, 2008), only a single published living donor study focused on Latinos (Dominguez, Gonzalez, Morales Otero, et al., 1991). As a result, considerable formative research was necessary prior to campaign development and implementation. Findings from our studies with members of the general Latino population provide some insight into Latino knowledge, attitudes, and behaviors regarding living organ donation.

The results of six focus groups conducted in Spanish with Spanish-dominant Hispanic non-donors with favorable attitudes toward organ donation are illustrative (Alvaro et al., 2008). While participants reported substantial exposure to organ donation information, they nonetheless felt that they were in need of more information and were rather unaware of even basic organ donation procedures. Not one participant knew how to go about being an organ donor. One especially relevant knowledge gap was that most participants were unaware that living donors could choose recipients. This is important in that one potential benefit of living organ donation is that Latinos could be quite receptive to live organ donation due to the choice component.

Another prominent knowledge gap was reflected in the fact that most participants reported that they knew somebody on dialysis yet very few reported that they knew someone who was in need of a kidney transplant. It is evident that the link between kidney failure and kidney transplantation is not common knowledge. Lastly, participants report mixed experiences with family discussion of organ donation with many expressing the difficulty of having such conversations in more traditional families. Even as living organ donation knowledge increased, participants did not feel capable of engaging in family discussions regarding living organ donation. In general, they agreed that it would be very difficult for them to approach a friend or family member if they ever found themselves in need of a kidney. They were uncertain as to how to broach the subject. Nor did they feel confident in their abilities to answer specific questions that may be asked.

This qualitative data complements the results of a large telephone survey conducted as part of the same project (Siegel et al., 2008). A total of 1,253 Latinos in three southwestern USA communities took part in a 10-minute Spanish-language telephone survey assessing living organ donation knowledge, attitudes, and behaviors. Survey results indicate that while attitudes toward living organ donation are overwhelmingly positive, knowledge deficits and beliefs about family and religion serve as barriers to donation (Siegel, et al., 2008). For example, 80% of the sample was in favor of living organ donation; however, over 59% felt they could not be living donors due to religion and over 54% believed living donation would be contrary to the wishes of their families. Perhaps most relevant to public education goals is the finding that 47% did not have any idea about how one goes about being a living donor. Data from this study also indicated that, while respondents were quite willing to both offer a kidney and accept a kidney, they were not very comfortable in discussing living donation as an option if they were to find themselves in need of a kidney transplant.

The campaign

In order to address the barriers noted above in relation to a non-patient population, a Spanish-language media campaign was developed then launched in southern Arizona in two waves: summer 2004 (July 16th - October 25th) and spring 2005 (March 2nd - April 30th).

Based on formative research, a slogan was arrived at and featured in all campaign ads. The slogan, "Atrevete" was a challenge to "step up" and brace oneself to do something about the kidney shortage in the local Hispanic community. The actual campaign ads were based on our formative research and developed locally by a Spanish-owned agency. Ads consisted of four 30-sec TV ads and two 60-sec radio ads encouraging information calls to a Spanish-language telephone hotline.

TV ads. Two ads focused on the disproportionate number of local Hispanics on dialysis. One featured a photo-montage local dialysis patients with narration connecting dialysis to kidney disease, noting the disproportionate number of Hispanics both affected and awaiting transplantation. The second ad inter-cut footage of dialysis patients with that of a local kidney recipient singing, golfing, and spending time with his family (the recipient narrates). This series drew on focus group data indicating lack of awareness: of the link between dialysis-kidney need, that live donors choose intended recipients, and a focus on real people. The series also served to emphasize that everyday Latinos in the local community did in fact actually receive transplants—this was not an experience reserved for the wealthy, celebrities, or the majority population.

Another two ads focused on donor-recipient pairs discussing their experience. One related the story of a male donating a kidney to a female cousin. The second featured an elderly woman who donated a kidney to her sister 20 previously—both, now elderly, are shown to be active and enjoying life. This series was informed by focus group data reflecting a desire to see real people and, even more, curiosity about transplantation outcomes for recipients and donors.

Radio ads. Two ads addressed the dialysis-kidney disease link, the disproportionate number of Hispanics affected and awaiting a kidney transplant, and that potential live donors could select their intended recipient.

Campaign Outcomes. The campaign was evaluated via a quasi-experimental design (Alvaro et al., 2010) and results were positive. The campaign was successfully implemented and attained exposure rates greater than 60% were achieved with a modest media budget. In terms of impact, analyses of community-wide impact pre- to post-campaign (relative to a comparison site) indicated significant differences in donation intentions. Analyses on exposure intensity suggest exposure to campaign advertisements was strongly related to organ donation intentions. Respondents reporting campaign exposure were significantly more likely to report pro-donation behavioral intentions. Moreover the same analyses indicated a positive relationship between living donation attitudes and perceived living donation norms. Data on calls to the advertised hotline support a positive campaign impact; calls were received from 62 unique individuals requesting more information on how to become a living donor.

What's Next for Living Donation Campaigns?

As with our early campaigns addressing nonliving organ donation (Alvaro, Jones, Robles, and Siegel, 2006), the living donation campaign was implemented to ascertain, via a methodologically sound quasi-experimental design, whether a mass media campaign could positively impact perceptions of organ donation in the Latino population. This was accomplished. Variations in messaging were not yet a concern and, in fact, were beyond the purview of the funding agency and our budget; thus, the study provides no real evidence on what types of messages are best to increase living organ donation outcomes. It is left to future efforts to apply a messaging perspective to this exceedingly challenging organ donation context. While there are innumerable applied research possibilities in this context, our own research does highlight some possible avenues of exploration.

A first step could be to ascertain which messaging approaches are best suited to facilitate issue awareness and knowledge acquisition. At least among Latinos in the USA, the issue of living organ donation is typified by considerable deficits in awareness and knowledge; both among the general non-patient population (Alvaro et al., 2008) as well as among renal disease patients and their families (Siegel et al., 2011). Investigations into increasing living organ donation awareness or salience should consider both the executional elements as well as message content. Considerations of imagery, pacing, and tone would be examples of the former while the examination of information addressing the number of local individuals in need exemplifies the latter. Perhaps there may be even interesting and powerful interactions between the two message elements.

For example, as noted above, the Alvaro et al. (2010) campaign featured an initial ad highlighting the plight of Latinos on dialysis. Executional elements included vivid images of ill individuals on dialysis machines as well as a somber tone imparted both by music and narration. Pre-testing of the messages revealed that the ads were seen as shocking and somewhat disturbing—responses that may have facilitated awareness and message recall in the campaign. On the content level, this initial ad focused on the number of Latinos—both nationally and locally—that were currently on dialysis while noting that they were on dialysis due to kidney failure—thus in need of a kidney transplant. The executional elements were designed to complement this content and, the combination of the two may have been responsible for a considerable impact on awareness. Future research may be designed to investigate the separate and combined contributions of executional and content elements to increasing living donation awareness.

As noted, when it comes to knowledge regarding living transplantation, the Latino communities for which data exist, demonstrate remarkable deficits in the basic facts of the donation and transplantation process. Mass media campaigns could be marshaled to provide such basic information to the public. Here the challenge is to ascertain effective theory-based messaging approaches leading to knowledge retention and learning. Theory and research on Entertainment Education (or "Edutainment") (Singhal and Rogers, 1999) and narrative transportation (Green, Brock, and Kaufman) may be valuable in delineating important executional and content features of mediated messages that facilitate the attention to, and retention of, basic factual information.

Some of the advertisements featured in the Alvaro et al. (2010) living donor campaign may provide an example of these considerations. As noted, two TV ads focused on donor-recipient pairs (young male and female cousins and two elderly sisters) discussing their experience. The emphasis was using their stories to convey some very rudimentary information about transplantation outcomes for recipients and donors. Our study provides no way of ascertaining if different message approaches would result in better or worse outcomes but one can imagine multiple studies that could be designed to do just that. For example, drawing on research on narrative vs. statistical presentation of information (see Kopfman et al. 1998; Feeley et al. 2006) messages similar to ours could be compared with those taking a drier statistical approach.

Another avenue of research may draw on data indicating a considerable disconnect between renal patients and their families (Siegel et al., 2011). Patients feel family members should come forward for donor assessment without being asked while family members believe that patients would ask them in the event of a need for a living donor. It appears that each party is willing (to either donate or accept a donation) but, as luck would have it, both are expecting the other to act! Clarification of this situation would be beneficial and could be achieved by making this disconnect known among the target population.

This approach may be particularly palatable in that no persuasion is necessary – both parties are already in favor of living donation so the task is one of explicating the status quo. Our own current research is investigating the potential for providing patients with feedback from actual donors and patients regarding both their attitudes and expectations towards donating or accepting a donation (see also Delair, Feeley, Kim, et al. 2010). It may be that this patient-centered intervention could be adapted for more broad mass media dissemination—to widely promulgate the extant social normative perceptions regarding living donation.

CONCLUSION

We know that mass media campaigns focused on either nonliving or living donation can have a positive impact on donation outcomes. What has been generally lacking is been a clear understanding, based on theory and research, as to what may be reasonably expected from mass media campaigns and, how campaign messages may be constructed to maximize these outcomes. In an attempt to address the first consideration, this chapter has briefly highlighted a number of key theories setting expectations for mass media process and outcomes.

The second issue has attracted considerably more attention in this chapter due to it being far more rarely addressed in discussions of mass media effects in general, and organ donation campaigns in particular. Featured prominently throughout is the proposition that an emphasis on a messaging perspective where the content and relational features of campaign messages are rigorously studied in both efficacy and effectiveness trials is necessary to further our understanding of how campaigns may be maximized to achieve desired organ donation outcomes.

Researchers should build on the extant research base regarding message features, initiate new efficacy studies on heretofore unconsidered message features, and build on these efficacy studies by implementing effectiveness trials in real world contexts with actual donation behaviors as outcomes.

Of course, researchers in this domain cannot do this alone. In order for the necessary work to be completed organizations funding campaigns and behavioral science research in this area need to recognize that an emphasis on intervention implementation may result in individual successes while short-changing the accumulation of knowledge and understanding. The vexing nature of the problems, the dire consequences for those in need, and the very human desire to alleviate suffering need not be discarded in the pursuit of this understanding—effectiveness trials are in-fact applied studies impacting real people. Efficacy trials—by nature small and relatively inexpensive—can be encouraged (financially as well as philosophically) prior to funding of effectiveness trials.

However, the key is to determine the relative impact of one messaging approach vis-à-vis another—not simply to determine that a particular campaign works better than its absence. Messages matter.

References

Alvaro, E. M. and Siegel, J. T. (2010). Where have we been and where to next? A review and synthesis of organ donation media campaigns. In J. T. Siegel and E. M. Alvaro (Eds.) Understanding organ donation: Contributions from applied behavioral science, pp. 41-63. Hoboken, NJ: Wiley-Blackwell.

Alvaro, E. M., Siegel, J. T., Crano, W. D., and Dominick, A. (2010). A mass mediated intervention on Hispanic organ donation. *Journal of Health Communication*, 15, 374-387.

Alvaro, E. M., Siegel, J. T., Turcotte, D., Lisha, N., Crano, W. D., and Alexander, S. (2008). Hispanic living kidney donation: A qualitative examination of barriers and opportunities. *Progress in Transplantation,* 18, 243-250.

Alvaro, E. M., Jones, S. P., Robles, A. S., and Siegel, J. T. (2006). Hispanic organ donation: Impact of a Spanish-language organ donation campaign. *Journal of the National Medical Association,* 98, 1-8.

Andersen, P. A., and Guerrero, L. K. (1998). Principles of communication and emotion in social interaction. In P. A. Andersen and L. K. Guerrero (Eds.), Handbook of communication and emotion: Research, theory, applications, and contexts (pp. 49-99). San Diego, CA: Academic Press.

Anderson, D. R., Levin, S. R., and Lorch, E. P. (1977). The effects of TV program pacing on the behavior of preschool children. *Educational Technology and Research*, 25, 159-166.

Anker, A. E., and Feeley, T. H. (2011a). Asking the difficult questions: Message strategies used by organ procurement coordinators in requesting familial consent to organ donation. *Journal of Health Communication,* 16, 643-659.

Anker, A. E., and Feeley, T. H. (2011b). Difficult communication: Compliance-gaining strategies of organ procurement coordinators. *Journal of Health Communication,* 16, 372-392.

Bauer, R. A. (1964). The obstinate audience: The influence process from the point of view of social communication. *American Psychologist,* 19, 319-328.

Burgoon, M., Alvaro, E., Grandpre, J., and Voloudakis, M. (2003). Revisiting the theory of psychological reactance: Communicating threats to attitudinal freedom. In J. Dillard and M. Pfau (Eds.) The handbook of persuasion, pp. 213-232. Thousand Oaks: Sage.

Chaiken, S. (1980). Heuristic versus systematic information processing and the use of source versus message cues in persuasion. *Journal of Personality and Social Psychology*, 39, 752-766.

Cohen, E. L. (2010). The role of message frame, perceived risk, and ambivalence in individuals'decisions to become organ donors. *Health Communication,* 25, 758-769.

Crano, W. D., (2010). There's nothing so practical…theoretical translations and organ donation. In J.T. Siegel, and E.M. Alvaro (Eds.) Understanding Organ donation: Contributions from applied behavioral science. Hoboken, NJ: Wiley-Blackwell.

Crano, W. D. (2000). Milestones in the psychological analysis of social influence. *Group Dynamics: Theory, Research, and Practice,* 4, 68-80.

Crano, W. D., (2001). Directed social influence. In Forgas, J. P., Williams, K. D., and Wheeler, L. (Eds.), The social mind: Cognitive and motivational aspects of interpersonal behavior. (pp. 389-405). New York: Cambridge University Press.

Crano, W. D., and Prislin, R. (2006). Attitudes and persuasion. *Annual Review of Psychology,* 57, 345-374.

Crano, W. D., and Prislin, R. (2008). Attitudes and attitude change. New York: Psychology Press.

Crano, W. D., Siegel, J. T., and Alvaro, E. M. (2012). The Siren's Call: Mass Media and Drug Prevention. In J. Dillard and M. Pfau (Eds.) The Handbook of Persuasion (2nd Ed). Thousand Oaks: Sage.

Crano, W. D., Siegel, J. T., Alvaro, E., Patel, N. (2007). Overcoming Adolescents' Resistance to Anti-Inhalant Appeals. *Psychology of Addictive Behaviors,* 21, 516-524.

DeLair, S., Feeley, T. H., Kim, H., del Rio Martin, J., Kim-Schluger, L., Rudow, D. L. et al (2010). A peer-based intervention to educate liver transplant candidates about living donor liver transplantation. *Liver Transplantation*, 16, 42-48.

Dominguez, J. M., Gonzalez Z. A., Morales Otero L. A., et al. (1991). Knowledge and attitude about organ donation in a Hispanic population. *Transplant Proceedings,* 23, 1804–1806.

Durkin, S., and Wakefield, M. (2006). Maximizing the impact of emotive antitobacco advertising: Effects of interpersonal discussion and program placement. *Social Marketing Quarterly,* 3, 3 -14.

Feeley, T. H., Marshall, H. M., and Reinhardt, A. M. (2006). Reactions to narrative and statistical written messages promoting organ donation, *Communication Reports,* 19, 89-100.

Foley, M., and Duck, S. (2006). Relational communication. In O. Hargie (Ed.) The handbook of communication skills (3rd ed., pp. 427-450). New York: Sage.

Ford, L. A., and Smith, S. W. (1991). Memorability and persuasiveness of organ donation message strategies. *American Behavioral Scientist,* 34, 695-711.

Ganikos, M. (2010). Organ donation: An overview of the field. In J. T. Siegel, and E. M. Alvaro (Eds.) Understanding Organ donation: Contributions from applied behavioural science. Hoboken, N. J: Wiley-Blackwell.

Gerbner, G. (1969). Toward "Cultural Indicators": The analysis of mass mediated public message systems. *AV Communication Review,* 17, 137-148.

Gerbner, G., Gross, L., Morgan, M., and Signorielli, N. (1980). The mainstreaming of America: Violence profile #11. *Journal of Communication, 30,* 10-29.

Green, M. C., Brock, T. C., Kaufman, G. F. (2004). Understanding media enjoyment: The role of transportation into narrative worlds. *Communication Theory,* 14, 311-327.

Gonzalez, A. V., Siegel, J. T., Alvaro, E. M., and O'Brien, E. (2013). The effect of depression on physician-patient communication among Hispanic end-stage renal disease patients. *Journal of Health Communication*, 57, 27-34.

Gunther, A. C., Bolt, D., Borzekowski, D. L. G., Liebhart, J. L., and Dillard, J. P. (2006). Presumed influence on peer norms: How mass media indirectly affect adolescent smoking. *Journal of Communication,* 56, 52-68.

Hafstad, A. and Aaro, L. E. (1997). Activating interpersonal influence through provocative appeals: Evaluation of a mass media-based antismoking campaign targeting adolescents. *Health Communication,* 9, 253–272.

Hovland, C. I., Janis, I. L., and Kelley, H. H. (1953). Communication and persuasion. New Haven, CT: Yale University Press.

Kopfman, J. E., Smith, S. W., Yun, J. K., and Hodges, A. (1998). Affective and cognitive reactions to narrative versus statistical evidence organ donation messages. *Journal of Applied Communication Research,* 26, 279-300.

LaVail, K. H., Anker, A. E., Reinhart, A., and Feeley, T. H. (2010). The persuasive effects of audiovisual PSAs to promote organ donation: The mediating role of psychological reactance. *Communication Studies,* 61, 46-69.

Lazarsfeld, P. F., Berelson, B. R., and Gaudet, H. (1948). The people's choice. Columbia University Press: New York, USA.

Lee, A. Y., and Aaker, J. L. (2004). Bringing the frame into focus: the influence of regulatory fit on processing fluency and persuasion. *Journal of Personality and Social Psychology,* 86, 205-218.

Lindsey, L. L. M., and Yun, K. A. (2005). The relationship between narrative content variation, affective and cognitive reactions, and a person's willingness to sign an organ donor card. *Communication Research Reports,* 22, 253-263.

Marshall, H. M., and Feeley, T. H. (2006). A normative approach to shaping college students' attitudes toward organ donation. *Communication Studies,* 57, 435-453.

McCombs, M. and Shaw, D. (1972). The agenda-setting function of mass media. *Public Opinion Quarterly,* 36, 176-187.

McGuire, W. J. The communication/persuasion matrix. In: Lipstein, B., and McGuire, W. J., (Eds.) Evaluating Advertising: A Bibliography of the Communication Process. New York: Advertising Research Foundation, 1978.

McGuire, W. J. Attitudes and attitude change. In: Lindzey, G., and Aronson, E. (Eds.) The Handbook of Social Psychology. 3d ed. Vol. 2. New York: Random House, 1985.

McGuire, W. J.; Papageorgis, D. (1962). Effectiveness of forewarning in developing resistance to persuasion. *Public Opinion Quarterly*, 26, 24-34.

McQuail, D. (1971). Towards a sociology of mass communication. London: Collier - Macmillian.

Morton, T., and Duck, J. (2001). Communication and health beliefs: Mass and interpersonal influences on perceptions of risk to self and others. *Communication Research,* 28, 602–26.

Petty, R. E., and Cacioppo, J. T. (1986). The elaboration likelihood model of persuasion. In L. Berkowitz (Ed.), Advances in experimental social psychology (19, pp. 123-205). Orlando, FL: Academic Press.

Petty, R. E., Cacioppo, J. T., and Schumann, D. (1983). Central and peripheral routes to advertising effectiveness: the moderating role of involvement. *Journal of Consumer Research*, 10, 135-146.

Reinhart, A. M., and Anker, A. E. (2012). An exploration of transportation and psychological reactance in organ donation PSAs. *Communication Research Reports,* 29, 274-284.

Reinhart, A. M., Marshall, H., Feeley, T. H., and Tutzauer, F. (2007). The persuasive effects of message framing in organ donation: The mediating role of psychological reactance. *Communication Monographs,* 74, 229-255.

Schramm, W. (1982). Men, women, messages and media. New York: Harper and Row.

Selnow, G. W., and Crano, W. D. (1987) Planning, implementing, and evaluating targeted communication programs: A manual for business communicators. New York: Quorum Books.

Siegel, J. T., Alvaro, E. M., and Maurer, D. (2011). "Can you spare an organ?"Exploring Hispanic Americans' willingness to discuss living organ donation with loved ones. *Health Communication*, 6, 74-80.

Siegel, J. T., Alvaro, E. M., Pace-Jones, S., Crano, W. C., Lac, A., Ting, S. (2008). A quasi-experimental investigation of message appeal variations on organ donor registration rates. *Health Psychology,* 27, 170-178.

Siegel, J. T., Alvaro, E. M., Lac, A., Crano, W. D., Dominick, A. (2008). Intentions of becoming a living organ donor among Hispanics: A theoretical approach exploring differences between living and non-living organ donation. *Journal of Health Communication*, 13, 80-99.

Singhal, A. and Rogers, E. M. (1999). Entertainment-Education: A communication strategy for social change. New Jersey: Lawrence Earlbaum Associates.

Smith, S. W., Morrison, K., Kopfman, J. E., and Ford, L. A. (1994). The influence of prior thought and intent on the memorability and persuasiveness of organ donation messages. *Health Communication,* 6, 1-20.

Tian, Y. (2010). Organ donation on Web 2.0: Content and audience analysis of organ donation videos on YouTube. *Human Communication,* 25, 238-246.

Watzlawick, P., Beavin, J., Jackson, D. D. (1967). Pragmatics of human communication: a study of interactional patterns, pathologies, and paradoxes. New York: W. W. Norton and Company.

Weber, K., Martin, M. M., Members of COMM 401, Corrigan, M. (2006). Creating persuasive messages advocating organ donation. *Communication Quarterly,* 54, 67-87.

Winkel, F. W. (1984). Public communication on donor cards: A comparison of persuasive styles. *Social Science and Medicine,* 19, 957-963.

In: Organ Donation and Transplantation
Editor: Mary Anne Lauri

ISBN: 978-1-62948-257-6

Chapter 15

PROMOTING ORGAN DONATION THROUGH COMMUNICATION CAMPAIGNS

Thomas Hugh Feeley [*] ***and Z. Janet Yang*** [†]
University at Buffalo, The State University of New York, New York, US

ABSTRACT

This chapter first reviews the goals of organ donation campaigns along the continuum from informing an audience to mobilizing an audience, including increasing consent rates and targeting audience's readiness to change. Based on this review, critical elements of communication campaigns to promote deceased or cadaveric donation are introduced, such as informational appeals and narrative appeals, using Berlo's Source-Message-Channel-Receiver model of the communication process as an organizing model. The chapter concludes by discussing the challenges to organ donation campaign research and offering directions for future research. In particular, future research should aim at determining which messages and channels yield consistent effects within and across community contexts, learning about adults' sentiments toward donation, as well as promoting receiver's long-term attitude and behavior change.

INTRODUCTION

The concept of a communication campaign or any campaign for that matter (e.g., a political campaign) likely borrowed its name from the concept of a military campaign. In the military sciences a *campaign* represents a strategic and usually large-scale plan that includes a series of inter-related operations conducted within a larger war or conflict. The scope and duration of a given campaign can vary depending on the military goal and resources available, such as number of troops and supplies.

Similarly, a communication campaign is designed around a specific outcome or goal and campaign planners strategize messages and communication of messages toward realization of

[*] thfeeley@buffalo.edu
[†] zyang5@buffalo.edu

this goal. The campaign might be weeks, months or in rare cases years in duration. A communication campaign is a defined, strategic and time-bound operation within a larger initiative (or *war*) waged on targeted attitudes or behaviors of a target audience. For example, a school-based communication campaign to promote dental hygiene might include in-class presentations, posters and perhaps an assembly for all students that includes pro-hygiene messages (frequent brushing, flossing, regular checkups) during the fall term of 2013 at certain primary schools in a given area. The specific objective in a specific operation within a campaign site is consistent with the overall campaign goal that likely spans tens or perhaps hundreds of operations or sites and the campaign itself is often positioned within the larger and likely national campaign to promote oral health.

Many communication campaigns can be considered health communication campaigns as the target behavior of interest is related to personal well-being or community health. The goal of the current chapter is to review health communication campaigns designed to promote organ donation. More specifically, the current chapter reviews characteristics of organ donation campaigns, such the campaigns' messaging (i.e., message appeals) and modalities (i.e., channel reliance). Two earlier reviews of organ donation campaigns were instructive to the current effort. Feeley and Moon (2009) recently reviewed 23 organ donation campaigns and through meta-analytic procedures indicated campaigns were roughly 5% more successful than controls in meeting project goals (e.g., increasing knowledge or registration rates). A later chapter by Morgan (2012) reviewed campaigns along two dimensions: by theoretical models and by communication contexts. The reader is directed to these works to gain a wider perspective on the nature of organ donation campaigns.

On the Goals of Organ Donation Campaigns

The goals of organ donation campaigns vary greatly and this realization certainly suggests that any attempt to directly compare campaign successes results is somewhat artificial (e.g., Feeley & Moon, 2009). Consider two examples to bring this claim into greater focus. DeLair et al. (2010) used pamphlets written in five languages to inform liver transplant patients in New York about the living donation process. The goal of the campaign was to increase the number of patients who present for evaluation for living donation across the five transplant centers. A second campaign by Weber and Martin (2008) sought to increase the number of targeted college students to enroll on the state registry. Weber and Martin used both mediated messages and face-to-face messaging (i.e., presentations to classes) to appeal to students. As you can readily see, these two projects have quite distinct goals, appeal to two entirely different target groups and rely on distinct message appeals to influence receivers.

An important dimension to consider when considering campaigns to promote organ donation is what Rogers and Storey (1987) label as a campaign's *level of objective.* By level of objective, Rogers and Storey refer to a continuum bounded by *informing* an audience at one end and *mobilizing* an audience at the other end. The objective of persuading an audience would fall between these two anchors. Campaign objectives toward the mobilizing end of the continuum are considered a higher level of objective that requires lower level objectives to be achieved first. Thus, a campaign designed to *mobilize* individuals to communicate their donation intentions to next-of-kin (e.g., Feeley, Anker, Williams, & Vincent, 2010) requires these individuals to first be *knowledgeable* about donation and have positive attitudes (i.e., *persuasion*) regarding the value of deceased donation. Thus, a campaign may have a *lower-level* objective to increase first-year medical students' knowledge and self-efficacy toward donation (e.g., Feeley, Tamburlin, & Vincent, 2008) or a *higher-level* objective to mobilize DMV customers to enroll in the registry during the license renewal process (e.g., Rodrigue et al., 2012).

Related to the level of objective of a given communication campaign to promote donation is the relative *distance* of the campaign objective from the initial exposure to campaign messages. In an integrated review of the literature, Feeley (2007) proposed that the ultimate outcome of any campaign to promote organ donation is to increase the number of individuals who actually consent to donation if eligible. It is understood that a mere fraction of hospital deaths result in eligible transplantation, so the stakes for increasing consent are quite high. That is, with few opportunities for donors and procurable organs from brain death donors (i.e., an estimated 1% of hospital deaths), the need for consent and subsequent conversion is great.

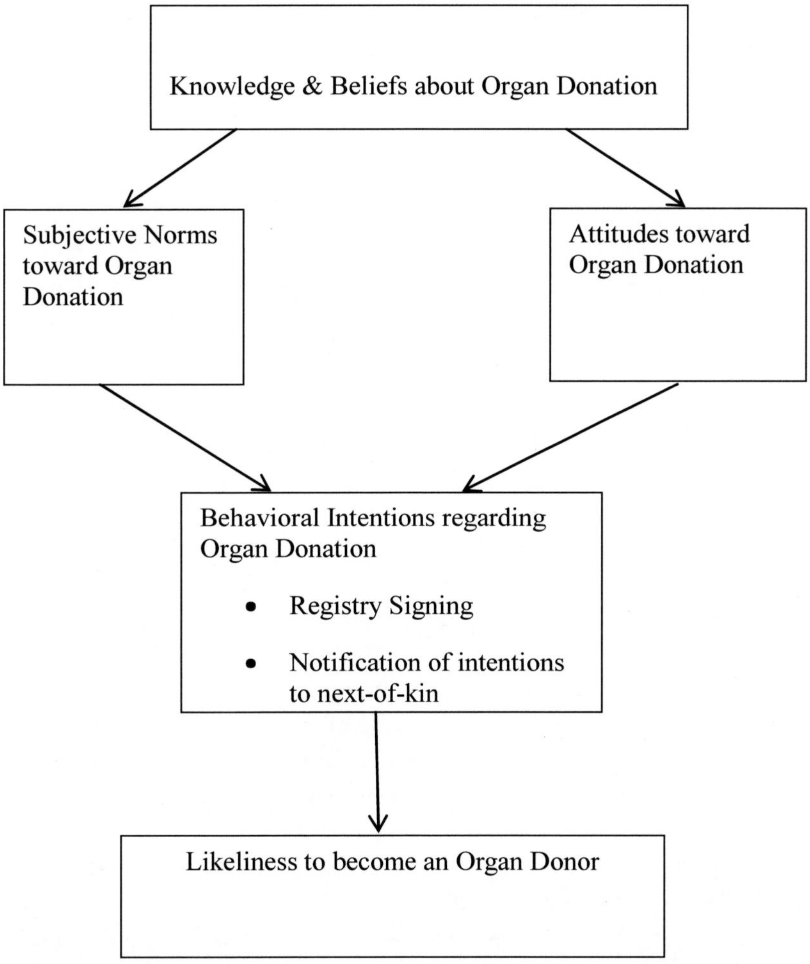

Figure 1. Model of Organ Donation Attitudes and Behaviors based on Theory of Reasoned Action (adopted from Feeley, 2007).

Understanding the need to increase conversion rates for donation, campaigns target factors that directly predict family and individual consent rates. These factors vary in their relative *strength* and distance to the donation decision. Considering Feeley's (2007) adapted model of theory of reasoned action (Fishbein & Ajzen, 1975), as depicted in figure 1, it is shown that family notification of one's donation intentions and documentation of donation intentions through a state registry are the closest and typically strongest predictors (using relative effect sizes) of donation (Rodrigue, Cornell, & Howard, 2006). Still further back in relative distance and predictive utility in Feeley's model is one's intentions to donate and an individual's perceptions of salient others' donation attitudes. These two factors (attitudes, subjective norms) are, in turn, predicted by attitudes toward donation and knowledge about the donation process.

Research and evaluation of organ donation campaigns vary in which factor or level of objective is targeted and many campaigns involve more than one objective. Consider one example from a study by Frates, Bohrer, and Thomas (2006) in California. The authors sought to increase consent rates (i.e., high-level objective) in the Los Angeles region through an advertising campaign targeting Hispanic adults in their designed Organ Procurement Organization region. The authors compiled consent rates over time (i.e., pre- and post-campaign) and also measured several lower- level objectives or antecedent factors, such as attitudes, family notification and enrollment in registry. Frates et al. (2006) learned that only a small portion of the sample recognized campaign messages, so they could not claim responsibility for increased consent rates due to their advertising campaign. Sound campaign evaluation protocol, as exemplified by Frates and colleagues, allows scholars to learn if a campaign worked (i.e., summative evaluation) and what aspects might be active ingredients accounting for why the campaign worked (i.e., formative evaluation).

The context of the campaign and a given target audience's readiness to change likely dictate the level of campaign objective one assumes. If an audience is positively disposed toward donation (i.e., positive attitudes), then a campaign might do well to target family notification of donation intentions or attempt to significantly increase the proportion of individuals who enroll on the state registry. By contrast, a campaign might confront a recalcitrant target audience who harbors negative attitudes toward the donation process and would be better served to debunk myths held by the audience and provide education on how the transplant process actually works. Any attempt to target a high-level outcome (e.g., signing organ cards) would likely meet resistance in the form of psychological reactance and campaign efforts would engender stronger attitudes *against* donation (cf. Reinhart, Marshall, Feeley, & Tutzauer, 2007).

With a discussion of the nature of campaign goals in the context of organ donation behind us, we turn attention to the critical elements of communication campaigns to promote donation. Before doing so, it is important to note that our discussion is reserved to campaigns to promote deceased or cadaveric donation and not living donation. This is not to suggest living donation is less important or devoid of campaign illustrations. The reality is opposite to this suggestion as the number of kidneys (and recently livers) recovered from living donors nearly parallels the number of organs procured from deceased donors. Our own computation using national data of donors reported from 1988 through November 24, 2012 (www.unos.org) indicates that 45% of all livers and kidneys donated were from living individuals. However, there is little evidence of communication campaigns seeking to promote living donation in the research literature.

The S-M-C-R Model of Communication

To adequately organize the research literature, we will adapt Berlo's (1960) S-M-C-R model of the communication process. The model was originally used to explain interpersonal communication processes and identifies source, message, channel and receiver features that help to explain and predict communication outcomes. For example, Berlo characterizes several source ingredients (e.g., skills, knowledge, attitudes, culture) that serve to help or hinder shared meaning and influence in communication. Where the original Berlo model deviates from the present treatment is in its discussion of channel characteristics, primarily due to its original emphasis on face-to-face communication. Berlo's channel characteristics are within the single channel of interpersonal communication and include the five senses whereas the current review considers multiple channels of communication that *mediate* meanings between senders and receivers.

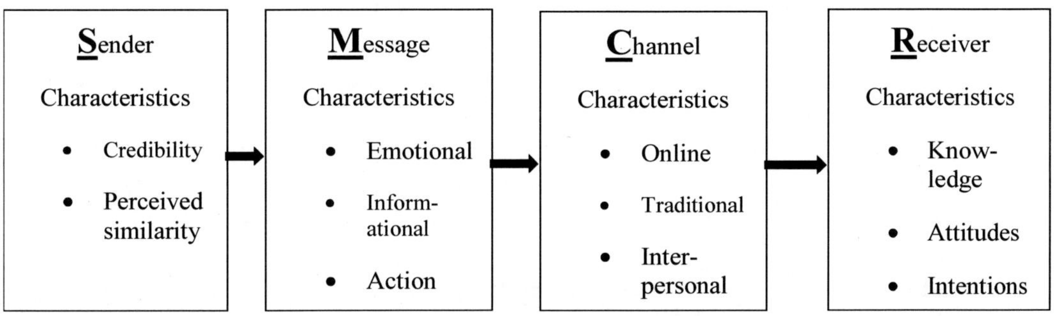

Figure 2. An S-M-C-R Communication Model of Organ Donation Campaigns (based on Berlo, 1960).

This model is an ideal organizing model to plot the primary elements of organ donation campaigns. As detailed in figure 2, each acronym in the model represents the source, the message, the channel, and the receiver in a given communication process. So for any given campaign, there is/are source(s) sending messages through one or more channels or medium/media to targeted message receivers.

It is understood that the model is somewhat simplistic, static, and limited in its ability to capture the dynamics and nuance of influence processes, such as campaigns; however, it still represents a parsimonious model for the purposes of the current chapter. We begin with a discussion of source or sender message factors related to organ donation campaigns.

Sender Characteristics

Organ donation campaigns can be considered a specific form of persuasive communication and as such a primary characteristic of any persuasive message is the credibility of the sender. The sender is relatively the least studied and featured element in donation campaigns. Promotional messages simply seem to appear in the public domain. Despite public relations efforts (e.g., "Donate Life" campaigns), the general public has little knowledge what an Organ Procurement Organization is or does in relation to the transplantation process. Thus, campaign efforts to feature the Organ Procurement

Organization as the message source have little to no effect on target audiences. The majority of published campaigns provide little mention if the campaign messages reveal the source(s) of the message. It is likely the case the regional Organ Procurement Organization (in the United States) sponsored the messages and at some point in the ad (usually at the end) the organization is revealed. Either way, the message source is not typically prevalently communicated to receivers. Two sender characteristics are often utilized in organ donation promotional ads and messages: source similarity and authority.

Source Characteristics

Generally speaking, we are more influenced by message senders who appear similar to us along several physical and attitudinal dimensions. We simply like people who are like us and using senders matched to receivers in age, ethnicity or affiliation is a common strategy in organ donation campaigns. A campaign by Feeley et al. (2009) in the New York City area exemplifies the sender similarity strategy. The authors used college students to promote organ donation among other college students on ethnically concentrated campuses and their surrounding communities.

It was hypothesized that targeted students would be more amenable to promotional messages sent by individuals similar to them in age and ethnicity. This peer-to-peer matching strategy (see also Feeley, Anker, Williams, & Vincent, 2010) posits that message senders would be better positioned to influence receivers who are similar to them, at the same time, targeted students would be more likely to attend to and ultimately yield to message appeals sent by their peers. Alternatively, it could be the case that students are somewhat immune to the "top-down" health promotion messages sent by state health officials, university officials and other distant authority figures whose good faith appeals may engender psychological reactance among students (Reinhart, Marshall, Feeley, & Tutzauer, 2007).

A second form of source similarity is to feature senders who live in the same geographic region as targeted receivers (and also may share similar demographic characteristics). An example from a recent campaign to promote donation in Michigan illustrates this principle. Harrison et al. (2010) used multiple methods to promote the Michigan Organ Donor Registry, including billboards and print messages featuring pictures of individuals from the intervention counties targeted. Messengers attempted to localize the donation problem to their areas of Michigan, used profile pictures, named their hometown and explained how they were affected by donation positively. To further emphasize the similarities between sources and receivers, written messages reinforced this relationship, such as, "Someone like you saved Charlie's life" (p. 702). A second benefit of using local donation narrative appeals is their ability to increase the vested interest of audience members. The concept of donating an organ is a distant concept, especially to young health adults. Any efforts to increase the vested interest of audience members will likely strengthen the weak relationship between individuals' reported attitudes toward donation and their donation-consistent behaviors, such as signing the registry and communicating donation intentions to family members (Anker, Feeley, & Kim, 2010).

The second factor in the Berlo model has to do with message characteristics and the content of what senders state or write in an effort to promote donation in a given audience. We turn attention to this factor next.

Message Characteristics

Like source characteristics, the literature is somewhat cryptic in what messages are used to promote donation. For example, Cosse and Weinberger (2000) conducted a campaign in Richmond Virginia using traditional media (over $70 million spent) and the only reference of message content was a brief mention of the theme of the campaign, "Organ and Tissue Donation: Share your life, share your decision" (p. 297). Other campaigns (e.g., Salim et al., 2011) simply report that messages addressed culturally sensitive issues surrounding the transplant process. Thus, it is still unclear which messages are more influential than other messages in promoting donation and increasing behavioral outcomes associated with consent to donation.

The studies that report message characteristics can be organized around three appeals: informational, narrative, and call to action. The ensuing discussion will describe each of these three appeals, but before doing so, it is important to note that many messages use one or more of these appeals in combination. For example, a message might tell a story of a teen who received a life-saving liver transplant (i.e., narrative appeal) and then indicate how one can support donation by signing their respective state registry (i.e., call to action). Or, this same message might indicate the number or proportion of state residents who have already signed the registry before or after the call to action (i.e., informational appeal).

Informational Appeals

Informational appeals to promote donation are often educational in their approach. That is, messages attempt to provide information about the need for donation, information about the organ allocation process (i.e., how organs are distributed), and/or provide information about the donation process (e.g., medical treatment for eligible donors). The need to educate receivers about donation cannot be overstated as most adults know little about donation and what they know is often based upon fictional accounts depicted in popular media (Quick, Kim, & Meyer, 2009; Morgan et al., 2008). Recent research also indicates that medical students know little about the organ transplantation process (Feeley, Tamburlin, & Vincent, 2008).

The challenge of educating and informing a given target group is formidable as the topic of donating an organ is hardly a topic that dominates conversation in the break room or in coffee shops. Also, donation stories are not commonplace in newspapers or on television (Feeley & Vincent, 2007; Quick et al., 2009). Thus, creativity in how organ donation information is conveyed and selectivity in where messages are located are critical considerations when conducting promotional campaigns. The level of dosage is important and campaigns need to rely on multiple messages using various media to influence target individuals.

Morgan et al. (2002), in one of the first documented worksite campaigns reported in the literature, used several informational messages to promote organ donation among employees of a large organization. For example, daily facts about donation were communicated through the company's intranet and educational in-service presentations attempted to detail the organ donation process to employees. The use of multiple media and multiple messages marks most campaigns in organ donation.

Perhaps the most common informational appeal used in campaigns is the use of messages that seek to debunk myths that individuals hold about donation. For example, a common myth harbored by many is that medical treatment is compromised for individuals who are eligible to donate and whose intentions to donate are known by medical staff. A second myth indicates that organ donation is inconsistent with religious beliefs (Morgan et al., 2008). Related to this, Morgan and colleagues (2002) used billboards placed on roads leading into and out of the targeted organization to reduce common misconceptions surrounding donation.

In a subsequent mass-scale worksite campaign, Harrison et al. (2011a) used brochures and other media that featured messages to dispel myths about donation. In a rare study that sought to compare the efficacy of message appeal conditions, Siegel, Alvaro, Crano, Lac, Ting, & Jones (2008) used counterarguments to fend off commonly referenced reasons individuals report for not signing the state organ donor registry. For example, one poster informed Arizona residents that state registry was the *only* method to become an organ donor. The supposition behind informational appeals is that identifying the facts surrounding donation will serve to increase public sentiments toward donation. Indirect evidence suggests that those with greater knowledge about donation also are more likely to report positive attitudes toward donation and intentions to become an organ donor (e.g., Feeley, 2007; Feeley & Servoss, 2005; Morgan & Cannon, 2003).

A study in 2007 by Reinhart and colleagues compared message framing and message reactions using written persuasive appeals to encourage organ donor registry signing among three samples of college students. Their findings provide formative information for informational appeals with relation to using differently valenced appeals – specifically, the use of positively framed materials (i.e., detailing benefits of becoming an organ donor) engendered more donation-friendly reactions when compared to messages using negatively framed materials (i.e., discussion of negative ramifications of not becoming a donor). Evidence from these studies indicates that negatively framed messages create psychological reactance on the part of message recipients because of the perceived manipulative intent. Thus, messages might go further if they focus on the benefits of organ donation for both donor families and recipients.

Narrative Appeals

A common message strategy in organ donation relies on narrative appeals or appeals that rely on stories or singular anecdotes to illustrate the benefits of transplantation. A campaign by Frates et al. (2006) illustrates this principle. After interviewing families who either agreed to or denied consent to donate, the authors created advertisements that featured actual donation stories in the targeted communities in Southern California. One ad featured a young patient who is awaiting a life-saving transplant who is shown recalling her childhood dreams and desire to live on to realize these dreams.

The benefit of narrative appeals is their ability to gain the attention of message receivers and theoretically transport the viewer/listener into the storyline to better empathize with individuals in need of organ donation. In many ways narrative appeals potentially make transplantation more real to receivers and in so doing increase individuals' sense of urgency to respond to the message, by increasing involvement or reducing feelings of guilt associated with not donating (Anker & Feeley, 2011; Marshall et al., 2008).

Consider a second ad used by Alvaro, Jones, Robles, and Siegel (2006) in an effort to promote donation among Hispanics in two counties in Arizona. One advertisement, among many used across media, features a paramedic attempting to save the life of a victim (donor) at the scene of a car accident and the scene quickly flashes to a hospital room where an organ recipient is surrounded by family members after a recent transplant surgery. This ad is similar to many in organ donation campaigns in that it uses a storyline to: (1) gain and sustain the attention of the audience members, (2) illustrate the benefits of transplantation, and (3) model the transplant process.

Campaigns that use individual accounts of donation stories are particularly influential. Harrison et al. (2010) relied on volunteers representing the local Organ Procurement Organization to promote donation to DMV customers in counties in the state of Michigan. Volunteers shared their personal donation stories to customers waiting to make the transaction. Weber and Martin (2008) used guest speakers to present for 15 minutes to college classes about their personal donation experience and to appeal to audience members to consider donation.

Many campaigns rely on mixed-messaging to promote donation by using certain message appeals in concert with certain media. A campaign may run quick radio ads providing short informational bits on donation and how one can register, while at the same time air 15-second ads that feature a donation story. Thus, it is nearly impossible to tease out which message appeal is more persuasive in shaping attitudes and intentions to donate. Two studies in the literature directly tested the persuasive effects of narrative versus statistical appeals (i.e., informational appeals that rely on statistics or numbers) to promote donation. A first study by Kopfman et al. (1998) exposed university students first to a statistical message promoting donation, then to a narrative message promoting donation and findings advantaged the statistical message along several dependent factors including message reactions.

Feeley, Marshall and Reinhart (2006) corrected an important methodological concern in the Kopfman study and controlled for receivers' baseline attitudes toward donation and found different results. First, Feeley et al. (2006) found time order to matter significantly such that messages presented first yielded a greater number of thoughts, especially positive thoughts about donation. Apparently, after responding to the first vignette, students reported all they have to say on the topic of donation. Second, narrative appeals were more persuasive than statistical appeals in producing more favorable reactions to vignettes when compared to an actual message taken from a newspaper story. However, when directly comparing narrative versus statistical appeals, there was no significant difference (see Reinhart, 2006 for a review). In summary, it is unclear which appeal is more persuasive and the preferred messaging technique is likely the combination of the two.

Call to Action

A common and important component of message strategies is to mobilize action and behavioral commitment to donation in the form of signing the organ registry and communicating one's commitment to next-of-kin. Some messages attempt to motivate action when the topic of donation is salient and use strong language, such as, "your procrastination could be deadly. Later is now!" (Siegel et al., 2008, p. 172). Others use campaign tag lines such as "Show us your heart" or "Tell us now" to promote action and signing (Harrison et al.,

2010, p. 702). Call to action is a direct method to address frequently cited reasons for not donating (e.g., "I would donate, but am unsure how to"; Feeley & Servoss, 2005; Feeley et al., 2012; Marshall & Feeley, 2006).

It is vital to note that message strategies must be considered in relation to other factors in Berlo's S-M-C-R model. One important determinant is the channel(s) used to deliver messages designed to promote donation. Certain channels (e.g., interpersonal) are more conducive for narrative appeals where other channels (e.g., posters) are better for informational appeals or a call to action. We turn to channel characteristics in the next section.

Channel Characteristics

Communication campaigns are best recalled by their channel characteristics; that is, one recounts a "direct mail campaign" or "advertising campaign" and the like. The case of organ donation is no different and the evolution of organ donation campaigns parallels the changes in communication technology. Early campaigns (e.g., Cosse & Weinberger, 2000, whose campaign took place in 1994) rely on communication channels such as billboards, TV and radio whereas more recent campaigns use social media platforms such as Facebook, Google and Websites (Salim et al., 2010; Stefanone et al., 2012).

More commonly however is the use of multiple media to permeate the message through a target audience. Although there are rare cases of reliance on single channels to promote donation, most efforts attempt to diversify their attack and use traditional mass media and interpersonal communication channels. If we return to our initial metaphor of military campaigns one might consider mass mediated channels as the air attack whereas interpersonal channels as the ground attack.

A recent campaign undertaken by Harrison and colleagues (2010) brings this last point into focus. The goal of the Harrison et al. campaign was to increase the percentage of Michigan residents who sign the state organ donor registry upon visiting their respective Department of Motor Vehicle (DMV) office. Toward this end, campaign ads were taken out on billboards and on radio ads to educate residents and shape attitudes toward the registration process. The mass mediated messages served to prime audience members before their periodic DMV visit. The DMV is the primary portal by which individuals in the United States enroll in the state registry. Although one may sign up online in most states, this method represents only a fraction of new registrants.

The primary channel elements of the Harrison et al. DMV campaign were designed to influence customers during their visit. The elements included point of decision-making materials (POD) and interpersonal interaction on-site. POD materials included posters, clerk cards, and footprint stickers strategically placed on the floors of DMV offices. Clerk cards were small cards placed on clerks' counters where customers complete their transactions. The final interpersonal channel had volunteers interact with customers waiting to complete transactions. Similar DMV campaigns (see Rodrigue et al., 2012) rely on multiple channels of communication to introduce or reinforce the donation message to customers.

Two Channel Dimensions

The various channels used to promote organ donation can be organized along two dimensions. The first dimension is the level of interactivity between senders and receivers – more interactive campaigns allow receivers to ask questions, voice concerns and interact in real time with senders. For example, discussing the transplantation process with a volunteer at a local DMV office would be a highly interactive channel whereas exposure to a radio ad would be considered a message low on interactivity. Stated differently, some campaign channels can be considered one-way messages, some allow two-way communication and some fall between these two. For example, one could send a promotional email to 50 individuals and certainly any given receiver could respond to the email but this is done asynchronously.

A second dimension has to do with the potential *reach* of a campaign. Mass communication channels allow senders to potentially reach more individuals whereas interpersonal channels are restricted to smaller groups or single individuals and theoretically have less reach. A promotional message sent on Facebook to a user's friends might reach potentially thousands whereas this same message sent over email to one friend would reach only one. However a Facebook page and user group with a formidable number of members would allow high reach and a relatively high level of interactivity among campaign message receivers.

Due to the nature of organ donation and its appeal to receivers, it is important that communication campaigns are sensitive to the limits of mass media, in particular new media in its ability to mobilize passive audience members to act upon their donation intentions. For example, Stefanone et al. (2012) recently reached a critical mass of individuals in New York through Google and Facebook advertising, but only a fraction of those individuals were persuaded to visit the project's website and sign the state's electronic organ donor registry. Balanced with reach is the *impact* of a campaign and this only measured through a campaign's ability to achieve its stated goals and objectives. Also of important concern is the profile of the target audience – some receivers rely primarily on new media (e.g., college-aged adults) whereas many (e.g., older adults) still read traditional print media and listen to radio. As always, each component of Berlo's model is interdependent on the other components for success.

Often organ donation campaigns rely on events to promote the cause of donation. For example, in a study by Feeley et al. (2009), student campaigners scheduled events in high traffic areas on college campuses in New York to raise awareness for donation. Morgan et al. (2002) scheduled lunches for employees at a large organization to promote donation through use of short presentations delivered by volunteers from the local Organ Procurement Organization. Events are typically used to reinforce the overall campaign message and are not typically the campaign itself. Events allow access to large numbers of individuals and typically provide convenient means to complete paper and pencil registration forms. In the case of Siegel et al. (2008), their campaign relied on kiosks to enlist new state donor registrants in Arizona.

Receiver Characteristics

Communication campaigns almost invariably target a group of individuals for one of two reasons: they have been identified as either an easy or difficult-to-sway audience. For organ donation, a campaign might target college students due to formative research that identified students as reporting pro-donation attitudes and intentions to donate (Feeley, 2007; Feeley & Servoss, 2005). Alternatively, campaigns target a specific group that traditionally reports negative beliefs toward donation or whose signing rates are disproportionately lower than other groups. A prime example of this is campaigns that specifically target Hispanics in Arizona and California (Frates et al., 2006; Alvaro et al., 2006; Salim et al., 2011). These campaigns feature pilot work that identifies knowledge deficits and beliefs based upon an incorrect interpretation of the transplantation process. After identifying these beliefs, campaigns set out to use messages and media tailored to targeted audiences in a given geographical area.

Profiling adults' sentiments toward transplantation is not as straightforward as one might think. For example, many authors (e.g., Feeley, 2007; Gallup, 2005) report positive attitudes toward donation, but a closer examination of the items that tap into attitudes clouds the picture. A more conservative interpretation of these studies would indicate that the majority of adults surveyed report positive attitudes toward the concept of deceased organ donation, but few surveys measure individuals' personal feelings toward becoming a future organ donor. The varied signing rates and less than ideal consent rates indicate that Americans are somewhat hesitant and uncomfortable with the concept of donating organs. Anti-donation beliefs are particular concerning in communities with a higher proportion of Hispanic or African-American residents.

Receiver characteristics are the singular quality of any given campaign that makes efforts to promote donation difficult. The majority of adults simply do not have organ donation on their radar, so messages through advertisements or otherwise often do not get noticed. Generally speaking, campaigns have three tasks – they must gain the attention of audiences, they must be processed, and ultimately they must motivate individuals to act upon their attitudes. These challenges are not easy to overcome and the goal is to increase individuals' vested interest in organ donation (Anker et al., 2009; Crano, 1997) by strengthening attitudes and increasing self-efficacy toward donation. Or, as one recent model (Anker & Feeley, 2011) frames it, campaigns must increase individuals' sense of *personal responsibility* to do something about the public health concern posed by donation.

CONCLUSION

There are many expositions of communication campaigns to promote donation in the health, communication and general social science literature (see Feeley & Moon, 2009; Morgan, 2012 for reviews). The overall conclusion is that campaigns produce small effects in terms of changing, shaping and reinforcing receivers' attitudes and behaviors related to organ donation. While these campaigns are descriptive and well-intended, there are more questions than answers regarding why and when campaigns work in achieving their stated objectives (e.g., increase registry signing rates). First and foremost, it is still unclear which campaign characteristics (or combination of characteristics) work best to promote organ donation.

There is preliminary evidence that campaigns show effectiveness in certain contexts such as the workplace (Harrison et al., 2011a; Morgan et al., 2002), on college campuses (Feeley et al., 2010; Feeley et al., 2011), and at Motor Vehicles Offices (Harrison et al., 2011b; Rodrigue et al., 2012). However, each campaign relies on different campaign messages, different channels of communication, and yields different effect sizes across campaign objectives, such as signing rates, knowledge gains and attitude change. Research would go far to determine which messages and channels yield consistent effects within and across community contexts. Pulling this thread further, campaign research could better assess dosage effects or the number of exposures required to obtain a certain effect.

In terms of receiver characteristics and formative research on adults' sentiments toward donation, it would be important to learn how individuals come to know about organ transplantation. Surveys (e.g., Marshall & Feeley, 2006) ask individuals to list what they know and what sources account for their donation knowledge, however this is an overly simplistic method of studying organ donation knowledge. Clearly what we come to know about any given phenomenon is a spiraling process (Slater, 2007) whereby certain knowledge and curiosities lead to greater exposure to media messages about the topic and knowledge accumulates below our level of consciousness. Accounts of what we know and how we know it may also suffer from recall bias or receivers' desire to sound plausible on a survey or to an interviewer.

A formative barrier to greater campaign impact and traction is receiver vested interest in the topic of donation. The topic of donation is both temporally and psychologically distant to most individuals who are not mindful of death, let alone death in a manner that would bring deceased donation. Organ donation is still a rare event and so few deaths result in transplantation, one estimate we have heard repeatedly is 1 out of every 100 hospital deaths. This reality must be at the fore when planning a campaign, as what topics are important to the message source are sometimes immaterial to the message receiver. A sobering realization is the following: the majority of messages designed to promote organ donation go unnoticed or fail to shape beliefs or plans in relation to donation. Clearly our work is before us in the promotion of donation, both living donation and deceased donation.

Finally, campaigns to promote donation should strive to achieve long-term goals with respect to organ donation that extend far beyond the temporal limitations of a given campaign. Thus, messages should endeavor to promote central processing on the part of message receivers whenever possible (Petty & Cacioppo, 1984). A campaign goal should be, at a minimum, to strengthen individuals' resolve about organ donation and a likely consequence of this stronger resolve is a greater number of advocates for the cause who discuss donation among salient others and colleagues.

REFERENCES

Anker, A. E., & Feeley, T. H. (2011). Are non-participants in prosocial behavior merely innocent bystanders? *Health Communication, 26*(1), 13-24.

Anker, A. E., Feeley, T. H., & Kim, H. (2010). Examining the attitude-behavior relationship in prosocial donation domains. *Journal of Applied Social Psychology, 40*(6), 1293-1324.

Alvaro, E.M., Jones, S.P., Robles, A.S.M., & Siegel, J. (2006). Hispanic organ donation: Impact of a Spanish-Language organ donation campaign. *Journal of the National Medical Association, 98*, 28-35.

Berlo, D.K. (1960). *The process of communication*. Holt, Rinehart, & Winston: New York.

Cosse, T.J., & Weisenberger, T.M. (2000). Words versus actions about organ donation: A four-year tracking study of attitudes and self-reported behavior. *Journal of Business Research, 50*, 297-303.

Crano, W. D. (1997). Vested interest, symbolic politics, and attitude-behavior consistency. *Attitudes and Social Cognition, 72*(3), 485–491.

DeLair, S., Feeley, T.H., Kim, H., Martin, J., Kim-Schluger, L., Rudow, D.L., Orloff, M., Sheiner, P.A., & Teperman, L. (2010). A peer-based intervention to educate liver transplant candidates about living donor liver transplantion. *Liver Transplantation, 16, 42-48.*

Feeley, T.H. (2007). College students' knowledge, attitudes, and behaviors regarding organ donation. *Journal of Applied Social Psychology, 37,* 243-271.

Feeley, T.H., Anker, A.E., Watkins, B. Rivera, J., Tag, N., & Volpe, L. (2009). A peer-to-peer campaign to promote organ donation among racially diverse college students in New York City. *Journal of National Medical Association, 101,* 1154-1162.

Feeley, T.H., Anker, A.E., Williams, C.R., & Vincent, D.E. (2010). A multi-campus classroom intervention to promote organ and tissue donation. In E. Alvaro & J. Siegel (Eds.). *Applied psychology and organ donation: Implementing and evaluating health behavior interventions*. Lawrence Erlbaum Associates.

Feeley, T.H., Marshall, H., & Reinhart, A.M. (2006). Reactions to Narrative and Statistical Written Messages Promoting Organ Donation. *Communication Reports, 19,* 89-100.

Feeley, T.H., & Moon, S. (2009). A Meta-Analytic Review of Communication Campaigns to Promote Organ Donation. *Communication Reports, 22,* 63-73.

Feeley, T.H., & Servoss, T.J. (2005). College students as potential organ donors: Reasons for low signing rates. *Journal of Health Communication, 10,* 237-250.

Feeley, T.H., & Vincent, D.E. (2007). How Organ Donation is Represented in Newspaper Articles in the United States. *Health Communication, 21,* 125-131.

Feeley, T. H., Tamburlin, J., & Vincent, D. E. (2008). An Educational Intervention for First-Year Medical Students on Organ and Tissue Donation. *Progress in Transplantation, 18,* 103-108.

Fishbein, M. & Ajzen, I. (1975). *Belief, attitude, and behavior: An introduction to theory and research*. Reading, MA: Addison-Wesley Publishing.

Frates, J., Bohrer, G.G., & Thomas, D. (2006). Promoting organ donation to Hispanics: The Role of the Media and Medicine. *Journal of Health Communication, 11*, 683-698.

Gallup Organization. (2005). *National Survey of Organ and Tissue Donation Attitudes and Behaviors.* ftp://ftp.hrsa.gov/organdonor/survey2005.pdf. Retrieved November 2, 2005.

Harrison, T.R., Morgan, S.E., Chewning, L.V., Williams, E.A., Barbour, J.B., DiCorica, M.J., & Davis, L.A. (2011a). Revisiting the worksite in worksite in health campaigns: Evidence from a multisite organ donation campaign. *Journal of Communication, 61*, 535-555.

Harrison, T.R., Morgan, S.E., King, A.J., DiCorcia, M.J., Williams, E.A., Ivic, R.K., & Hopeck, P. (2010). Promoting the Michigan organ donor registry: Evaluating the impact of a multifaceted intervention utilizing media priming and communication design. *Health Communication, 25*, 700-708.

Harrison, T.R., Morgan, S.E., King, A.J., & Williams, E.A. (2011b). Saving lives branch by branch: The effectiveness of driver licensing bureau campaigns to promote organ donor registry sign-ups to African Americans in Michigan. *Journal of Health Communication, 16*, 805-819.

Kopfman, J. E., Smith, S., Ah Yun, J. ., & Hodges, A. (1998). Affective and cognitive reactions to narrative versus statistical evidence organ donation messages. *Journal of Applied Communication Research, 26*, 279-300.

Marshall, H. & Feeley, T.H. (2006). Attitudes toward organ donation: A test of injunctive norms. *Communication Studies 57,* 435-453.

Marshall, H. M., Reinhart, A., Feeley, T. H., Tutzauer, F., & Anker, A. E. (2008). Comparing college students' value-, outcome-, and impression-relevant involvement in health–related issues. *Health Communication, 23,* 171-183.

Morgan, S.E. (2012). Public communication campaigns to promote organ donation: Theory, design and implementation (pp. 219-230). In R.E. Rice & C.K. Atkin (Eds)., *Public communication campaigns*. Sage: Los Angeles.

Morgan, S.E., & Cannon, T. (2003). African Americans' knowledge about organ donation: Closing the gap with more effective persuasive message strategies. *Journal of the National Medical Association, 95*, 1066-1071.

Morgan, S. E., Miller, J. & Arasaratnam, L.A. (2002). Signing cards, saving lives: An evaluation of the Worksite Organ Donation Promotion Project. *Communication Monographs, 69*, 253-273.

Morgan, S.E., Stephenson, M.T., Harrison, T.R., Afifi, W.A., & Long, S. D. (2008). Facts versus 'feelings' How rational is the decision to become an organ donor? *Journal of Health Psychology, 13*, 644-658.

Petty, R.E., & Cacioppo, J.T. (1984). The effects of involvement on responses to argument quantity and quality: Central and peripheral routes to persuasion. *Journal of Personality and Social Psychology, 46*, 69-81.

Quick, B.L., Kim, D.K., & Meyer, K. (2009). A 15-year review of ABC, CBS, and NBC news coverage of organ donation: Implications for organ donation campaigns. *Health Communication, 24*, 137-145.

Reinhart, A.M. (2006). *Comparing the persuasive effects of narrative versus statistical messages: A meta-analytic review*. Doctoral Dissertation. Proquest Dissertations & Theses.

Reinhart, A.M., Marshall, H.M., Feeley, T.H., & Tutzauer, F. (2007). The persuasive effects of message framing in organ donation: The mediating role of psychological reactance. *Communication Monographs, 74*, 229-255.

Rodrigue, J. R., Cornell, D. L., & Howard, R. J. (2006). Organ donation decision: Comparison of donor and nondonor families. *American Journal of Transplantation, 6*, 190-198.

Rodrigue, J.R., Krouse, J., Carroll, J., Giery, K.M., Fraga, Y., and Edwards, E. (2012). A Department of Motor Vehicles intervention yields moderate increases in donor designation rates. *Progress in Transplantation, 22*, 18-24.

Rogers, E.M., & Storey, D. (1987). Communication campaigns. In C.R. Berger & S.H. Chaffee (Eds), *Handbook of communication science* (pp. 817-846. Newbury Park, CA: Sage.

Salim, A., Berry, C., Ley, E.J., Schulman, D., Navarro, S., & Chan, L.S. (2011). Utilizing the media to help increase organ donation in the Hispanic American population. *Clinical Transplantation, 25*, E622-E628.

Siegel, J.T., Alvaro, E.M., Crano, W.D., Lac, A., Ting, S., & Jones, S.P. (2008). A quasi-experimental investigation of message appeal variations on organ donation registration rate. *Health Psychology, 27*, 170-178.

Slater, M. D. (2007). Reinforcing spirals: The mutual influence of media selectivity and media effects and their impact on individual behavior and social identity. *Communication Theory, 17*, 281-303.

Stefanone, M., Anker, A.E., Evans, M., & Feeley, T.H. (2012). Click to "Like" Organ Donation: The Use of Online Media to Promote Organ Donor Registration. *Progress in Transplantation, 22,* 168-174.

Weber, K., & Martin, M.M. (2008). *Designing and evaluating the campus organ donor project*. Paper presented to meeting of National Communication Association, San Diego, CA.

INDEX

A

B

C

D

E

F

G

H

K

L

M

N

O

P

Q

R

S

T